UNDERSTANDING CANADIAN PRESCRIPTION DRUGS

UNDERSTANDING CANADIAN PRESCRIPTION DRUGS

A Consumer's Guide to Correct Use

DOROTHY L. SMITH, PHARM. D.

KEY PORTER BOOKS

Canadian Cataloguing in Publication Data

Smith, Dorothy L.
Understanding Canadian prescription drugs

ISBN 1-55013-129-X

1. Drugs - Canada - Dictionaries. 2. Drugs - Canada - Safety measures - Dictionaries. 3. Drugs - Administration. I. Title.

RS51.S55 1989 615'.1 C88-095381-0

Key Porter Books Limited
70 The Esplanade
Toronto, Ontario
M5E 1R2

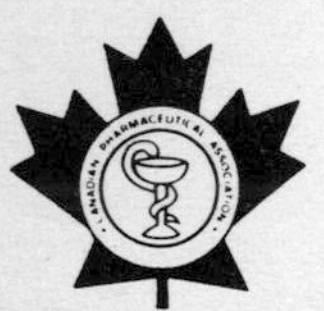

This logo is the trademark of the Canadian Pharmaceutical Association - the national professional association of pharmacists.

Jacket photo: Greg Eligh
Typesetting: Caltsoudas Inc.

Printed and bound in Canada

89 90 91 92 93 6 5 4 3 2 1

To my mother, Mrs. Edna Smith, who repeatedly urged me to write a home reference book on Canadian prescription drugs. My sincere thanks for recognizing the need for this book. Your continuous encouragement to pursue my goal of helping people learn how to take their medications correctly has been truly invaluable.

CONTENTS

FOREWORD	ix
ACKNOWLEDGEMENTS	xi
ADVISORY BOARD	xiii
INDEX	xxiv
ARE YOU TAKING YOUR MEDICINES CORRECTLY?	1
HOW TO USE THIS BOOK	4
GENERIC DRUGS	12
HOW TO ADMINISTER MEDICATIONS	15
Oral Liquid Medicines	15
How to Use an Oral Liquid Syringe	15
How to Use a Medicine Dropper	19
How to Use a Medicine Spoon	20
Buccal Tablets	20
Sublingual Tablets	21
Eye Drops	22
Eye Ointments	24
Ear Drops	25
Nose Drops	27
Nasal Sprays	28
Inhalers	29
Topical Preparations for the Skin	34
How to Use Creams, Ointments, Gels, Solutions and Lotions	34
How to Use Aerosol Sprays	34
How to Use Transdermal Patches	35
Rectal Suppositories	37
Rectal Creams	38
Vaginal Creams, Ointments and Gels	38
Vaginal Tablets, Ovules and Inserts	39
Vaginal Suppositories	40
PRESCRIPTION DRUG INSTRUCTIONS	41
APPENDIX A. Foods Rich in Potassium	385
APPENDIX B. General Instructions for Patients with Diabetes	387
APPENDIX C. Tips to Detect Tampering	389

Foreword

The Canadian Pharmaceutical Association is the national voluntary association for pharmacists. Pharmacists are on the "front lines" in the distribution of medicines to patients and are aware of the drug information needs of patients.

Because the human body is very complex and modern medicines are potent, it is important to have an understanding of both the benefits and risks of our medication usage. It is also important to remember that medicines may act differently on different individuals or even affect the same person differently at different times. Consequently, those of us who use medications may feel a need for additional drug information for our particular situations. This book will be an aid in answering many of your general questions.

We also encourage you to ask your pharmacist about any additional drug information you may need. Pharmacists are well-trained and accessible. I recommend that you take advantage of this by taking your specific questions on your medications to your pharmacist.

Leroy Fevang
Executive Director
Canadian Pharmaceutical Association

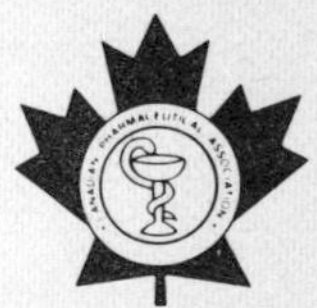

Acknowledgements

This is truly a book for Canadians prepared by Canadians, and it has been one of the most enjoyable books I have written. It gave me an opportunity to work once again with many of my colleagues in Canada. Their willingness to work with me under very tight deadlines has now made it possible for Canadians to have their own home reference book on prescription drugs. Many Canadian consumers are using books that have been written on American prescription drugs, but Canadian medications are different from American medications in many ways. For example, a Canadian medication may have exactly the same brand name as an American medication but contain different ingredients, have different uses, different storage requirements, and even different times and methods of administration.

A very special thank you goes to Dr. Linda Hensman who offered to take a leave of absence from her hospital responsibilities to help me research the hundreds of medications listed in this book. As always, it was a pleasure working with Linda, and I look forward to many more years of professional collaboration.

I am indebted to the many pharmacists and physicians who agreed to serve as members of the Professional Advisory Board. They represented every area of practice as well as every province. This was one of the best boards I have ever had the pleasure to work with, and I would like to thank each of them for giving priority to the manuscript in spite of their own busy schedules and summer vacations. A very special thank you goes to Dr. Eleanor Vogt who helped me during the final review stage of the Advisory Board comments. Ellie's contribution to the book was invaluable and demonstrated her commitment to helping consumers better understand their medications.

Appreciation is also expressed to several other people: to Anne Ribler for the painstaking efforts she took to ensure the accuracy of the word processing and the final printout; to Brian Buchman who duplicated the manuscript several times during the various stages; to Nancy Howard for the excellent medical illustrations she prepared for the book; and to Dr. James Kuperberg who graciously volunteered his time to help us meet the final deadline. Gratitude is also expressed to the pharmaceutical companies for responding so quickly to my requests for information. I sincerely appreciated the advance copy of the 1988 "Compendium of Pharmaceutical Sciences" as well as the assistance given to me on numerous occasions by the Canadian Pharmaceutical Association.

I do not think anyone can ever anticipate in advance the teamwork that will be required to complete a book. The team we had for this book was superb. I am deeply indebted to all of you. Thank you for being so willing to invest your time, knowledge and expertise. Now the book is complete and belongs to the Canadian people. We hope that it will help individuals take their prescription drugs in a more knowledgeable manner.

Dr. Dorothy L. Smith

ADVISORY BOARD

PATIENT EDUCATION CONSULTANT

PROFESSIONAL ADVISORY BOARD

Fenwick Medical Centre
Halifax, Nova Scotia
and
Sessional Lecturer
College of Pharmacy
Dalhousie University
Halifax, Nova Scotia

Barry S. Phillips, B.Sc.Phm.
Community Pharmacy/Owner
Shoppers Drug Mart
Jane Finch Mall
Downsview, Ontario

Neelan Pillay, M.B.Ch.B, F.C.P.(SA), M.R.C.P.(UK), F.R.C.P.C.
Head and Program Director
Section of Neurology
Health Sciences Centre
University of Manitoba
and
Director, Seizure Clinic
Director, Evoked Potentials Laboratory
Health Sciences Centre
University of Manitoba
Winnipeg, Manitoba

Laura-Lynn Pollock, B.Sc.(Pharm)
Senior Instructor & Chairman
Division of Clinical Pharmacy
Faculty of Pharmaceutical Sciences
University of British Columbia
and
Coordinator
Ambulatory Care Pharmacy Services
University Hospital-Shaughnessy Site
Vancouver, British Columbia

Arlene I. Ponting, B.Sc.(Pharm)
Coordinator, Continuing Pharmacy Education
Faculty of Pharmacy and Pharmaceutical Sciences
University of Alberta
Edmonton, Alberta

Bob Pritchard, B.Sc.Phm.
Coordinator of Public and Professional Information
Shoppers Drug Mart
Ontario

Anna W. Przybylo, B.Sc.(Pharm), Pharm.D.
Clinical Pharmacist
Obstetrics, Gynecology, Neonatology
Health Sciences Centre
Winnipeg, Manitoba

Melanie J. Rantucci, B.Sc.Pharm., M.Sc.Phm.
Tutor in Clinical Pharmacy
Faculty of Pharmacy
University of Toronto
Toronto, Ontario
and
Pharmacist
Silvercreek Pharmacy
Mississauga, Ontario

Ronald A. Remick, M.D., F.R.C.P.(C)
Associate Professor and Assistant Head
Department of Psychiatry
University of British Columbia
Vancouver, British Columbia

Alfred J. Remillard, B.Sc.(Micro), B.Sc.Pharm., Pharm.D.
Associate Professor of Pharmacy
College of Pharmacy
University of Saskatchewan
and
Associate Member of Medicine
Department of Psychiatry
University of Saskatchewan
Saskatoon, Saskatchewan

Debra J. Ricciatti-Sibbald, B.Sc.Phm.
President
Debary Dermatologicals
and

Lorna M. Teare, B.Sc.(Ph.)
Staff Pharmacist
Department of Pharmacy Services
Addiction Research Foundation
Toronto, Ontario

Patricia A. Thomson, B.S.P.
Pharmacy Department Head
Pinders Drugs - Grosvenor
Saskatoon, Saskatchewan
and
Dispensing Laboratory Assistant
College of Pharmacy
University of Saskatchewan
Saskatoon, Saskatchewan

Jacques Trottier, B.Sc.Phm.
Community Pharmacist/Owner
Victoria Pharmacy
Ottawa, Ontario
and
President
PROVIPHARM Inc.
Ottawa, Ontario

Louyse I. Trottier, B.Sc.Phm.
Community Pharmacist/Owner
Victoria Pharmacy
Ottawa, Ontario

Lynn R. Trottier, B.Sc.(Pharm)
Clinical Pharmacy Specialist, Geriatrics
University Hospital - UBC Site
Vancouver, British Columbia
and
Assistant Clinical Professor
Division of Clinical Pharmacy
Faculty of Pharmaceutical Sciences
University of British Columbia
Vancouver, British Columbia

C. Brian Tuttle, B.Sc.(Pharm), M.Sc.Phm.
Director of Drug Information Services
Provincial Drug Information Service
Camp Hill Hospital
and
Honorary Special Lecturer
College of Pharmacy
Dalhousie University
Halifax, Nova Scotia

Patricia A. Vassallo, B.Sc.(Pharm.)
Pharmacist
Westminster West End Pharmacy
New Westminster, British Columbia

Ronald H. Waller, B.Sc.(Pharm), M.Sc.(Pharm)
Community Pharmacist/Owner
Lakeside Clinical Pharmacy Ltd.
Kelowna, British Columbia

Dennis E. Walter, M.B.B.S.(London)
General Practitioner
Private Practice
Regina, Saskatchewan

Caroline Y. Wang, B.Sc., M.D.
General Practitioner and Staff Physician
Richmond General Hospital
Richmond, British Columbia

Trevor M. Watson, B.A., B.Sc.(Pharm)
Pharmacy Practitioner
Derma Apothecary Shop Ltd.
Vancouver, British Columbia
and
Member
Canadian Drug Advisory Committee
and
Chairman
Canadian Drug Scheduling Group (1982-1988)

James W. Watt, B.Sc.Phm.
Community Pharmacist/Owner
Sarnia Pharmacy Ltd.
Sarnia, Ontario

Donna M. Woloschuk, B.S.P.(Sask.), Pharm.D.
Oncology Specialty Resident

INDEX

Abenol Suppositories, 42-44
AC&C, 95-100
Accutane Roche, 254-258
ACEBUTOLOL, 330-336
ACETAMINOPHEN (ORAL), 42-44
ACETAMINOPHEN (RECTAL), 42-44
ACETAMINOPHEN-CAFFEINE-CODEINE, 45-48
ACETAMINOPHEN-CODEINE (ORAL), 45-48
ACETAMINOPHEN-OXYCODONE, 45-48
Acetaminophen Suppositories, 42-44
ACETOHEXAMIDE (ORAL), 48-52
Achromycin V, 355-359
ACYCLOVIR (ORAL), 52-54
ACYCLOVIR (TOPICAL), 55-57
Adalat, 181-185
Adalat P.A. 20, 181-185
Aerosporin Ophthalmic, 312-313
aging and color vision, 182
Ak-Sulf Eye Drops, 341-342
Aldactazide, 342-346
Aldactone, 342-346
Aldomet, 271-274
Aldoril, 271-274
Alka Butazolidin, 305-307
Alka-Phenylbutazone, 305-307
Alkabutazone, 305-307
Allerdryl, 186-188
Alloprin, 57-59
ALLOPURINOL (ORAL), 57-59
ALPRAZOLAM (ORAL), 60-62
Alupent Metered Aerosol, 246-250
Alupent Syrup, 246-250
Alupent Tablets, 246-250
AMCINONIDE (TOPICAL), 62-67
Amersol, 165-170
AMILORIDE (ORAL), 67-70
AMILORIDE-HYDROCHLOROTHIAZIDE, 67-70
AMINOPHYLLINE (ORAL), 359-363
AMINOPHYLLINE (RECTAL), 359-363
AMITRIPTYLINE, 56, 80, 141-142
AMITRIPTYLINE HCl (ORAL), 70-76
AMITRIPTYLINE-PERPHENAZINE (ORAL), 76-80
AMOBARBITAL (ORAL AND RECTAL), 81-85
AMOBARBITAL-SECOBARBITAL, 81-85
AMOXAPINE, 70-76
AMOXICILLIN-POTASSIUM CLAVULANATE, 85-88
AMOXICILLIN TRIHYDRATE (ORAL), 85-88
Amoxil, 85-88
AMPHETAMINE, 141-142
AMPICILLIN (ORAL), 88-91
Amytal, 81-85
Anacin with Codeine, 95-100
Anacin 3, 42-44
Anacin 3 Extra Strength, 42-44
Anafranil, 70-76
Anaprox, 165-170
Ancasal 8, 95-100
Ancasal 15, 95-100
Ancasal 30, 95-100
Ansaid, 165-170
APO-Acetaminophen, 42-44
Apo-Allopurinol, 57-59
Apo-Amitriptyline, 70-76
Apo-Amoxi, 85-88
Apo-Ampi, 88-91
Apo-Benztropine, 107-110
Apo-Carbamazepine, 121-124
Apo-Chlorax, 127-129
Apo-Chlordiazepoxide, 60-62
Apo-Chlorpropamide, 48-52
Apo-Chlorthalidone, 223-226
Apo-Cimetidine, 143-145
Apo-Cloxi, 88-91
Apo-Diazepam, 60-62
Apo-Dipyridamole, 188-191
Apo-Doxy, 194-197
Apo-Erythro Base, 197-202
Apo-Erythro-ES, 197-202
Apo-Erythro-S, 198-202
Apo-Fluphenazine, 137-143
Apo-Flurazepam, 214-216

Apo-Furosemide, 204-208
Apo-Haloperidol, 216-220
Apo-Hydro, 223-226
Apo-Hydroxyzine, 232-235
Apo-Ibuprofen, 165-170
Apo-Imipramine, 71-76
Apo-Indomethacin, 235-238
Apo-ISDN, 250-254
Apo-K, 313-315
Apo-Lorazepam, 60-62
Apo-Methazide, 271-274
Apo-Methyldopa, 271-274
Apo-Metoprolol, 330-336
Apo-Metoprolol (Type L), 330-336
Apo-Metronidazole, 278-280
Apo-Naproxen, 165-170
Apo-Nifed, 181-185
Apo-Nitrofurantoin, 287-289
Apo-Oxazepam, 60-62
Apo-Pen-VK, 299-301
Apo-Perphenazine, 137-143
Apo-Phenylbutazone, 305-307
Apo-Piroxicam, 165-170
Apo-Prednisone, 110-114
Apo-Procainamide, 319-321
Apo-Propranolol, 330-336
Apo-Quinidine, 338-341
Apo-Ranitidine, 143-145
Apo-Sulfamethoxazole, 352-355
Apo-Sulfatrim, 352-355
Apo-Sulfatrim DS, 352-355
Apo-Sulfatrim Pediatric, 352-355
Apo-Sulfisoxazole, 352-355
Apo-Tetra, 355-359
Apo-Thioridazine, 137-143
Apo-Tolbutamide, 48-52
Apo-Triazide, 372-376
Apo-Trifluoperazine, 137-143
Apo-Trimip, 71-76
Apresoline, 220-223
Aristocort, 110-114
Aristocort C, 64-67
Aristocort D, 64-67
Aristocort R, 64-67
ASA, 95, 97, 98, 340, 375
ASA-BARBITURATE (ORAL), 92-95
ASA-BARBITURATE-CAFFEINE, 92-95
ASA-BARBITURATE-CAFFEINE-CODEINE, 92-95
ASA-BARBITURATE-CODEINE, 92-95
ASA-CAFFEINE-CODEINE (ORAL), 95-100
ASA-CODEINE, 95-100
ASA-OXYCODONE, 96-100
Asasantine, 188-191
Asendin, 70-76
aspirin burn, 97
Atarax, 232-235
Atasol, 42-44
Atasol Forte, 42-44
Atasol-8, 45-48
Atasol-15, 45-48
Atasol-30, 45-48
ATENOLOL, 330-336
ATENOLOL-CHLORTHALIDONE, 331-336
Athrombin-K, 379-383
Ativan, 60-62
ATROPINE, 56, 141-142
ATROPINE-SCOPOLAMINE-HYOSCYAMINE-PHENOBARBITAL (ORAL), 100-103
Aventyl, 71-76
Axid, 143-145
Azo-Gantrisin, 352-355

BACAMPICILLIN, 88-91
Baciguent, 312-313
BACITRACIN, 312-313
bacterial infections, transmitted by pets, 87
bacterial infections, transmitted by toothbrushes, 351
Bactrim, 352-355
Bactrim DS, 352-355
bad-tasting medicines, 91
baking soda, 275
Barriere-HC, 63-67
Beben, 63-67
BECLOMETHASONE, 62-67
BECLOMETHASONE (INHALATION), 103-105
BECLOMETHASONE (NASAL), 105-107
Beclovent Inhaler, 103-105

BECLOVENT ROTACAPS, 103-105
BECONASE, 105-107
BECONASE AQUEOUS NASAL SPRAY, 105-107
bedridden people, 318
bee stings, 169
BELLADONNA, 56
BENADRYL, 186-188
BENDROFLUMETHIAZIDE, 223-226
BENSYLATE, 107-110
BENTYLOL, 170-174
BENTYLOL DOSPAN, 170-174
BENTYLOL WITH PHENOBARBITAL, 170-174
BENYLIN COUGH SYRUP, 186-188
BENYLIN DECONGESTANT, 186-188
BENYLIN DIETETIC (SUGARLESS), 186-188
BENYLIN DM, 186-188
BENYLIN DM-D, 186-188
BENYLIN DM-D-E, 186-188
BENZTROPINE, 141-142
BENZTROPINE MESYLATE (ORAL), 107-110
BETACORT SCALP LOTION, 63-67
BETADERM, 63-67
BETADERM SCALP LOTION, 63-67
BETAGAN, 363-366
BETALOC, 330-336
BETALOC DURULES, 330-336
BETAMETHASONE, 63-67
BETAMETHASONE (ORAL), 110-114
BETAXOL HCl, 363-366
BETNELAN, 110-114
BETNESOL, 110-114
BETNOVATE, 63-67
BETOPTIC, 363-366
BIQUIN DURULES, 338-341
birth control pills, 80, 284
bladder control, loss of, 226-227
BLEPH-10 LIQUIFILM, 341-342
BLOCADREN, 331-336
blood pressure, 121, 208, 223
BONAMINE, 269-271
BRICANYL AEROSOL, 247-250
BRICANYL TABLETS, 247-250
BROMAZEPAM, 60-62
BROMPHENIRAMINE (ORAL), 114-117
BROMPHENIRAMINE MALEATE-PHENYLEPHRINE-PHENYLPROPANOLAMINE, 114-117
BROMPHENIRAMINE-PHENYLEPHRINE-PHENYLPROPANOLAMINE-ACETAMINOPHEN, 115-117
BROMPHENIRAMINE-PHENYLEPHRINE-PHENYLPROPANOLAMINE-CODEINE, 115-117
BROMPHENIRAMINE-PHENYLEPHRINE-PHENYLPROPANOLAMINE-DEXTROMET-HORPHAN, 115-117
BROMPHENIRAMINE-PHENYLEPHRINE-PHENYLPROPANOLAMINE-GUAIFENESIN, 114-117
BROMPHENIRAMINE-PHENYLEPHRINE-PHENYLPROPANOLAMINE-GUAIFENESIN-CODEINE, 115-117
BROMPHENIRAMINE-PHENYLEPHRINE-PHENYLPROPANOLAMINE-GUAIFENESIN-HYDROCODONE, 115-117
BRONALIDE AEROSOL, 103-105
bulimia, 176
BUTABARBITAL, 81-85
BUTAZOLIDIN, 305-307
BUTISOL SODIUM, 81-85

C2 BUFFERED WITH CODEINE, 95-100
C2 WITH CODEINE, 95-100
caffeine in beverages, 84
Canadian and American medications, 114
Canadian Medic-Alert, 6
cancer test kits, 365
CANESTEN, 150-152
CANESTEN 1, 150-152
CANESTEN 1 COMBI-PAK, 150-152
CANESTEN 3, 150-152
CAPOTEN, 118-120
CAPTOPRIL, 56
CAPTOPRIL (ORAL), 118-120

CARBAMAZEPINE (ORAL), 121-124
CARBOLITH, 264-267
CARDIOQUIN, 338-341
CARDIZEM, 181-185
CATAPRES, 145-149
CECLOR, 59, 124-126
CEDOCARD-SR, 250-254
CEFACLOR (ORAL), 124-126
CEFADROXIL, 124-126
CELESTODERM-V, 63-67
CELESTODERM-V/2, 63-67
CELESTONE, 110-114
CELONTIN, 208-211
CEPHADRINE, 124-126
CEPHALEXIN MONOHYDRATE, 124-126
CEPOREX, 124-126
C.E.S., 129-134
CETAMIDE EYE OINTMENT, 341-342
chemotherapy, 371
chewable tablets, 120
child-proof caps, 274
children, giving medicine to, 127, 173, 190, 201
CHILDREN'S BENYLIN-DM-D, 186-188
CHLOR-TRIPOLON, 134-137
CHLOR-TRIPOLON DECONGESTANT SYRUP, 134-137
CHLORDIAZEPOXIDE, 56, 80
CHLORDIAZEPOXIDE-CLIDINIUM (ORAL), 127-129
CHLORDIAZEPOXIDE HCI, 60-62
CHLOROTRIANISENE (ORAL), 129-134
CHLORPHENIRAMINE MALEATE (ORAL), 134-137
CHLORPHENIRAMINE MALEATE-PHENYLEPHRINE, 134-137
CHLORPHENIRAMINE-PHENYLPROPANOLAMINE, 134-137
CHLORPHENIRAMINE-PHENYLPROPANOLAMINE-DEXTROMETHORPHAN, 134-137
CHLORPHENIRAMINE-PHENYLPROPANOLAMINE-GUAIFENESIN, 134-137
CHLORPROMAZINE, 56, 80, 141-142
CHLORPROMAZINE HCl (ORAL AND RECTAL), 137-143
CHLORPROPAMIDE, 48-52
CHLORTHALIDONE, 56, 223-226
CHOLEDYL, 359-363
CHOLEDYL SA, 359-363
CIMETIDINE, 56, 143-145, 154
CLAVULIN, 85-88
CLINORIL, 165-170
CLOBETASOL PROPIONATE, 63-67
CLOBETASONE, 63-67
CLOMIPRAMINE, 70-76
CLONAZEPAM, 60-62
CLONIDINE (ORAL), 145-149
CLONIDINE-CHLORTHALIDONE (ORAL), 145-149
CLORAZEPATE DIPOTASSIUM, 60-62
CLOTRIMAZOLE (TOPICAL), 150-152
CLOTRIMAZOLE (VAGINAL), 150-152
CLOXACILLIN, 88-91
CO-BETALOC, 331-336
coatings, 11
COGENTIN, 107-110
color of medicines, 184
COMBID, 321-324
COMBIPRES, 145-149
CONJUGATED ESTROGENS, 129-134
contact lenses, discolored by drugs, 354
COPTIN, 352-355
CORDARONE, 59
CORGARD, 331-336
CORIUM, 127-129
CORONEX, 250-254
COROPHYLLIN, 359-363
CORTACET, 63-67
CORTATE, 63-67
CORTEF, 63-67, 110-114
CORTICREME, 63-67
CORTISONE, 110-114
CORTISPORIN EYE DROPS, 312-313
CORTISPORIN EYE OINTMENT, 312-313
CORTODERM, 63-67
CORTONE, 59, 110-114
CORYPHEN-CODEINE, 95-100
CORZIDE, 331-336
COUMADIN, 59, 379-383

CROMOGLYCATE SODIUM (INHALATION), 154-157
CROMOGLYCATE SODIUM (NASAL), 157-159
CROMOGLYCATE SODIUM (OPHTHALMIC), 159-161
CROMOGLYCATE SODIUM (ORAL), 152-154
C2 Buffered with Codeine, 95-100
C2 with Codeine, 95-100
CYCLOBENZAPRINE (ORAL), 161-163
Cyclocort, 62-67
CYPROHEPTADINE HCl (ORAL), 163-164
Cytomel, 258-261

Dagenan, 352-355
Dalmane, 214-216
Darbid, 245-246
Darvon-N, 327-330
Darvon-N with ASA, 327-330
Darvon-N Compound, 328-330
Day-Barb, 81-85
Decadron, 110-114
Deltasone, 110-114
DEMECLOCYCLINE, 190
Depakene, 376-379
Dermovate, 63-67
Deronil, 110-114
DESICCATED THYROID, 258-261
DESIPRAMINE, 56, 70-76, 80
DESONIDE, 63-67
DESOXIMETASONE, 63-67
Desyrel, 71-76
Detensol, 330-336
DEXAMETHASONE, 110-114
Dexasone, 110-114
DiaBeta, 48-52
Diabinese, 48-52
diarrhea, 173
DIAZEPAM, 56, 60-62, 80
DICLOFENAC (RECTAL), 165-170
DICLOFENAC SODIUM (ORAL), 165-170
Diclophen, 170-174
DICLOXACILLIN, 88-91
DICYCLOMINE HCl (ORAL), 170-174
DICYCLOMINE HCl-PHENOBARBITAL, 170-174
DIETHYLPROPION (ORAL), 174-176
DIFLORASONE, 63-67
DIFLUCORTOLONE, 63-67
DIFLUNISAL (ORAL), 176-179
DIGOXIN, 234
DIGOXIN (ORAL), 179-181
Dilantin Capsules, 307-312
Dilantin Infatabs, 307-312
Dilantin-30 Suspension, 307-312
Dilantin-125 Suspension, 307-312
DILTIAZEM (ORAL), 181-185
diluents, 11
Dimelor, 48-52
Dimetane, 114-117
Dimetane Expectorant, 114-117
Dimetane Expectorant-C, 115-117
Dimetane Expectorant-DC, 115-117
Dimetapp, 114-117
Dimetapp-A, 115-117
Dimetapp-A Pediatric, 115-117
Dimetapp-C, 115-117
Dimetapp with Codeine, 115-117
Dimetapp-DM, 115-117
Dimetapp Oral Infant Drops, 114-117
DIPHENHYDRAMINE COMPOUNDS, 186-188
DIPHENHYDRAMINE HCl (ORAL), 186-188
Diprolene, 63-67
Diprosone, 63-67
DIPYRIDAMOLE (ORAL), 188-191
DIPYRIDAMOLE-ASA, 188-191
disintegrants, 11
DISOPYRAMIDE (ORAL), 191-194
Diuchlor H, 223-226
diuretics, 141-142
DIVALPROEX SODIUM, 376-379
Dolobid, 176-179
Donnagel, 59
Donnatal, 59, 100-103
Dopamet, 271-274
double doses, 234
DOXEPIN, 70-76
DOXYCYCLINE, 190
DOXYCYCLINE (ORAL), 194-197

Drenison, 63-67
Drenison Tape, 63-67
Dristan Long Lasting Capsules, 134-137
driving performance, affected by medication, 99
drug dependence, 83
drug interactions, 197, 243-244, 354, 358, 381
dry mouth, 75, 113, 136
Duralith, 264-267
Duretic, 223-226
Duricef, 124-126
Dyazide, 372-376
Dynapen, 88-91
Dyrenium, 372-376

E-Mycin, 197-202
E-Pam, 60-62
Ectosone Mild, 63-67
Ectosone Regular, 63-67
Ectosone Scalp Lotion, 63-67
Edecrin, 204-208
EES 200, 197-202
EES 400, 197-202
EES 600, 197-202
Elavil, 70-76
Elavil Plus, 76-80
Elixophyllin, 359-363
Eltroxin, 258-261
emergency phone numbers, 338
Emex, 274-277
Emo-Cort, 63-67
Empracet-30, 45-48
Empracet-60, 45-48
Emtec-30, 45-48
ENALAPRIL, 118-120
Endocet, 45-48
Endodan, 96-100
epileptic seizures, 311
EPINEPHRINE HYDROCHLORIDE, 2%, 354
EPINEPHRYL BORATE, 1%, 354
Epival, 376-379
Eryc 125, 197-202
Eryc 250, 197-202
Erythrocin, 198-202
Erythromid, 197-202
ERYTHROMYCIN BASE, 197-202
ERYTHROMYCIN ESTOLATE, 197-202
ERYTHROMYCIN ETHYL SUCCINATE, 197-202
ERYTHROMYCIN ETHYLSUCCINATE-SULFASOXAZOLE (ORAL), 202-204
ERYTHROMYCIN PRODUCTS (ORAL), 197-202
ERYTHROMYCIN STEARATE, 198-202
Estinyl, 129-134
Estrace, 129-134
Estraderm Patch, 129-134
ESTRADIOL, 129-134
ESTRADIOL (TRANSDERMAL), 129-134
ESTROGENS (VAGINAL), 129-134
ESTROPIPATE, 129-134
ETHACRYNIC ACID, 204-208
ETHINYL ESTRADIOL, 129-134
ETHOSUXIMIDE (ORAL), 208-211
Etrafon-A, 76-80
Etrafon-D, 76-80
Etrafon-F, 76-80
Etrafon 2-10, 76-80
Euglucon, 48-52
Eumovate, 63-67
Exdol, 42-44
Exdol Strong, 42-44
Exdol-8, 45-48
Exdol-15, 45-48
Exdol-30, 45-48
eye drops, 258, 315

FAMOTIDINE (ORAL), 143-145
Fastin, 174-176
Feldene, 59, 165-170
Feldene Suppositories, 165-170
FENOPROFEN, 95
FENOPROFEN CALCIUM (ORAL), 165-170
Fiorinal, 92-95
Fiorinal-C 1/4, 92-95
Fiorinal-C 1/2, 92-95
Fivent Inhaler, 154-157
Flagyl, 278-280

FLECAINIDE (ORAL), 211-214
FLEXERIL, 161-163
FLORONE, 63-67
FLUCLOX, 88-91
FLUCLOXACILLIN, 88-91
FLUMETHASONE PIVALATE, 63-67
FLUNISOLIDE, 103-107
FLUOCINOLONE ACETONIDE, 63-67
FLUOCINONIDE, 63-67
FLUODERM, 63-67
FLUOLAR, 63-67
FLUONIDE, 63-67
FLUPHENAZINE HCl, 137-143
FLURANDRENOLIDE, 63-67
FLURAZEPAM (ORAL), 214-216
FLURBIPROFEN (ORAL), 165-170
FLUTONE, 63-67
food-drug interactions, 242-243, 284
FORMULEX, 170-174
FROBEN, 165-170
FUROSEMIDE (ORAL), 204-208
FUROSIDE, 204-208

GANTANOL, 352-355
GARDENAL, 81-85
GBH, 261-264
glove compartments, storing medicines in, 50
GLUCOPHAGE, 48-52
GLYBURIDE, 48-52
GRISEOFULVIN, 244
GUANETHIDINE, 56

HALCINONIDE, 63-67
HALCION, 214-216
HALDOL, 216-220
HALOG, 63-67
HALOPERIDOL (ORAL), 216-220
halves of tablets, 117, 230
heat exhaustion, 140-141
HEPARIN, 80
HEXADROL, 110-114
high blood pressure, 121
HISTANTIL, 325-327
HISTASPAN-P, 134-137
HYDERM, 63-67
HYDRALAZINE, 56
HYDRALAZINE (ORAL), 220-223
HYDROCHLOROTHIAZIDE, 141-142
HYDROCHLOROTHIAZIDE (ORAL), 223-226
HYDROCODONE AND PHENYLTOLOXAMINE-RESIN COMPLEXES (ORAL), 228-232
HYDROCORTISONE, 63-67, 110-114
HYDROCORTISONE-NEOMYCIN, 63-67
HYDRODIURIL, 223-226
HYDROXYZINE HCl (ORAL), 232-235
HYGROTON, 223-226

IBUPROFEN, 95
IBUPROFEN (ORAL), 165-170
ILOSONE, 197-202
IMIPRAMINE, 56, 71-76, 80, 141-142
IMODIUM, 267-269
IMPRIL, 71-76
incontinence, 227-228
INDAPAMIDE, 223-226
INDERAL, 330-336
INDERAL LA, 330-336
INDERIDE, 331-336
INDOCID, 235-238
INDOCID SR, 235-238
INDOCID SUPPOSITORIES, 235-238
INDOMETHACIN, 95
INDOMETHACIN (ORAL), 235-238
INDOMETHACIN (RECTAL), 235-238
INSOMNAL, 186-188
insulin, 51, 154
INTAL NEBULIZER, 154-157
INTAL SPINCAPS, 154-157
INTRABUTAZONE, 305-307
IONAMIN, 174-176
ISOCARBOXAZID, 141-142
ISOCARBOXAZID (ORAL), 238-244
ISOPROPAMIDE (ORAL), 245-246
ISOPROTERENOL (INHALATION AND SUBLINGUAL), 246-250
ISOPTIN, 181-185
ISOPTO-CETAMIDE EYE DROPS, 341-342
ISORDIL, 250-254
ISOSORBIDE DINITRATE (ORAL), 250-254

ISOSORBIDE DINITRATE (SUBLINGUAL), 250-254
ISOTRETINOIN (ORAL), 254-258
Isuprel Mistometer, 246-250
Isuprel Sublingual Tablets, 246-250

K-Long, 313-315
K-Lor, 59, 313-315
K-Lyte, 313-315
K-Lyte/C1, 313-315
K-Med, 313-315
K-10, 313-315
Kalium Durules, 313-315
Kao-Con, 59
Kaochlor, 313-315
Kaochlor-20 Concentrate, 313-315
Kaon, 59, 313-315
Kato, 313-315
Kay-Ciel, 313-315
KCI 5%, 313-315
Keflex, 59, 124-126
Kemadrin, 59
Kenacort, 110-114
Kenalog, 64-67
Kenalog Spray, 64-67
KETOPROFEN, 95
KETOPROFEN (ORAL), 165-170
KETOPROFEN (RECTAL), 165-170
Koffex, 59
Kwellada, 261-264

labels, 65
LABETALOL, 330-336
lanolin, topical application, 232
Lanoxin, 179-181
Lanoxin Pediatric Elixir, 179-181
Largactil, 137-143
Lasix, 204-208
laxatives, 238
Lectopam, 60-62
Ledercillin-VK, 299-301
Lenoltec with Codeine No. 1, 45-48
Lenoltec with Codeine No. 2, 45-48
Lenoltec with Codeine No. 3, 45-48
Lenoltec with Codeine No. 4, 45-48
Levate, 70-76
LEVOBUNOLOL HCl, 363-366
LEVOTHYROXINE SODIUM (ORAL), 258-261
Librax, 127-129
Librium, 60-62
Lidemol, 63-67
Lidex, 63-67
Lidocaine, 190
LINDANE (TOPICAL), 261-264
LIOTHYRONINE, 258-261
LIOTRIX, 258-261
Lithane, 264-267
LITHIUM CARBONATE (ORAL), 264-267
Lithizine, 264-267
Locacorten, 63-67
Lomine, 170-174
LOPERAMIDE (ORAL), 267-269
Lopresor, 330-336
Lopresor SR, 330-336
LORAZEPAM (ORAL and SUBLINGUAL), 60-62
Lozide, 223-226
Ludiomil, 71-76
Lyderm, 63-67

Macrodantin, 287-289
MAPROTILINE, 71-76
Marplan, 238-244
Maxeran, 274-277
Maxitrol Eye Drops, 312-313
Maxitrol Eye Ointment, 312-313
Mazepine, 121-124
MECLIZINE HCl (ORAL), 269-271
medicine cabinets, 47
Medihaler-Iso Inhaler, 246-250
Medilium, 60-62
Medrol, 110-114
Medrol Topical, 64-67
MEFENAMIC ACID, 95
Megacillin, 299-301
Mellaril, 137-143
MEPHENYTOIN, 307-312
MEPROBAMATE, 56
Mesantoin, 307-312
MESORIDAZINE, 137-143
Metaderm, 63-67
METFORMIN, 48-52

METHOTRIMEPRAZINE, 137-143
METHSUXIMIDE, 208-211
METHYCHLOTHIAZIDE, 223-226
METHYLDOPA, 56
METHYLDOPA (ORAL), 271-274
METHYLDOPA-CHLOROTHIAZIDE, 271-274
METHYLDOPA-HYDROCHLOROTHIAZIDE, 271-274
METHYLPREDNISOLONE, 64-67, 110-114
METHYLPREDNISOLONE-NEOMYCIN, 64-67
METOCLOPRAMIDE (ORAL), 274-277
METOLAZONE, 223-226
METOPROLOL, 330-336
METOPROLOL-HYDROCHLOROTHIAZIDE, 331-336
METRONIDAZOLE (ORAL), 278-280
Meval, 60-62
MEXILETINE, 366-369
Mexitil, 366-369
Micatin Cream, 280-284
Micatin Lotion, 280-284
MICONAZOLE NITRATE (TOPICAL), 280-284
MICONAZOLE NITRATE (VAGINAL), 280-284
Micro-K Extencaps, 313-315
Micro-K-10 Extencaps, 313-315
Midamor, 67-70
Milontin, 208-211
Minipress, 316-319
Minocin, 194-197
MINOCYCLINE, 190, 194-197
Mobenol, 48-52
Moditen, 137-143
Moduret, 67-70
Monistat, 280-284
Monistat Derm Cream, 280-284
Monistat 3 Dual-Pak, 280-284
Monistat 3 Vaginal Ovules, 280-284
Monistat 5 Tampons, 280-284
Monistat 7, 280-284
Monitan, 330-336
Monoamine Oxidase Inhibitors, 141-142, 238-244, 243
Motrin, 165-170
Multipax, 232-235
Myclo, 150-152

NADOLOL, 331-336
NADOLOL-BENDROFLUMETHIAZIDE, 331-336
Nadopen-V, 299-301
Nalcrom, 152-154
Nalfon, 165-170
Naprosyn, 165-170
Naprosyn Suppositories, 165-170
NAPROXEN, 95
NAPROXEN (ORAL), 165-170
NAPROXEN (RECTAL), 165-170
NAPROXEN SODIUM (ORAL), 165-170
Nardil, 238-244
nasal congestion, 220, 340
Natrimax, 223-226
Naturetin, 223-226
nausea from chemotherapy, 371
Naxen, 165-170
Nembutal, 81-85
Neo-Codema, 223-226
Neo-Cortef, 63-67
Neo-K, 313-315
Neo-Medrol Topical, 64-67
Neo-Metric, 278-280
Neosporin Eye and Ear Solution, 312-313
Neosporin Eye Ointment, 312-313
Nephronex, 287-289
Nerisone, 63-67
Nicorette, 284-287
NICOTINE RESIN COMPLEX (SMOKING CESSATION AID), 284-287
NIFEDIPINE, 181-185
Nitro-Bid, 295-299
NITROFURANTOIN (ORAL), 287-289
Nitroglycerin, 291-295
NITROGLYCERIN (ORAL), 289-291
NITROGLYCERIN (SUBLINGUAL), 291-295
NITROGLYCERIN (TRANSLINGUAL), 291-295

NITROGLYCERIN OINTMENT (TOPICAL), 295-299
Nitrol, 295-299
Nitrol Tsar Kit, 295-299
Nitrolingual Spray, 291-295
Nitrong, 295-299
Nitrong-SR, 289-291
Nitrostat, 291-295
NIZATIDINE, 143-145
Nobesine-75, 174-176
NORIPRAMINE, 59
Norpace, 191-194
Norpace CR, 191-194
Norpramin, 59, 70-76
NORTRIPTYLINE, 71-76, 80, 141-142
nose drops, 220
Nova-Rectal, 81-85
Novamoxin, 85-88
Novo-Ampicillin, 88-91
Novo-Hyalazin, 220-223
Novo-Nifedin, 181-185
Novo-Rythro Base, 197-202
Novo-Rythro Estolate, 197-202
Novo-Rythro Stearate, 198-202
Novobetamet, 63-67
Novobutamide, 48-52
Novobutazone, 305-307
Novochlorpromazine, 137-143
Novocimetine, 143-145
Novoclopate, 60-62
Novocloxin, 88-91
Novodipam, 60-62
Novodoparil, 271-274
Novoflupam, 214-216
Novoflurazine, 137-143
Novofuran, 287-289
Novohydrazide, 223-226
Novohydrocort, 63-67
Novohydroxyzin, 232-235
Novolente-K, 313-315
Novolexin, 124-126
Novolorazem, 60-62
Novomedopa, 271-274
Novomethacin, 235-238
Novometoprol, 330-336
Novonaprox, 165-170
Novonidazol, 278-280
Novopen-G-500, 299-301
Novopen-VK, 299-301
Novoperidol, 216-220
Novopheniram, 134-137
Novopirocam, 165-170
Novopoxide, 60-62
Novopramine, 71-76
Novopranol, 330-336
Novoprofen, 165-170
Novopropamide, 48-52
Novopropoxyn, 327-330
Novopropoxyn Compound, 327-330
Novopurol, 57-59
Novoquinidin, 338-341
Novoridazine, 137-143
Novosalmol, 247-250
Novosemide, 204-208
Novosorbide, 250-254
Novosoxazole, 352-355
Novospiroton, 342-346
Novospirozine, 342-346
Novotetra, 355-359
Novothalidone, 223-226
Novotriamzide, 372-376
Novotrimel, 352-355
Novotrimel DS, 352-355
Novotriptyn, 70-76
Novoxapam, 60-62
Nozinan, 137-143

Oestrilin Vaginal, 129-134
Ogen, 129-134
Opticrom, 159-161
Oradexon, 110-114
Orbenin, 88-91
ORCIPRENALINE (ORAL AND INHALATION), 246-250
Orinase, 48-52
Ornade, 134-137
Ornade-A.F., 134-137
Ornade-DM 10 Pediatric, 134-137
Ornade-DM 15, 134-137
Ornade-DM 30, 134-137
Ornade Expectorant, 134-137
Ortho Dienestrol Cream, 129-134
Orudis, 165-170
Orudis E-50, 165-170

Orudis E-100, 165-170
Orudis Suppositories, 165-170
ostomy odors, 261
ovulation test kits, 152
Ox-Pam, 60-62
OXAZEPAM, 60-62
OXPRENOLOL, 331-336
OXTRIPHYLLINE (ORAL), 359-363
Oxycocet, 45-48
Oxycodan, 96-100

Palaron, 359-363
Panadol, 42-44
Panadol Chewable, 42-44
Parnate, 238-244
Pediazole, 202-204
Pen-Vee, 299-301
Penbritin, 88-91
Penglobe, 88-91
PENICILLIN G, 243
PENICILLIN G POTASSIUM, 299-301
PENICILLIN V (ORAL), 299-301
PENICILLIN V POTASSIUM, 299-301
PENTAZOCINE, 80
PENTOBARBITAL, 81-85
PENTOXIFYLLINE (ORAL), 302-305
Pepcid, 143-145
Peptol, 143-145
Percocet, 45-48
Percocet-Demi, 45-48
Percodan, 96-100
Percodan-Demi, 96-100
Periactin, 163-164
Peridol, 216-220
Permitil, 137-143
PERPHENAZINE, 137-143
Persantine, 188-191
Pertofrane, 70-76
pharmacists, 44, 150, 381
Phenaphen, 92-95
Phenaphen No. 2, 92-95
Phenaphen No. 3, 92-95
Phenaphen No. 4, 92-95
Phenazine, 137-143
Phenbuff, 305-307
PHENELZINE, 141-142, 238-244
Phenergan, 325-327
PHENIRAMINE-PHENYLPROPANOLAMINE-PYRILAMINE, 134-137
PHENIRAMINE-PHENYLPROPANOLAMINE-PYRILAMINE-GUAIFENESIN, 134-137
PHENIRAMINE-PHENYLPROPANOLAMINE-PYRILAMINE-GUAIFENESIN-DEXTROMETHORPHAN, 134-137
PHENOBARBITAL, 81-85
PHENOTHIAZINES, 141-142
PHENOXYBENZAMINE, 56
PHENSUXIMIDE, 208-211
PHENTERMINE HCl, 174-176
PHENYLBUTAZONE (ORAL), 305-307
PHENYLBUTAZONE-ANTACIDS, 305-307
Phenylone Plus, 305-307
PHENYTOIN, 234
PHENYTOIN (ORAL), 307-312
Phyllocontin, 359-363
Phyllocontin-350, 359-363
PINDOLOL, 331-336
PINDOLOL-HYDROCHLOROTHIAZIDE, 331-336
PIROXICAM, 95
PIROXICAM (ORAL), 165-170
PIROXICAM (RECTAL), 165-170
PIVAMPICILLIN, 88-91
PMS Benztropine, 107-110
PMS Dopazide, 271-274
PMS Levazine, 76-80
PMS Metronidazole, 278-280
PMS Promethazine Syrup, 325-327
PMS Propranolol, 330-336
PMS Sulfasalazine, 348-351
PMS Sulfasalazine E.C., 348-351
PMS Theophylline Elixir, 359-363
PMS Thioridazine, 137-143
POLYMYXIN (OPHTHALMIC), 312-313
POLYMYXIN B-BACITRACIN, 312-313
POLYMYXIN B-GRAMICIDIN, 312-313
POLYMYXIN B-NEOMYCIN-COMBINATIONS, 312-313
POLYMYXIN B-NEOMYCIN-STEROID COMBINATIONS, 312-313

POLYSPORIN EYE/EAR DROPS, 312-313
POLYSPORIN EYE/EAR OINTMENT, 312-313
PONDOCILLIN, 88-91
POTASSIUM-ROUGIER, 313-315
POTASSIUM SANDOZ, 313-315
POTASSIUM SUPPLEMENTS (ORAL), 313-315
PRAZOSIN (ORAL), 316-319
PREDNISONE, 110-114
PREMARIN, 129-134
PREMARIN VAGINAL CREAM, 129-134
prescription records, 150, 381
prescription refills, 346
PROAVIL, 76-80
PROCAINAMIDE (ORAL), 319-321
PROCAN SR, 319-321
PROCHLORPERAZINE, 137-143
PROCHLORPERAZINE-ISOPROPAMIDE (ORAL), 321-324
PROLOID, 258-261
PROMAZINE, 137-143
PROMETHAZINE (ORAL), 325-327
PRONESTYL, 319-321
PRONESTYL SR, 319-321
PROPADERM, 62-67
PROPRANOLOL, 56, 80, 141-142
PROPRANOLOL (ORAL), 330-336
PROPRANOLOL-HYDROCHLOROTHIAZIDE, 331-336
PROPANTHELINE, 56
PROPOXYPHENE, 80
PROPOXYPHENE HCl (ORAL), 327-330
PROPOXYPHENE HCl-ASA-CAFFEINE, 327-330
PROPOXYPHENE NAPSYLATE, 327-330
PROPOXYPHENE NAPSYLATE-ASA, 327-330
PROPOXYPHENE NAPSYLATE-ASA-CAFFEINE, 328-330
PROTRIN, 352-355
PROTRIN DF, 352-355
PROTRIPTYLINE, 71-76, 141-142
PROTYLOL, 170-174
PULMOPHYLLINE, 359-363
PURINOL, 57-59
PVF, 299-301
PVF-K, 299-301

quack cures, 209
questions to ask pharmacists, 44
QUIBRON-T LIQUID, 359-363
QUIBRON-T/SR, 359-363
QUINAGLUTE DURA-TABS, 338-341
QUINATE, 338-341
QUINIDEX EXTENTABS, 338-341
QUINIDINE BISULFATE (ORAL), 338-341
QUINIDINE GLUCONATE, 338-341
QUINIDINE POLYGALACTURONATE, 338-341
QUINIDINE SULFATE, 338-341

RANITIDINE, 143-145
refrigerating medicines, 47
REGLAN, 274-277
RESERPINE, 56
RESTORIL, 214-216
RHINALAR, 105-107
RIFAMPIN, 354
RIVAL, 60-62
RIVOTRIL, 60-62
ROBIGESIC, 42-44
ROUBAC, 352-355
ROUBAC DS, 352-355
ROUNOX, 42-44
ROUNOX + CODEINE, 45-48
ROYCHLOR 10%, 313-315
ROYCHLOR 20%, 313-315
ROYONATE, 313-315
RYNACROM CARTRIDGES, 157-159
RYNACROM NASAL SOLUTION, 157-159
RYTHMODAN, 191-194
RYTHMODAN-LA, 191-194

SALAZOPYRIN, 348-351
SALAZOPYRIN EN-TABS, 348-351
SALBUTAMOL (ORAL AND INHALATION), 247-250
SARNA HC 1.0%, 63-67
S.A.S. ENTERIC-500, 348-351
S.A.S.-500, 348-351
SCOPOLAMINE, 141-142
SECOBARBITAL, 81-85

Seconal Sodium, 81-85
Sectral, 330-336
Seldane, 59
senility due to medicine, 154
Septra, 352-355
Septra DS, 352-355
Serax, 60-62
Serentil, 137-143
sharing medicines, 348
side effects, 124
Sincomen, 342-346
Sinequan, 70-76
642's, 327-330
692's, 327-330
Slo-Bid, 359-363
Slo-Pot 600, 313-315
Slow-K, 313-315
Slow-Trasicor, 331-336
smoking, and response to medication, 80-81
sodium bicarbonate, 275
Sodium Sulamyd Eye Drops, 341-342
Sodium Sulamyd Eye Ointment, 341-342
SODIUM SULFACETAMIDE (OPHTHALMIC), 341-342
Solazine, 137-143
Solium, 60-62
Som-Pam, 214-216
Somnol, 214-216
Somophyllin-T, 359-363
Somophyllin-12, 359-363
Sotacor, 331-336
SOTALOL, 331-336
Sparine, 137-143
Spasmoban, 170-174
Spasmoban-PH, 170-174
SPIRONOLACTONE, 56
SPIRONOLACTONE (ORAL), 342-346
SPIRONOLACTONE-HYDROCHLOROTHIAZIDE, 342-346
Stelazine, 137-143
Stemetil, 137-143
StieVaa, 369-372
stomach acid secretion, 223
storing medicines, 47, 50, 65
SUCRALFATE (ORAL), 346-348
Sulcrate, 346-348
Sulfadiazine, 351-355
SULFADIAZINE, 351-355
SULFADIAZINE-TRIMETHOPRIM, 352-355
SULFAMETHOXAZOLE, 352-355
SULFAMETHOXAZOLE-TRIMETHOPRIM, 352-355
SULFAPYRIDINE, 352-355
SULFASALAZINE, 354
SULFASALAZINE (ORAL), 348-351
Sulfex 10% Eye Drops, 341-342
SULFISOXAZOLE, 352-355
SULFONAMIDE-PHENAZOPYRIDINE PREPARATIONS, 352-355
SULFONAMIDE PREPARATIONS (ORAL), 351-355
SULINDAC, 95
SULINDAC (ORAL), 165-170
Supres, 271-274
Surgam, 165-170
Surmontil, 71-76
swallowing tablets, 136, 229, 336-337
Synalar, 63-67
Synamol, 63-67
Synthroid, 258-261
syrup-based medicines, 268

tablet halves, 117, 230
Tace, 129-134
Tagamet, 143-145
Tambocor, 211-214
tartrazine in drugs, 181
Tecnal, 92-95
Tecnal C 1/4, 92-95
Tecnal C 1/2, 92-95
Tegretol, 121-124
Tegretol-CR, 121-124
TEMAZEPAM, 214-216
Tempra, 42-44
Tempra Chewable, 42-44
Tempra Extra Strength, 42-44
Tempra Syrup, 42-44
Tenoretic, 331-336
Tenormin, 330-336
Tenuate, 174-176
Tenuate Dospan, 174-176

TERBUTALINE (ORAL AND INHALATION), 247-250
TERFLUZINE, 137-143
TETRACYCLINE, 197, 243
TETRACYCLINE HCl (ORAL), 355-359
TETRACYN, 355-359
THEO-DUR, 359-363
THEO-SR, 359-363
THEOCHRON, 359-363
THEOLAIR, 359-363
THEOLAIR SR, 359-363
THEOPHYLLINE, 80
THEOPHYLLINE (ORAL), 359-363
THIAZIDES, 56
THIORIDAZINE, 56
THIORIDAZINE HCl, 137-143
THYROGLOBULIN, 258-261
THYROID, 258-261
THYROID, 234
THYROLAR, 59, 258-261
THYTROPAR, 59
TIAPROFENIC ACID (ORAL), 165-170
TIMOLIDE, 331-336
TIMOLOL, 331-336
TIMOLOL (OPHTHALMIC), 363-366
TIMOLOL-HYDROCHLORO-THIAZIDE, 331-336
TIMOPTIC, 363-366
TOCAINIDE (ORAL), 366-369
TOFRANIL, 71-76
TOLBUTAMIDE, 48-52
TOLECTIN, 165-170
TOLMETIN, 95
TOLMETIN SODIUM (ORAL), 165-170
TONOCARD, 366-369
tooth discoloration, 358
toothbrushes as source of infection, 351
topical application of lanolin, 232
TOPICORT, 63-67
TOPSYN GEL, 63-67
TRANDATE, 330-336
transdermal patches, 37, 133, 302
TRANXENE, 60-62
TRANYLCYPROMINE, 141-142, 238-244
TRASICOR, 331-336
travelling, 51, 184-185, 276-277
TRAZODONE, 71-76
TRENTAL, 302-305
TRETINOIN (TOPICAL), 369-372
TRIADAPIN, 70-76
TRIADERM, 64-67
TRIAMCINOLONE, 64-67, 110-114
TRIAMED, 76-80
TRIAMINIC, 134-137
TRIAMINIC-DM, 134-137
TRIAMINIC EXPECTORANT, 134-137
TRIAMINIC ORAL INFANT DROPS, 134-137
TRIAMTERENE (ORAL), 372-376
TRIAMTERENE-HYDROCHLORO-THIAZIDE, 372-376
TRIANIDE MILD, 64-67
TRIANIDE REGULAR, 64-67
TRIAVIL, 76-80
TRIAZOLAM, 214-216
TRIDESILON, 63-67
TRIFLUOPERAZINE HCl, 137-143
TRILAFON, 137-143
TRIMIPRAMINE, 71-76
TRIPTIL, 71-76
TUINAL, 81-85
TUSSIONEX, 228-232
222, 95-100
222 FORTE, 95-100
282, 95-100
292, 95-100
293, 95-100
TYLENOL, 42-44
TYLENOL CHEWABLE, 42-44
TYLENOL WITH CODEINE ELIXIR, 45-48
TYLENOL WITH CODEINE NO. 2, 45-48
TYLENOL WITH CODEINE NO. 3, 45-48
TYLENOL WITH CODEINE NO. 4, 45-48
TYLENOL EXTRA-STRENGTH, 42-44
TYLENOL JUNIOR STRENGTH, 42-44
TYLENOL NO. 1, 45-48
TYLENOL NO. 1 FORTE, 45-48

UNICORT, 63-67
UNIPHYL, 359-363
URIDON, 223-226
urine color, 289
URITOL, 204-208
URO GANTANOL, 352-355

UROZIDE, 223-226

V-CILLIN K, 299-301
VALISONE SCALP LOTION, 63-67
VALIUM, 60-62
VALPROIC ACID, 376-379
VANCENASE NASAL INHALER, 105-107
VANCERIL ORAL INHALER, 103-105
VASOTEC, 118-120
VC-K 500, 299-301
VEGANIN, 45-48
VELOSEF, 124-126
VENTOLIN INHALER, 247-250
VENTOLIN NEBULES, 247-250
VENTOLIN ORAL LIQUID, 247-250
VENTOLIN RESPIRATOR SOLUTION, 247-250
VENTOLIN ROTACAPS, 247-250
VENTOLIN TABLETS, 247-250
VERAPAMIL, 181-185
VIBRA-TABS C-PAK, 194-197
VIBRAMYCIN, 194-197
VISCEROL, 170-174
VISKAZIDE, 331-336
VISKEN, 331-336
VISTACROM, 159-161
vitamin A, 327
VITAMIN A ACID, 369-372
VIVOL, 60-62
VOLTAREN, 165-170
VOLTAREN S.R., 165-170
VOLTAREN SUPPOSITORIES, 165-170
vomiting from chemotherapy, 371

WARFARIN, 234
WARFARIN POTASSIUM (ORAL), 379-383
WARFARIN SODIUM, 379-383
WARFILONE, 379-383
WESTCORT, 63-67
WINPRED, 110-114

XANAX, 59, 60-62

ZANTAC, 59, 143-145
ZAPEX, 60-62
ZARONTIN, 208-211
ZAROXOLYN, 223-226
ZOVIRAX, 52-57
ZYLOPRIM, 57-59

UNDERSTANDING CANADIAN PRESCRIPTION DRUGS

ARE YOU TAKING YOUR MEDICINES CORRECTLY?

Research shows that one of every two prescription drugs is not being taken correctly. Modern medicines can be very effective in curing and preventing diseases or relieving the symptoms of many medical conditions. They can save many days previously lost from work and return a person to work earlier — IF THEY ARE TAKEN CORRECTLY. If not taken correctly, modern medicines can become less effective and, even worse, may cause unnecessary adverse effects. It has been estimated that:

- 50% of patients (including children) are not taking their prescription drugs correctly.
- 30% of prescription drugs are being misused in a manner that poses a serious threat to the patient's health.
- 60% of patients cannot identify their medicines.
- 40% of patients receive drugs prescribed by two or more doctors.
- 12% of patients take other people's drugs.
- 3-30% of hospital admissions are due to incorrect use of drugs by patients at home.
- Only 54% of authorized repeat prescriptions are actually refilled.

I have always felt that if a medication is important enough to be prescribed for a patient, it is important enough to be explained to the patient. In order for a prescription drug to be effective, it must be:

Properly PRESCRIBED by the PHYSICIAN

▽

Properly DISPENSED by the PHARMACIST

▽

AND

▽

Properly ADMINISTERED by the PATIENT

If the patient does not take the medicine correctly, all the care taken by the physician and the pharmacist is significantly negated. In addition, millions of dollars spent on prescription drugs are being wasted due to incorrect use of prescription drugs by patients at home. *The responsibility of the patient in the drug therapy is just as important as that of the physician and pharmacist.*

For several years, I have been concerned with the high number of errors that patients make when taking prescription drugs. One of the most common reasons for these errors is a lack of information. The directions on a prescription label are almost always incomplete and do not provide enough information for a person who is responsible for treating him- or herself or a family member. "Take 1 capsule every 6 hours" and "Take as directed" are inadequate instructions.

Before people can be expected to take a drug correctly, they must know the *exact times* to take the medicine, know how to administer it and *how long* to take it. Before they can avoid drug interactions with food, alcohol, nonprescription drugs or other prescription drugs, they must first know what these interactions are. Before they can *manage* or handle a harmless but annoying side effect, they must know what the symptoms of the side effect are. Finally, since every drug carries a risk, patients must know which symptoms of an adverse drug reaction should prompt them to call their doctor.

In addition to the need for more information about prescription drugs, patients need information that is PRACTICAL, CONCISE and that they can UNDERSTAND. It is the intent of this book to provide the patient with a translation of complicated medical terminology into easy-to-understand language.

The purpose of this book is to provide the consumer with essential information on the most commonly prescribed drugs in Canada. It cannot be emphasized too greatly that these medication instructions are general in nature and *are to be used only under the direction and guidance of a health care professional.* Every patient is special because of his or her medical condition, other medications that may have been prescribed, daily activities and age. It is often necessary to adjust the drug therapy depending upon these factors. The medication instructions in this book have been carefully prepared in cooperation with a review board of distinguished Canadian physicians and pharmacists. The content of the instructions was based on the official pharmaceutical manufacturers' literature, the *Compendium of Pharmaceuticals and Specialties 1988*, the medical literature and the recommendations of the physicians and pharmacists who reviewed the manuscript.

The next time you receive a prescription or if you are presently taking a prescription drug, it is important that you understand the correct method of taking it. Only in this way can you receive the most benefit from your drug treatment. If you have any questions at all about your medications, do not hesitate to ask your doctor or pharmacist. The contents of the drug monographs are not intended to take the place of the patient's doctor or pharmacist. The author and publisher cannot be responsible for errors in publication or any consequences arising from the use of the information contained herein.

Your physician and pharmacist are providing you with the best drug treatment available — but YOU must UNDERSTAND HOW TO TAKE YOUR PRESCRIPTION DRUGS in order to receive the most benefit. It is the wish of everyone involved in the preparation of this book that you will find the information helpful and that you have a speedy recovery.

Dr. Dorothy L. Smith

HOW TO USE THIS BOOK

I. READ THE PRESCRIPTION LABEL

Determine the name of the medicine on the prescription label. If you have difficulty with the spelling of the drug name, check with your pharmacist.

II. INDEX

Turn to the Index at the front of the book to find the medicine you are interested in and the page number in this book that discusses the drug and how to take it. Then turn to that page.

III. SPECIFIC DRUG INSTRUCTIONS

GENERIC NAME

All of the medicines included in the book are arranged alphabetically under the generic name for each drug.

All drugs have a generic name. The generic name is the standard drug name that is recognized by health professionals and scientific organizations.

BRAND NAMES

The most commonly prescribed brand names (or trade names) are listed in alphabetical order.

The brand name is the name that the pharmaceutical manufacturer gives to its brand of the drug. If a drug is still protected by the patent granted to the original manufacturer, only one brand name will appear. However, if the patent protection has expired, other companies can manufacture that generic drug and give each of their products a different name. Some manufacturers prefer to sell their products under the generic name. Other manufacturers prefer to market their drug products under a trade name that is unique to their company. This is why there is sometimes only one brand name for a generic drug and at other times there are several brand names.

This is the only consumer book that provides general information on the most commonly prescribed generic drugs as well as additional information on the specific brand you are taking. With many drug products, the specific brand instructions are extremely important.

Special instructions for brand names are indicated throughout the book. For example, in the monograph for "ERYTHROMYCIN," some brands of this antibiotic have special administration instructions. Whenever a brand of medicine has special instructions, the names of those brands will be indicated in the following way:

> *If you were prescribed* APO-ERYTHRO BASE, E-MYCIN, ERYC, ERYTHROMID, NOVORYTHRO BASE:

It is very important to know which brand of medicine you are taking. If you have any questions, ask your pharmacist.

Purpose

The drug monographs contain a description of the usual purpose(s) of each medicine.

Before a person takes a prescription drug, it is important to understand the reason the drug has been prescribed. Only approved uses of the drugs are included. Investigational or experimental uses of a drug are not included. If you do not understand why a particular medicine has been prescribed for you, ask your doctor.

Allergies/Warnings

The drug monographs contain the most common allergy warnings. If you have ever had an allergic reaction to any of the drugs listed in the warning, do not take the medicine. Call your doctor or pharmacist.

It is important to tell your physician and pharmacist if you are allergic to any medicines, foods or color dyes (for example, tartrazine). This will help prevent you from receiving a prescription for a drug to which you may be allergic. Some medicines are closely related to each other in chemical structure, and you could experience an allergic reaction if you were allergic to one of the medicines and later received the other similar medicine. Some medicines are flavored or colored with ingredients to which some people are allergic.

The drug monographs also contain selected warnings for medical conditions in which the drug may be contraindicated or which may require special dosage calculations and/or special monitoring by the physician.

Some people have a history of medical conditions that could make them more susceptible to developing adverse effects with certain drugs. For example, a person who has an ulcer should not receive a prescription for a drug that can irritate the ulcer. If you have any of the medical conditions listed, be sure that your doctor knows before you take any of the medicine. As a general rule, be sure to tell every physician you are seeing the names of any drugs you are allergic to, all drugs you are taking and the medical conditions for which you are being or have been treated. Complete the Medicine Card in this book and carry it in your wallet next to your driver's license. Consider joining Canadian Medic-Alert (293 Eglinton Avenue East, Toronto, Ontario M4P 2Z8 or phone (416) 481-5171) and wear one of the Medic-Alert necklaces or bracelets that will contain your medical and drug history. Ask your physician or pharmacist for the Medic-Alert application form.

How to Use This Medicine

Time of Administration

Each drug monograph provides recommendations regarding the time(s) that the specific drug should be taken.

Ask your pharmacist to suggest exact times that will fit in with your daily meals and work schedule. Try to follow these times as closely as possible. For example, if you are prescribed a medicine that is to be taken "three times a day," the day (24 hours) should be divided into three equal time periods. The doses should be spaced 8 hours apart (24 hours/day divided by 3 doses/day = 8 hours apart). Then, determine the exact times you should take the medicine so that it interferes the least amount possible with your daily activities. For example, one person may be able to take the medicine at 7 A.M.-3 P.M.-10 P.M. and another person may find a 9 A.M.-5 P.M.-12 midnight schedule to be better. The times you take the medicine can be flexible, but ask your pharmacist for advice because some medicines should not be taken at meals and others must be taken with food.

Many parents ask if they must wake their child up during the middle of the night to give them a dose of the medicine. This depends on the specific medicine and the child's illness. Many times, a convenient schedule can be planned that does not interfere with the child's sleep.

Some drugs must be taken on an empty stomach (1 hour before or 2 hours after eating food) in order to be absorbed completely. In contrast, other drugs that are irritating to the stomach should be taken immediately after eating some food to help prevent stomach upset.

In special circumstances, these times may have to be changed by your doctor or pharmacist depending on your medical condition or other drugs you are taking. People who have liver or kidney problems metabolize and excrete some medicines differently, and it may be necessary for the doctor to alter the dosage schedule of some of their medicines. Some people may be taking another prescription medicine that will make it necessary to change the normal times of administration of these drugs so that they are not taken at the same time and will not interact with each other.

How to Administer

Instructions for the correct method of administering a drug are included whenever necessary.

In addition, the section How to Administer Medications contains instructions for the administration of:

- Liquid Medicines
  - How to Use an Oral Liquid Syringe
  - How to Use a Medicine Dropper
  - How to Use a Medicine Spoon
- Buccal Tablets
- Sublingual Tablets
- Eye Drops
- Eye Ointments
- Ear Drops
- Nose Drops
- Nasal Sprays
- Inhalers
- Topical Preparations for the Skin
  - How to Use Creams, Ointments, Gels, Solutions, and Lotions
  - How to Use Aerosol Sprays
  - How to Use Transdermal Patches
- Rectal Suppositories
- Rectal Creams
- Vaginal Creams, Ointments and Gels
- Vaginal Suppositories
- Vaginal Tablets, Ovules and Inserts

Special Instructions

Length of Therapy

It is important to know how long you should take the prescribed medicine. Many people make the mistake of stopping a medicine before the treatment is completed. This can prevent the medicine from providing the full benefit and may result in unnecessary adverse complications.

Pregnancy/Breastfeeding

Warnings regarding the use of each medicine during pregnancy and breastfeeding are included. Women who are pregnant or breastfeeding should not take any medicines or home remedies without consulting their doctor or pharmacist.

Drug Interactions

Warnings regarding the use of the prescribed medicine with certain foods and/or nonprescription drugs are included.

Some foods (including milk and fruit juices) can interfere with the absorption of some drugs into the blood and decrease their effectiveness. For example, the antibiotic tetracycline should not be taken with milk or dairy products because the antibiotic will bind with the calcium in these dairy products and prevent the body from absorbing some of the antibiotic. As a result, the antibiotic will be less effective. Many of these interactions can be avoided by simply avoiding those specific foods during the time (usually 2 or 3 hours) the drug is being absorbed or, in some cases, by avoiding the foods during the entire drug treatment.

Many people make a mistake in thinking that medicines they can buy without a prescription aren't "drugs." All over-the-counter products contain drugs and many are capable of interacting with prescription medicines. A person taking a prescription medicine should never self-medicate with any nonprescription drug without first checking with his or her doctor or pharmacist.

This book does not contain information on prescription drug interactions with other prescription drugs. It is the responsibility of the physician (before prescribing the drug) and the pharmacist (before dispensing the drug) to review the individual drug therapy of each patient. There are too many other factors to consider, such as the medical condition of the patient, to even attempt to cover this area in a comprehensive, safe and accurate manner. If you are taking any other medications, consult with your pharmacist or doctor regarding the safety of the combination.

Alcohol

Warnings are included regarding the dangers of drinking alcoholic beverages while taking certain prescription drugs.

It is generally not a good idea to drink alcoholic beverages while taking any drug. However, alcoholic beverages are definitely contraindicated with some medicines because they can interact with the drug and cause potentially serious side effects.

Special Precautions

This book contains information on how to manage commonly occurring side effects and provides advice on when to consult your doctor or pharmacist. Special attention has been given to translating the technical medical names of these symptoms into easy-to-understand language.

Every medicine can cause side effects. People should know which side effects a drug commonly causes and what precautionary measures they can take either to avoid or manage the side effect if it occurs. For example, if a medicine commonly causes drowsiness, dizziness or blurred vision, people should be careful driving an automobile, flying an airplane or operating electrical equipment until they know how they will respond to the drug.

When to Call Your Doctor

Selected warning signs that should prompt the patient to call the doctor are included for each drug.

Patients should always call their doctor or pharmacist if they feel that the drug is not "agreeing" with them or if they develop some symptoms that they have never experienced before and that they feel may be due to the drug.

In addition, there are warning signs with some medicine that should prompt a person to seek medical advice. This can help ensure that the person continues to receive the maximum benefit from the treatment. It may be necessary for the doctor to adjust the dose of the medicine or to prescribe another drug that does not cause the same problem.

Allergic Reactions

Always call your doctor or go to the nearest hospital emergency department if you think you are allergic to a medicine. The more common signs of an allergic reaction are a skin rash, hives, itching, swelling of the face or difficulty in breathing.

Refills

Dangerous side effects can develop with some medicines if they are stopped suddenly. This book contains reminders with these drugs to call the pharmacist for a refill 2 or 3 days before the medicine will be used up.

Storage

Special storage instructions are included.

In general, a cool dry place is the best storage place for most medicines. It is important not to store prescription drugs in the bathroom medicine cabinet. The bathroom often becomes hot and steamy and the heat and humidity can destroy some drugs or make them less effective.

Some medicines must be stored in the refrigerator while others should be stored at room temperature. If a person takes a medicine that has deteriorated because of improper storage, the drug could become less effective and, in some cases, dangerous.

Never take a medicine that is outdated. The expiration date will appear on the prescription label if the medicine is expected to become outdated in a short time period. If you have any questions about the expiration date of a prescription drug, call your pharmacist.

Miscellaneous

These prescription drug instructions are general in nature and may have to be altered by your doctor or pharmacist because of your medical condition or other drugs you may be taking. The instructions are selective and do not cover all possible uses, actions, precautions, side effects or interactions.

If you have any questions about the medicine you are taking, ask your doctor or pharmacist. Sometimes, a question that you may think is very unimportant can be very important to your health.

IV. MEDICINE CARDS

Four Medicine Cards are included in this book and it is recommended that you or anyone in your family taking prescription drugs complete the card and carry it in the wallet or purse. The Medicine Card could help save your life if you were ever in an accident. The doctors treating you would know immediately what allergies you have, which drugs you have been taking and the phone numbers of your doctors and pharmacist.

V. APPENDICES

APPENDIX A contains a listing of foods that are high in potassium. This is important for some patients taking diuretics (water pills).

APPENDIX B contains general instructions for diabetics on diet, foot care and treatment of hypoglycemia and hyperglycemia.

APPENDIX C contains tips to detect tampering of medicines that can be purchased without a prescription.

What Is in a Tablet Other Than the Drug?

In addition to the medicine, tablets may contain the following ingredients.

Diluents (such as lactose, starch or dextrose) to add bulk and make the tablet large enough to be handled and ensure a constant size.

Disintegrants (such as starch) to speed up the rate at which the tablet will break down and dissolve in the body.

Coatings to protect the tablet from light, air and moisture, to disguise an unpleasant taste and to add color. Some coatings contain tartrazine (a yellow dye) and people who are hypersensitive to tartrazine should tell their doctor so that another medicine can be prescribed.

Some coatings are specially designed to protect the tablet from dissolving in the stomach fluids or to pass through the stomach and into the small intestine intact. These are called enteric coatings. Tablets with enteric coatings should not be chewed or given with milk or antacids because this may remove the protective coating on the tablet.

Long-acting tablets and capsules are formulated to provide two or three doses over a long period of time. This eliminates the need for the person to take a medicine so often. However, if these medicines are crushed or chewed, all of the medicine would be released at one time and the person would receive too much of the medicine at that time. Side effects or toxicity could result.

GENERIC DRUGS

- *Generic and brand name drugs are simply two ways of naming pharmaceutical products.*

When a drug is first discovered, it is known by its chemical name or generic name, also called the "active ingredient." The pharmaceutical company that discovered the drug then gives the drug a special brand name or trade name. This brand name medicine will be the only product available in Canada until the patent expires. After the patent has expired, the drug can be copied and marketed by other pharmaceutical companies. The copies of the original product are usually marketed under the generic name or a new brand name. Therefore, after a patent has expired, the medicine may be available both as the original brand name and several generic copies.

- *Generic and brand name drugs are similar but NOT exactly the same.*

Generic and brand name products must be alike only as far as the ACTIVE ingredients (the actual drug) are concerned. This can represent as little as 10% of a tablet or capsule.

The remaining 90% is composed of INACTIVE INGREDIENTS—such as starch, lactose, sugar, lubricants, preservatives, dyes, and flavoring agents. These ingredients are needed to bind the drug particles together so that the tablet or capsule will disintegrate (break apart) after it is swallowed, and subsequently dissolve in the blood. They also make the product large enough so that a person can easily pick it up. Inactive ingredients are generally considered to be "trade secrets" and the various manufacturers must select their own inactive ingredients and manufacturing processes.

- *More than one company often manufactures the same generic drug.*

Some provincial governments cover the costs of prescription drugs under the terms of a provincial drug plan. The provincial formulary or list of covered drugs may contain several products with the same active ingredient(s) but made by different manufacturers. Provincial laws vary but in most provinces, the pharmacist may legally substitute a generic or the least expensive product with the same active ingredient(s) for the prescribed medication unless the physician or patient specifically requests otherwise. This means that a patient could receive a different company's product if the provincial drug list changed and the pharmacy adjusted its stock accordingly.

• *There is no question that all drugs—brand name as well as generic—are of high quality.*

All drugs must be approved by the federal government before they can be marketed. However, differences may exist not only between the brand name drug and a generic, but from generic to generic because of the different inactive ingredients and the manufacturing processes used by each company. Differences can also exist between brand name drug products.

There have been isolated reports that when some patients were switched between different manufacturers' products of the SAME DRUG (generic or brand name drugs) at refills, they experienced a change in the incidence of side effects and/or in the effectiveness of the drug products in controlling their symptoms. These reports have sparked a call for well-designed research studies.

• *A very complex issue*

Generic drugs are safe and effective and may save the patient money as long as they are used wisely. For most conditions (i.e. colds, infections, pain, etc.), problems will probably not arise when one product is substituted for another. However, repeated substitution of different manufacturers' products may be inadvisable for:

- *chronically ill patients with life threatening conditions such as high blood pressure, blood clots, heart disease, thyroid disease and asthma;*
- *patients receiving medications with doses that must be kept within a narrow therapeutic range. Examples include:*

  Medicines for seizures (anticonvulsants)
  Heart medicines
  Thyroid medicines
  Insulins
  Blood thinners (anticoagulants)
  Birth control pills
  Long-acting or sustained release products

A patient should probably stay on the SAME MANUFACTURER'S PRODUCT (regardless of whether it is a brand name medicine or a generic product) for any of these chronic conditions or medications. This is a very complex medical and scientific issue and until the questions are all answered, it would be wise to discuss any questions you have with your doctor and pharmacist. Depending on your medical condition and the drugs you are being prescribed, they may recommend the same manufacturer's product for each refill.

Provincial laws vary but several provinces require the pharmacist to type the name of the drug and its manufacturer on the prescription label. This is a valuable law since it assures that a person will know the name of the medicine and will be able to request the same manufacturer's product each time the prescription medicine is refilled. If the name of the manufacturer does not appear on the label, just ask the pharmacist.

- *Ask Questions*

Ask your doctor or pharmacist if you are being prescribed a medication in which it would be wise to stay on the same manufacturer's product at each refill. Ask how much your prescription will cost if you purchase the brand name product or one of the generic products. Remember, you have the right to request a particular manufacturer's product, but you may have to pay the difference in price between the two products.

The cost of the medicine you purchase is only one factor. It is also important to consider your need for the wide range of monitoring and counseling services that pharmacists can offer. Have all your prescriptions dispensed at the same pharmacy so that the pharmacist can keep accurate medication records for you and provide you with the professional advice you need in order to take your medicines correctly.

HOW TO ADMINISTER MEDICATIONS

ORAL LIQUID MEDICINES

The best way to administer liquid medicines is by using an *oral liquid syringe, medicine dropper* or a *medicine spoon.*

If your doctor has prescribed liquid medicine for you, follow the instructions for using the oral liquid syringe, the medicine spoon, or medicine dropper.

Do not use household teaspoons or tablespoons because they are not accurate enough.

When a prescription indicates that "1 teaspoon" of a medicine should be administered, this means that 1 teaspoon is equal to 5 ml of liquid. However, household teaspoons range in size from 2.5 ml to 9.7 ml. Studies have also shown that the volume of liquid measured using the same teaspoon varies greatly depending upon the person using the spoon.

Do not use the same syringe or medicine spoon to administer medicine to another person. Germs could be transferred to the other person.

How to Use an Oral Liquid Syringe

- Measurc the correct amount of medicine either using a plastic adapter or measuring directly from a medicine cup.

ORAL LIQUID SYRINGE WITH ADAPTER

- Wet the plastic bottle adapter with warm water. Press the adapter into the mouth of the medicine bottle.
    - Remove the cap from the tip of the oral liquid syringe.
    - Fit the tip of the syringe into the adapter.
    - Turn the markings on the syringe toward you so that you will be able to read them.
    - The plunger rod should be pushed down completely into the syringe barrel.
    - Turn the bottle (with the adapter and syringe connected) upside down.
    - The barrel of the syringe is calibrated. Slowly pull down the plunger to the correct dosage mark on the barrel of the syringe.

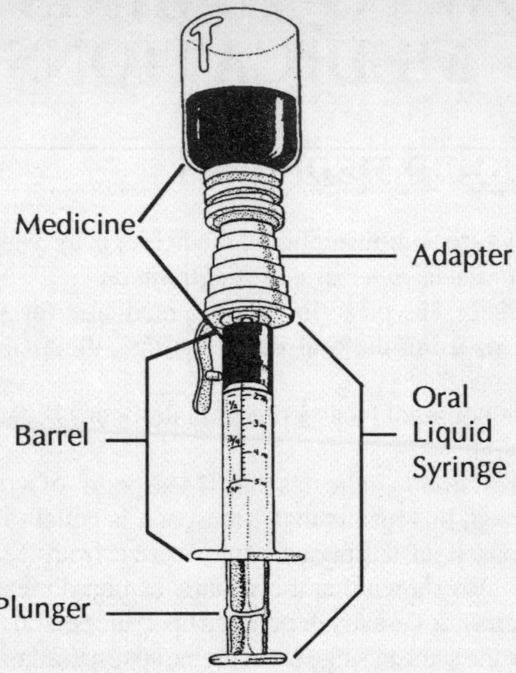

Oral liquid syringe with adapter

- Overfill the syringe a small amount (approximately 1 ml). This will help remove any bubbles and ensure that an accurate dose is being measured.
- Pull the plunger back until the line on the plunger is level with the correct dosage amount indicated on the outside of the oral liquid syringe.
- Remove the syringe from the adapter.

ORAL LIQUID SYRINGE WITHOUT ADAPTER

- Pour a small amount of the liquid medicine into a clear container (a cup or a small glass).
- Remove the cap from the tip of the syringe.
- Turn the markings on the syringe toward you so that you will be able to read them.
- The plunger rod should be pushed down completely into the syringe barrel.
- Place the tip of the syringe into the medicine.

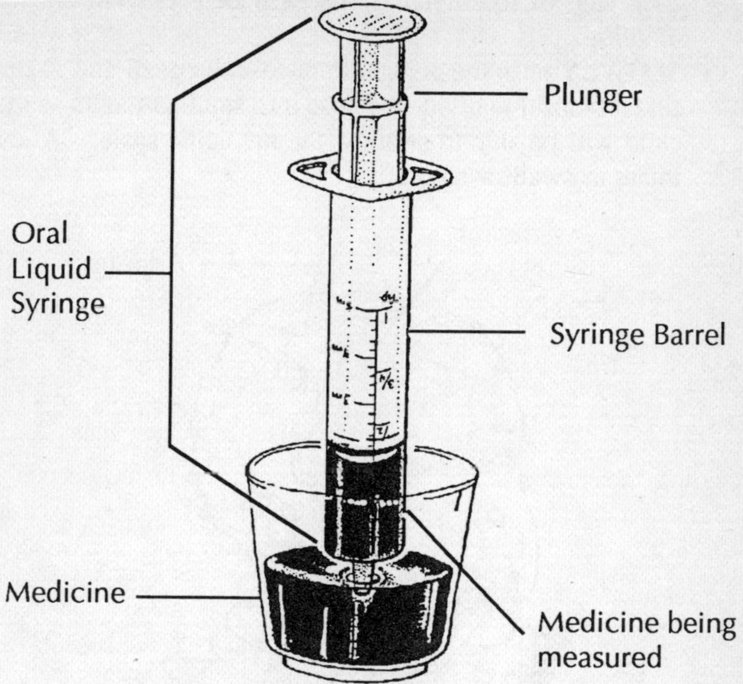

Oral liquid syringe without adapter

- The barrel of the syringe is calibrated. Slowly pull the plunger up to the correct dosage mark of the barrel of the syringe.
- Overfill the syringe a small amount (approximately 1 ml). This will help remove any bubbles and ensure that an accurate dose is being measured.
- Pull the plunger up until the line on the plunger is level with the correct dosage amount indicated on the outside of the oral liquid syringe. You may wish to mark this line with a piece of tape.
- Remove the syringe from the liquid.

- *For an infant:*
    - If the medicine is being given to an infant, the infant's head should be well supported with one hand while the infant is held in the lap. Be sure the infant's head and shoulders are raised.
    - Gently press down on the chin with your thumb in order to open the infant's mouth.
    - Point the tip of the oral liquid syringe to the inside cheek or the

back side of the mouth. This will help prevent choking or drooling.

- SLOWLY push the plunger to release the medicine. You may find it helpful to divide the dose into small amounts so that the child will be able to swallow the medicine easier. Allow the infant to swallow naturally.

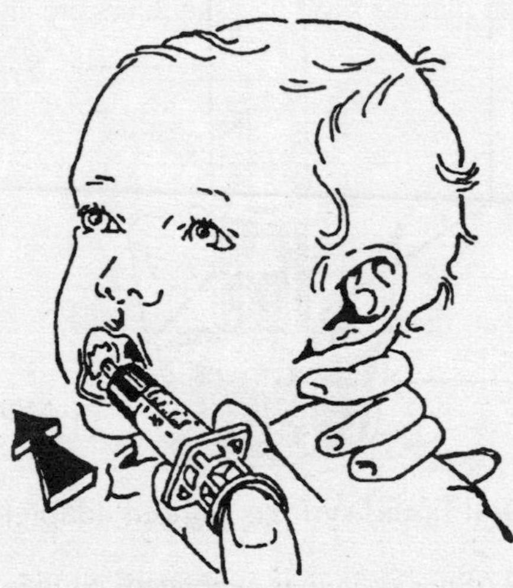

Administering medicine to an infant using an oral liquid syringe

- *For a child or adult:*
  - Have the person sit upright and point the tip of the oral liquid syringe to the inside cheek or the back side of the mouth. This will help prevent choking or drooling.
  - SLOWLY push the plunger rod to release the medicine. Allow the person to swallow naturally.
  - Ask your pharmacist if drinking some water after taking the medicine is okay.
- Rinse the oral liquid syringe with warm water. The plunger rod may be removed. Dry the plunger rod thoroughly.
- Replace the storage cap on the syringe. Keep the storage cap away

from children since they could swallow the cap. Store the oral liquid syringe in a cool, dry place.

How to Use a Medicine Dropper

- Withdraw the correct amount of medicine from the bottle by squeezing the bulb of the dropper. If the dropper is calibrated, check that you have the correct dose by holding the dropper upright and looking at it at eye level.
- Hold the infant so that his head and shoulders are slightly elevated.

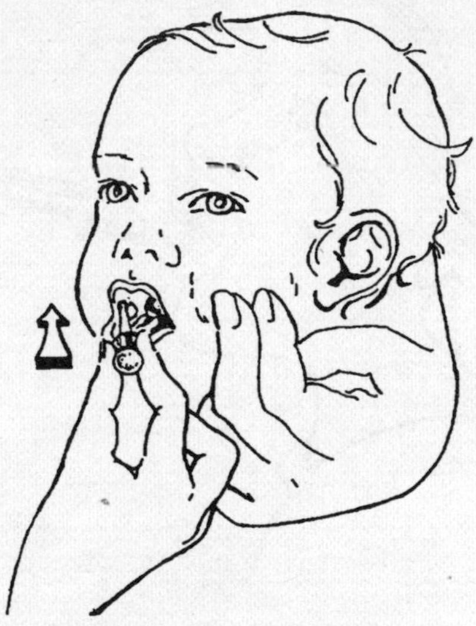

Using a medicine dropper

- Press down gently on the infant's chin with thumb to open the infant's mouth. If the infant will not open his mouth, try stroking the side of his cheek.
- Drop the prescribed number of drops into the infant's mouth. If you are using a calibrated dropper, place the dropper between the infant's cheek and gum to help prevent him from spitting out the medicine. Allow the child to swallow naturally.
- Ask your pharmacist if giving the child some water to drink after taking the medicine is okay.
- Rinse the medicine dropper with warm water after each use and shake gently to remove any drops of water.

How to Use a Medicine Spoon

- Pour the liquid medicine into the medicine spoon to the correct dosage line.
- Have the child or adult sit upright and *slowly* tip the spoon forward to release the liquid medicine. Allow the person to swallow naturally.

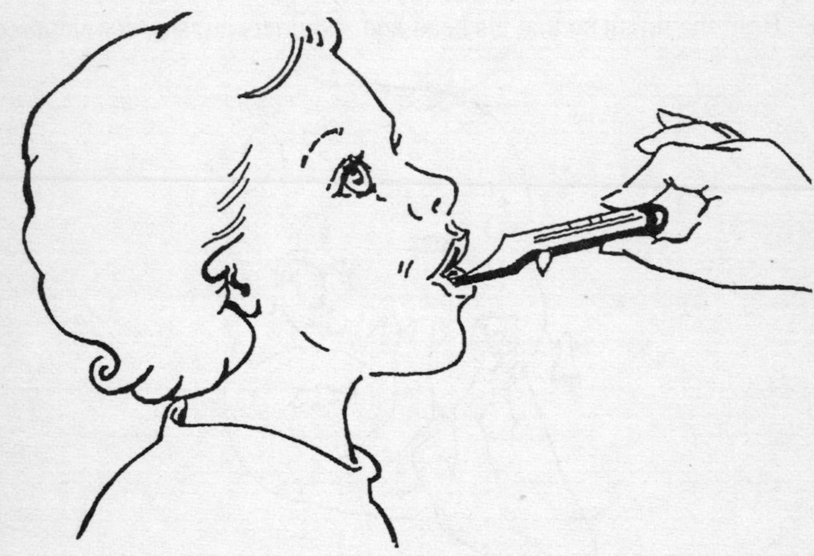

Using a calibrated medicine spoon

- Encourage the child or adult to suck all the medicine from the spoon so that the entire dose is administered.
- Ask your pharmacist if giving the person some water to drink after taking the medicine is okay.
- Rinse the medicine spoon with warm water after each use.

BUCCAL TABLETS

- Place a tablet *in the pouch* between the cheek and the teeth. Close your mouth and let the tablet dissolve completely. *Do not swallow or chew* the tablet since this type of tablet works faster when it is absorbed through the lining of the mouth.

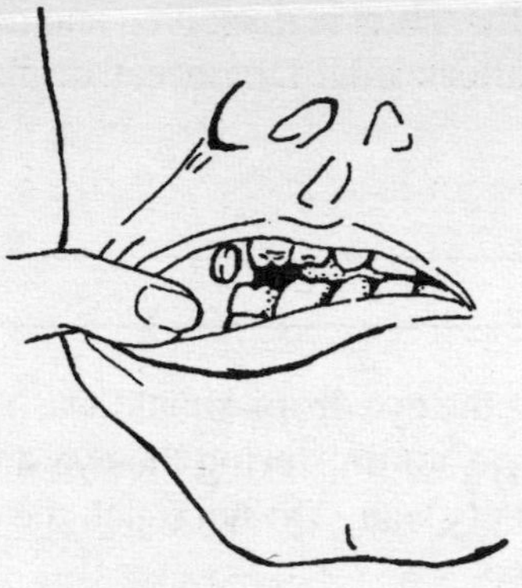

Buccal tablet dissolving in pouch of cheek

- Try not to swallow until the tablet is dissolved and do not rinse your mouth for a few minutes. Do not eat, drink or smoke while the tablet is dissolving.

SUBLINGUAL TABLETS

- Place a tablet *under your tongue* and let it dissolve completely. *Do not swallow or chew* the tablet since this type of tablet works faster when it is absorbed through the lining of the mouth.

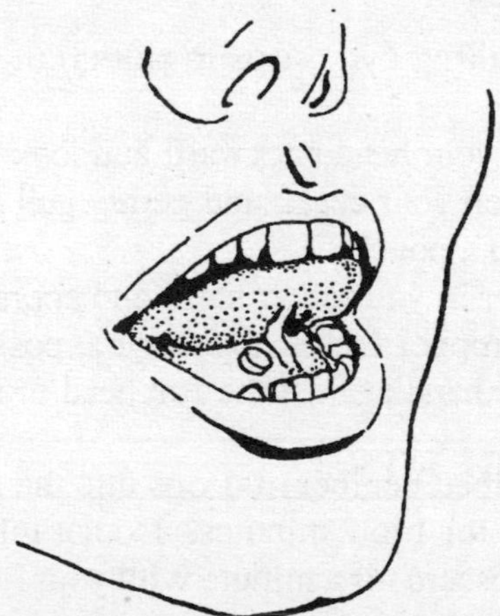

Sublingual tablet dissolving
under the tongue

- Try not to swallow until the tablet is dissolved and do not rinse your mouth for a few minutes afterwards. Do not eat, drink or smoke while the tablet is dissolving.

EYE DROPS

- The person administering the eye drops should wash his or her hands with soap and water before administering the eye drops.
- The eye drops must be kept clean. Do not touch the dropper against the face or anything else.

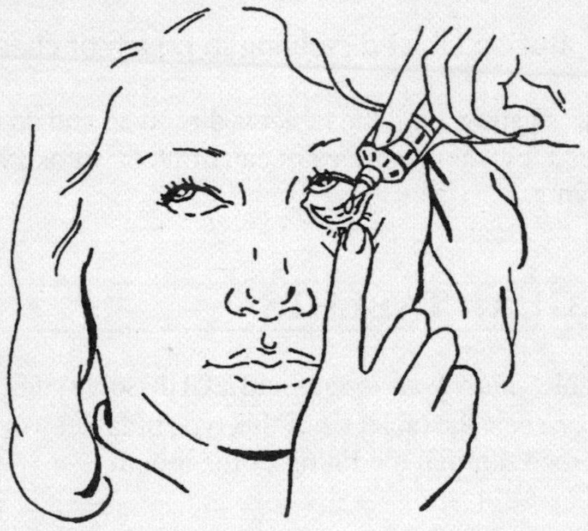

Instilling eye drops in pouch of eyelid

- Lie down or tilt your head backward and look up at the ceiling.
- Rest your hand on your cheek and gently pull down the lower lid of your eye to form a pouch.
- Hold the dropper in your other hand and approach the eye from the side. Place the dropper as close to the eye as possible without touching it. Resting your hand against the forehead or nose may help steady your hand.
- Place the prescribed number of drops into the *pouch* of the eye.
- Close your eyes for 1 to 2 minutes. Do not rub them.
- Apply gentle pressure for a minute with your fingers to the bridge of the nose and the inner corner of the eye to prevent the eye drops from being drained from the eye.

- Try not to blink more often than usual and do not close the eyes tightly after you have instilled the drops. This can remove the medicine from the place on the eye where you want the medicine to work.
- Blot the excess solution around the eye with a tissue.

Alternative (Closed Eyes) Method

If you have difficulty instilling eye drops with your eyes open, check with your doctor or pharmacist to see if you can use the following method:

- Lie down on your back and close your eyes.
- Place the prescribed number of drops on the eyelid in the corner of the eye nearest the nose. (This is called the inner canthus.)
- Then blink your eyes and the drops will fall naturally into the eyes as the eyelids are opened. You may wish to tilt the head slightly to the outside to help the drops run in.
- Wipe off any remaining drops on the eyelids with a clean tissue.

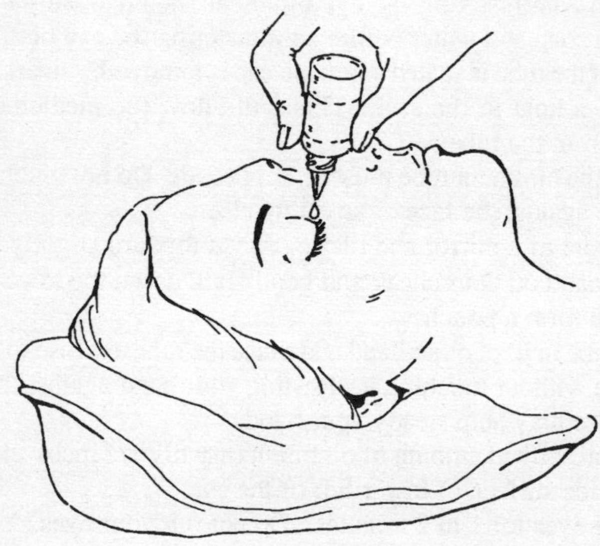

Instilling eye drops using
the closed eyes method

NOTE: The CLOSED EYES METHOD may be particularly helpful in administering eye drops to children.

If necessary, have someone else administer the eye drops for you.

If you are using more than one kind of eye drop, wait at least 5 minutes before instilling the second kind.

Some eye drops may blur the vision for a few minutes after using them. Do not drive a car or operate dangerous machinery or do jobs that require you to be alert until your vision has cleared.

Call your doctor if the condition for which the eye drops are being used persists or becomes worse or if the drops cause itching or burning for more than just a few minutes after use. Many eye drops sting for a short time after use.

Keep the eye drop bottle tightly closed when not in use. Do not use the eye drops if they change in color or in any other way after being purchased. Do not use outdated eye drops as they could be contaminated or ineffective.

EYE OINTMENTS

- The person administering the eye ointment should wash his or her hands with soap and water before administering the eye ointment.
- If the top of the tube is sealed when the cap is removed, invert the cap and pierce a hole in the seal. This will allow the medicine to be squeezed from the tube.
- The tip of the ointment tube must be kept clean. Do not touch the tip of the tube against the face or anything else.
- Stand in front of a mirror and tilt your head forward slightly.
- Rest your hand on your cheek and gently pull down the lower lid of your eye to form a pouch.
- Hold the tube in your other hand and place the tube as close to the eye as possible without touching it. Resting your hand against the forehead or nose may help steady your hand.
- Place the prescribed amount of ointment (usually 1/2 inch) along the pouch (inside surface of lower lid) of the eye.
- Close your eyes for 1 to 2 minutes. Do not rub your eyes.
- Wipe off any excess ointment around the eye with a tissue.
- Clean the tip of the ointment tube with a tissue.

If necessary, have someone else administer the eye ointment for you.

Vision may be blurred for a few minutes after applying the ointment. Do not drive a car or operate dangerous machinery or do jobs that require you to be alert until your vision has cleared.

Call your doctor if the condition for which the eye ointment is being used persists or becomes worse or if the ointment causes itching or burning for more than just a few minutes after use. Some eye ointments sting for a short time immediately after use.

Keep the eye ointment tube tightly closed when not in use. Do not use outdated eye ointments as they could be contaminated or ineffective.

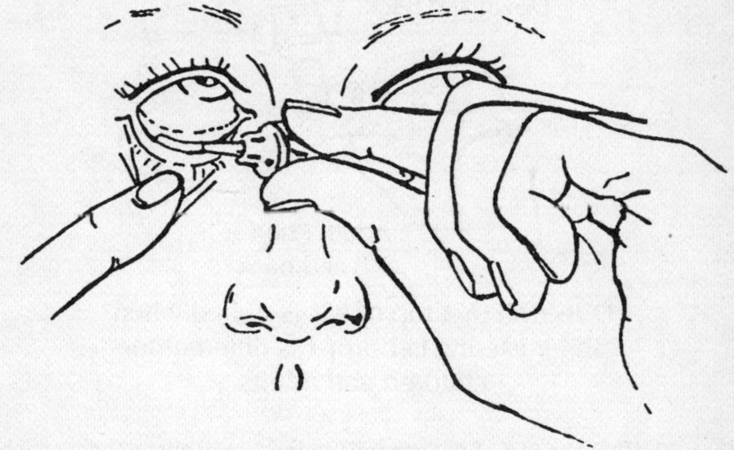

Placing prescribed dose of eye ointment in pouch of lower eyelid

EAR DROPS

- Warm the ear drops to body temperature by holding the bottle in your hands for a few minutes. Do *not* heat the drops in hot water because this could cause pain and dizziness.
- The person administering the ear drops should wash his or her hands with soap and water.
- The ear drops must be kept clean. Do not touch the dropper against the ear or anything else that could contaminate it.
- Shake the bottle before use if necessary.
- Tilt your head or lie on your side so that the ear you are treating is facing up.
- In *adults and children over 3 years*, gently pull the top of the ear *up and back.*
- In *children under 3 years*, gently pull the top of the ear *down and back.*

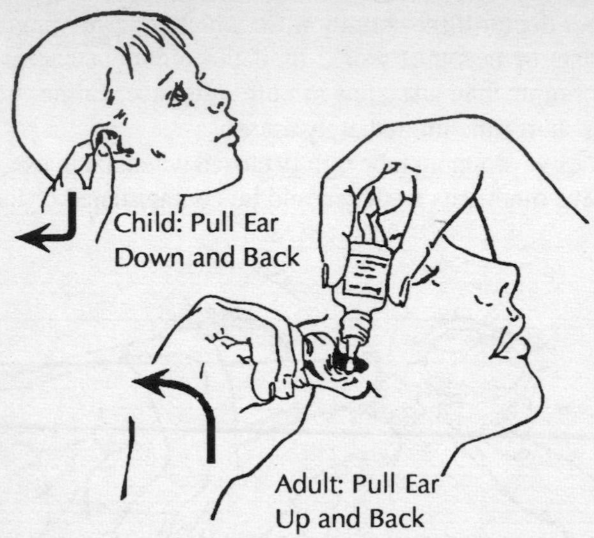

Direction that top of ear is pulled when administering ear drops is different for children and adults

Note: Pulling the top of the ear will help to straighten the ear canal so that the ear drops can reach the eardrum.

- Place the prescribed number of drops into the ear. Do not insert the dropper into the ear canal as it may cause injury.
- Remain in the same position for a short time (5-10 minutes) after you have administered the drops. This will allow the ear drops to run down into the ear canal.
- Dry the ear lobe if there are any ear drops on it.

If you must administer drops in both ears, wait about 5 to 10 minutes before placing the drops in the second ear. This will help keep the medicine in the ear canal of the first ear for at least 5 to 10 minutes before you have to tilt your head to put drops in the other ear. It is generally not recommended that cotton be placed in the ear after the ear drops have been instilled because the cotton can soak up the drug.

Do not use the ear drops more frequently or in larger quantities than prescribed by your doctor.

Do not use the ear drops if they change in color or change in any way after being purchased.

Call your doctor if the condition for which these ear drops are being used persists or becomes worse or if the ear drops cause itching or burning for more than just a few minutes after use.

Do not use this medicine at the same time as any other ear medicine without the approval of your doctor. Some medicines cannot be mixed.

These instructions may be altered by your doctor or pharmacist because of your medical condition or the specific medicine in the ear drops.

NOSE DROPS

- Blow your nose gently to clean the nostrils.
- Sit in a chair and tilt your head backward or lie down on a bed with your head extending over the edge of the bed or lie down and place a pillow under your shoulders so that your head is tipped backward.

For *children:* Let the head hang over the edge of a table, bed or parent's lap and follow the same procedure.

For *infants:* While holding the child on your lap, tilt the child's head slightly backward and use your hand to support the child's head.

- Insert the dropper into the nostril about 1/3 inch and drop the prescribed number of drops into the nose.

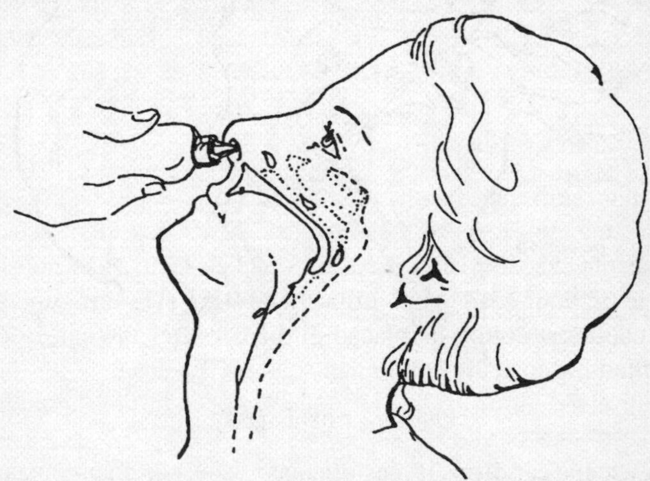

Administering nose drops

- Try not to touch the inside of the nose with the dropper as it will probably make you sneeze and will contaminate the dropper.
- Immediately bend your head forward toward your knees. Stay in this position for a few seconds and then sit upright. The drops will then trickle down the back of the throat.
- Repeat for the other nostril if necessary.
- Remain in the same position for at least 5 minutes.

Clean the plastic nasal piece with warm water after each use. Dry well.

NASAL SPRAYS

- Blow your nose gently to clean the nostrils.
- Sit upright with your head slightly forward.
- Shake the container.
- Insert the spray tip firmly into the nostril. The spray tip should be pointed at the *back* and *outer side* of the nose to obtain the best results. Close the other nostril by pressing your finger on the side of it.

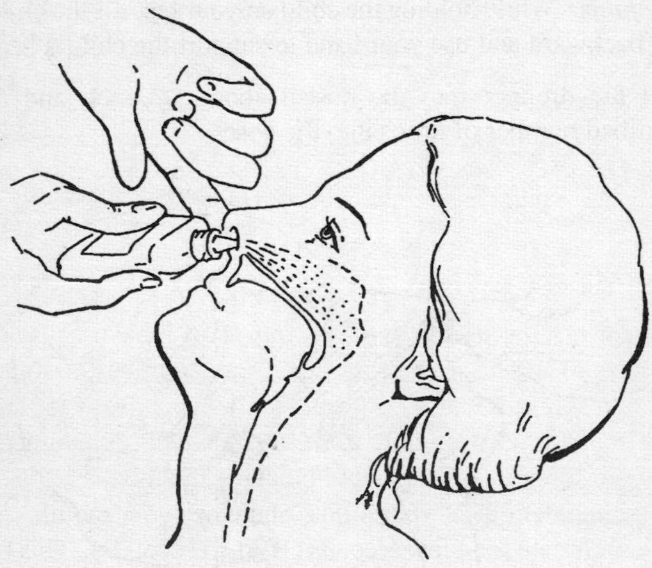

Using a nasal spray

- With your mouth closed, sniff gently and squeeze the bottle to release a firm, quick spray.

- Remove the spray tip from your nostril. Bend your head forward for a few seconds to allow the spray to spread over the nasal membranes. Then tilt the head upright or backward and the spray will trickle down the back of the throat.
- Hold your breath a few seconds and then breathe out through your mouth.
- Repeat for the other nostril if necessary.

Clean the plastic nasal piece with warm water after each use. Dry well.

INHALERS

If troubled with mucous or phlegm in the lungs, try to clear your chest as completely as possible before using this medicine. This will help the drug to reach more deeply into your lungs.

Hold the inhaler according to the specific instructions for that drug contained on the label or in the package.

Shake the container well each time before use.

There are 2 basic methods of using medicine in inhalers. Follow whichever method has been recommended by your doctor.

METHOD I. CLOSED-MOUTH INSTRUCTIONS

- Breathe out fully and place the lips tightly around the mouthpiece. The mouthpiece should be over the tongue and well into the mouth.
- Tilt the head slightly back.
- Start to breathe in slowly and deeply through the mouth. At the middle of a deep breath in, press down the top of the inhaler as far as it will go to release a "puff." By starting to breathe in before inhaling the medicine, you will help to prevent the medicine from staying in the mouth and you will get more of the medicine into the lungs.
- Keep your tongue down to avoid blocking the mist.
- Take the inhaler out of your mouth and close your mouth.
- Hold your breath for a few seconds (10 to 15 seconds). This helps the medicine to reach the tiny air passages in the lungs where its action is needed. Breathe out through your nose slowly.
- Check your technique in front of a mirror. If you see a white mist es-

caping into the air, you may not be breathing in correctly or your lips may not be sealed around the mouthpiece.

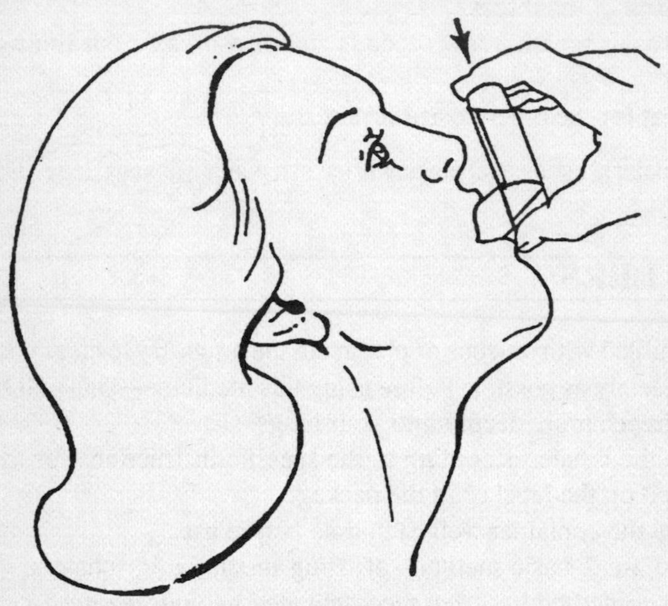

Closed-Mouth Method: The angle at which the inhaler must be held depends on the specific product

Closed-Mouth Method Using an Inhaler Aid

If a person is having difficulty coordinating his or her breathing and inhaling the medicine, inhaler aids are now available. One example is the Aerochamber. The inhaler aid (also called Extender Device or Spacer) is designed to be attached to the inhaler and has a chamber in which the spray from the inhaler is deposited. The person then breathes through the inhaler aid rather than directly from the inhaler. Because of the new additional space between the mouth and the inhaler, the patient has a few more seconds to inhale the medication after it has been released into the device. This makes it possible for the patient to inhale the medication more slowly and thus help the drug reach more deeply into the lungs.

Inhaler aids also allow time for the propellants in the spray to evaporate. This makes the particles of medication travel more slowly and there is less chance the medication will be deposited on the back of the throat.

Each brand of inhaler aid is slightly different. Be sure you understand how to correctly use the brand you have purchased. It is also important to select a device that will fit the specific inhaler you are using. Not all inhaler aids will fit all inhalers.

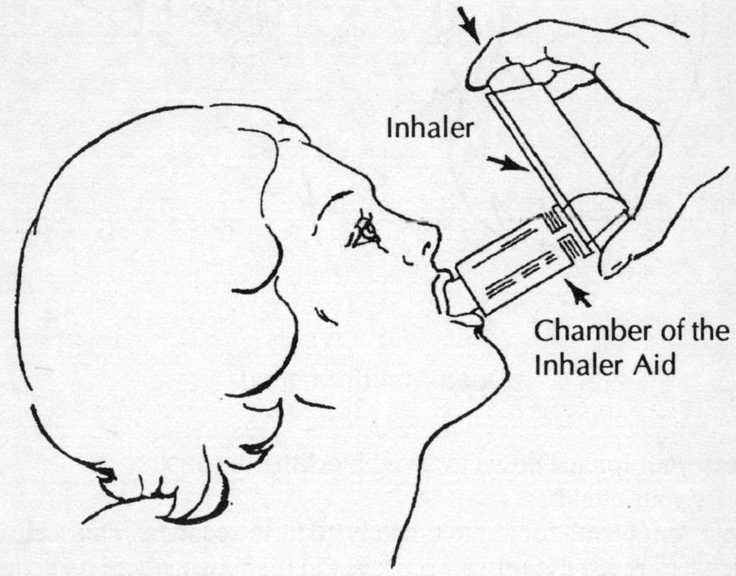

Using an inhaler aid attached
to the inhaler

METHOD II. OPEN-MOUTH INSTRUCTIONS

- Open your mouth.
- Place the tip of the pressurized inhaler approximately 1 inch in front of your opened mouth.
- Breathe out through your mouth as completely as possible.
- Start to breathe in slowly and deeply through your mouth. In the middle of a deep breath in, press down the top of the inhaler as far as it will go to release a "puff." By starting to breathe in before you release a "puff," you will help to prevent the medicine from staying in the mouth and will get it to the lungs.

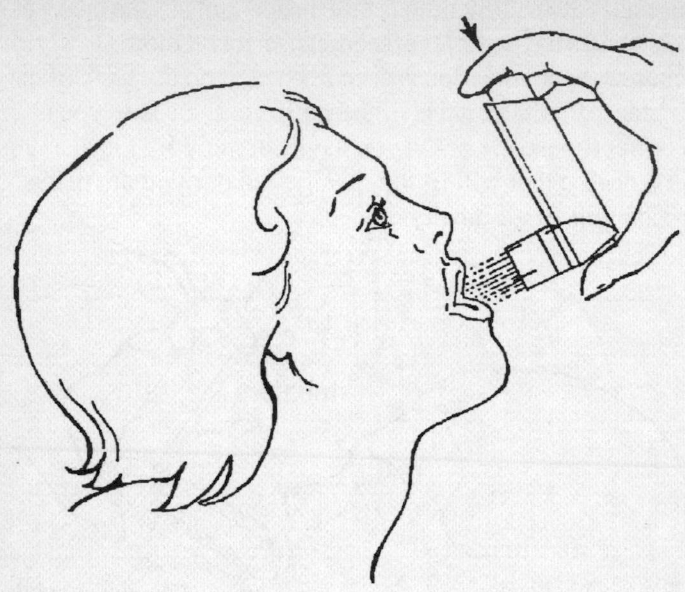

Open-Mouth Method

- Keep your tongue down to avoid blocking the mist.
- Close your mouth.
- Hold your breath for approximately 10 to 15 seconds. This helps the medicine to reach the tiny air passages in the lungs where its action is needed. Then breathe out through your nose slowly.

FOR BOTH METHODS:

If your doctor has prescribed 2 "puffs," wait at least 30 seconds between "puffs" so that the valve pressure in the inhaler can build up.

Rinse your mouth with warm water after you have inhaled the medicine. This will help prevent your mouth and throat from becoming dry.

The mouthpiece of the inhaler should be kept clean and dry.

Failure to follow these instructions carefully can cause your medicine not to work properly or completely.

These instructions may be altered by your doctor or pharmacist because of your medical condition or the specific medicine in the inhaler.

Store the inhaler at room temperature. Do not place it in hot water or near radiators, stoves or other sources of heat. Do not puncture, burn, or incinerate the container (even when it is empty).

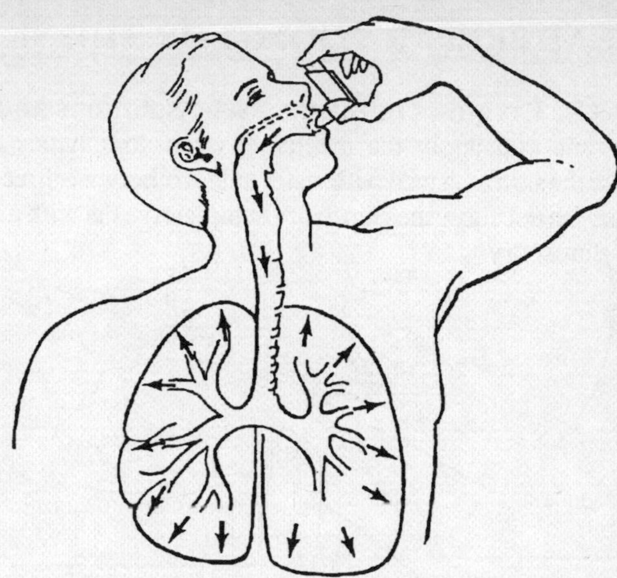

When medicine is inhaled correctly,
it reaches the tiny air passages in the lungs.

HOW TO DETERMINE THE AMOUNT OF MEDICINE LEFT IN AN AEROSOL INHALER

The amount of medicine remaining in an aerosol container may be checked by a very simple method:

- Place the aerosol inhaler in a container of water that is at room temperature.

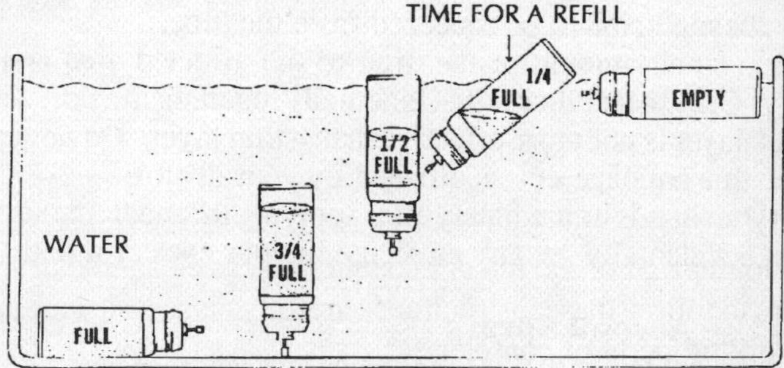

- If the aerosol inhaler is full, it will sink to the bottom. If it is empty, it will float on top of the water. A partially filled inhaler will float at an angle as shown in the diagram.

Reference: *Canadian Pharmaceutical Journal*

TOPICAL PREPARATIONS FOR THE SKIN

How to Use Creams, Ointments, Gels, Solutions and Lotions

- Each time you apply the medicine, wash your hands and gently cleanse the skin area well with water unless otherwise directed by your doctor. Do not allow the skin to dry completely. Pat with a clean towel until almost dry.

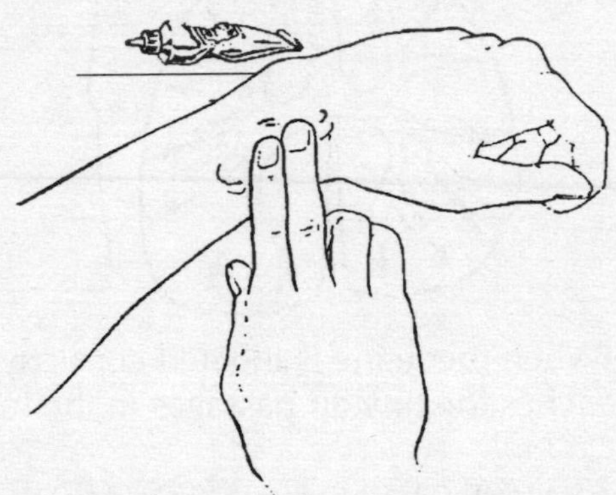

Applying an ointment

- If you were prescribed a lotion, shake the bottle well before using.
- If you were prescribed a cream, ointment or gel and if the top of the tube is sealed, invert the cap and pierce a hole in the seal. This will allow the medicine to be squeezed from the tube.
- Apply a small amount of the drug to the affected area and spread lightly. Only the medicine that is actually touching the skin will work. A thick layer is not more effective than a thin layer. Do not cover the area with a bandage unless directed by your doctor.
- Wash your hands immediately after applying the medicine so that you do not accidentally get any medicine in your eyes or mouth.

How to Use Aerosol Sprays

- Shake the container well each time before using.
- Cleanse the affected area well with water unless otherwise directed by your doctor. Do not allow the skin to dry completely. Pat with a clean towel until slightly damp.
- Hold the container straight up and about 15 to 20 cm (6 to 8 inches) away from the skin.

- Spray the affected area for 1 to 3 seconds.
- Shake the container well between sprays.

Do not spray into the eyes, nose or mouth and try to avoid inhaling the vapors.

Do not smoke while using the spray and do not use near an open flame, fire or heat.

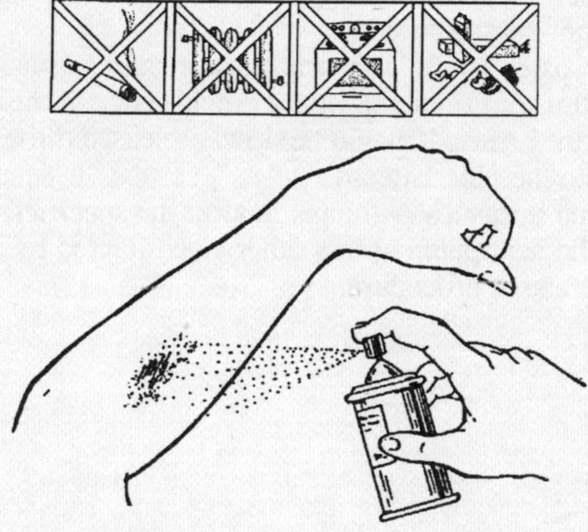

Using an aerosol spray

Do not place the aerosol container in hot water or near radiators, stoves or other sources of heat. Do not puncture or incinerate the container (even when it is empty). Do not store at temperatures greater than 50° C or 120° F.

Do not use the spray near food.

How to Use Transdermal Patches

- Apply the patch at the same time(s) so that the level of the medicine in your body is constant.
- Apply to a non-hairy area of the body. Some patches must be applied to certain parts of the body (e.g. behind the ear). Check with your pharmacist.
- Do not apply the patch over cuts, scrapes or areas with calluses or scars because this can change the absorption of the drug through the skin.
- Do not apply the patch on skin folds or wear under tight clothing since the patch may fall off.
- Do not use the same spot all the time but rotate to different areas. This will help prevent skin irritation.

- Wash your hands with soap and water before applying the patch. Dry hands completely.
- Cleanse the area chosen with soap and water. Rinse and wipe the area completely dry with a clean tissue.
- Do not apply a patch directly after showering, bathing or swimming. Wait until you are sure the skin is completely dry.
- Open the package and remove and throw away the protective backing. Do not touch the inside (sticky side) because the medicine is in this area. Do not cut the patches.
- Attach the patch to the skin and press firmly in place for 10 to 15 seconds. Run your finger along the outside edge of the patch to seal it.
- The medicine in the patch will be slowly released through the skin and directly into the bloodstream.
- Remove and throw away the patch after the specified time or before applying the next patch unless otherwise directed by your doctor.
- Repeat the above procedure.

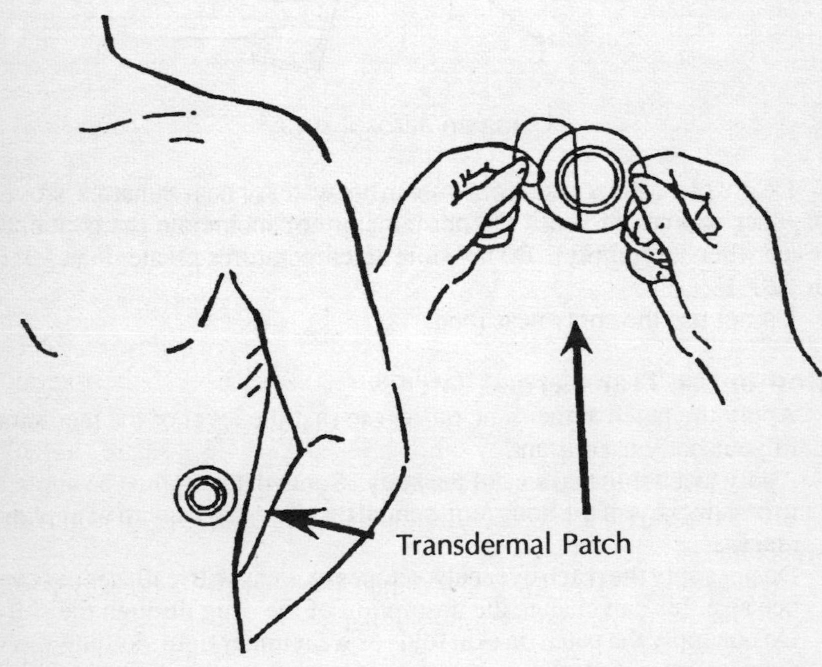

Applying a transdermal patch

Leaking Microwave Oven Causes Burn Under Transdermal Patch

The *New England Journal of Medicine* has reported that a leaking microwave oven was implicated in a case of a second-degree burn in a 51-year-old man with angina pectoris. The man had been using a transdermal patch containing nitroglycerin for several months without any ill effects. He had been applying the patches to his chest, and went to his doctor when he developed a burn on the chest which was of the size and shape of the patch containing the medication.

The man related that he had been sitting near a microwave oven that was in operation when he first began to feel warmth in the area of the patch. By the time he was able to pull the patch off, a second-degree burn had occurred.

The microwave was checked and found to have a leak. It was assumed that the microwave radiation heated the adhesive strip of aluminized (metallic) plastic in the transdermal patch and caused the burn.

Patients wearing transdermal patches that have metallic components should be very careful sitting in front of operating microwave ovens that might be leaking.

RECTAL SUPPOSITORIES

- Remove the wrapper from the suppository.
- If the suppository is too soft, chill it *before* removing it from the foil wrapper by placing it under cold running water or in the refrigerator for a few minutes.
- Moisten the suppository by dipping it quickly into some cool water.
- Lie on your side and raise your knee to your chest.
- Insert the suppository with the tapered (pointed) end first into the rectum.
- Remain lying down for a few minutes so that the suppository will dissolve in the rectum. Wash your hands.
- Try to avoid having a bowel movement for at least 1 hour so that the drug will have time to work.

Rectal suppositories are more effective if they are used when the bowels are empty. If possible, try to insert the suppositories after a bowel movement. Check with your doctor or pharmacist if you have any questions about the best time(s) to use the suppositories.

Suppositories should generally be stored in a cool place. Do not store them in the refrigerator, however, unless directed by your pharmacist.

RECTAL CREAMS

How to Apply to Rectal Skin Area

- Bathe and dry the rectal area.
- If the top of the tube is sealed when the cap is removed, invert the cap and pierce a hole in the sealed top. This will allow the medicine to be squeezed from the tube.
- Apply a small amount of the cream to the rectal area and spread lightly. Only the cream that is touching the skin will work. A thick layer of cream is not more effective than a thin layer of cream.

How to Insert Cream into Rectum

- Attach the plastic applicator to the opened tube of cream.
- A small amount of lubricant, such as petroleum jelly (e.g. Vaseline) or some of the cream may be placed on the outside of the applicator.
- Lie on your side and raise your knee to your chest.
- Insert the applicator tip into the rectum and gently squeeze the tube to deliver the cream.
- Remove the applicator from the rectum and wash the applicator with warm, soapy water. Dry well.
- Replace the cap on the tube of cream.

VAGINAL CREAMS, OINTMENTS AND GELS

- Remove the cap from the tube of cream.
- If the top of the tube is sealed when the cap is removed, invert the cap and pierce a hole in the sealed top. This will allow the medicine to be squeezed from the tube.
- Screw the applicator to the tube.
- Squeeze the tube until the applicator plunger is fully extended. The applicator will now be filled with medicine. If your doctor has prescribed a smaller dose, fill it to the level indicated.
- Unscrew the applicator by the cylinder.
- Apply a small amount of cream to the outside of the applicator.
- Lie on your back with your knees drawn up and spread apart.

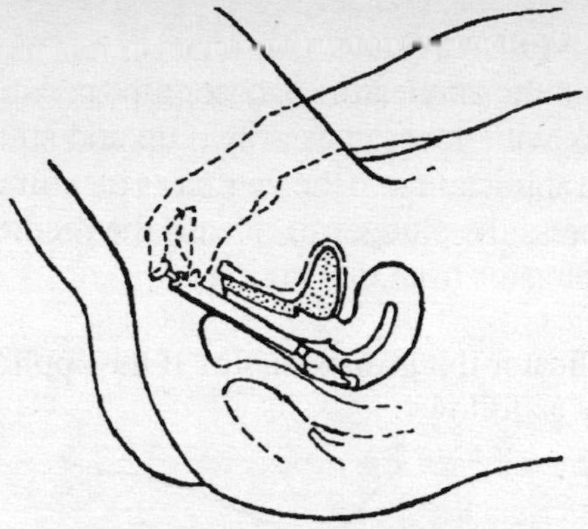

Insertion of vaginal cream
using an applicator

- Hold the filled applicator by the cylinder and gently insert it into the vagina as far as it will comfortably go without using force.
- While still holding the cylinder, push the plunger to deposit the cream into the vagina.
- While keeping the plunger depressed, remove the applicator from the vagina.

Discard the applicator if it is disposable. If the applicator is reusable, clean it thoroughly as follows:

CLEANING THE APPLICATOR
- After each use, take the applicator apart by holding the cylinder and the top of the plunger and pull to separate them. Generally, a "pop" is heard as they separate. Note: Some applicators have screw tops.
- Wash both sections of the applicator thoroughly with warm water and soap and rinse thoroughly. Sterilization of the applicator is unnecessary and extremely hot water should not be used on plastic applicators since it could soften them.
- Dry the applicator. Reassemble by dropping the plunger back into the cylinder as far as it will go.

VAGINAL TABLETS, OVULES AND INSERTS

- This is not an oral medicine and should not be swallowed.
- Remove the wrapper from the tablet. Quickly dip the tablet into some lukewarm water just to moisten it.
- Insert the wide end of the tablet high up into the vagina.

IF THERE IS AN APPLICATOR:

- Put the tablet into the applicator. Do not dip the tablet into water.
- Lie on your back with your knees drawn up and spread apart.
- Gently insert the applicator into the vagina as far as it will comfortably go and then depress the plunger to release the medication.
- Remove the applicator from the vagina.

Discard the applicator if it is disposable. If the applicator is reusable, clean it thoroughly as follows:

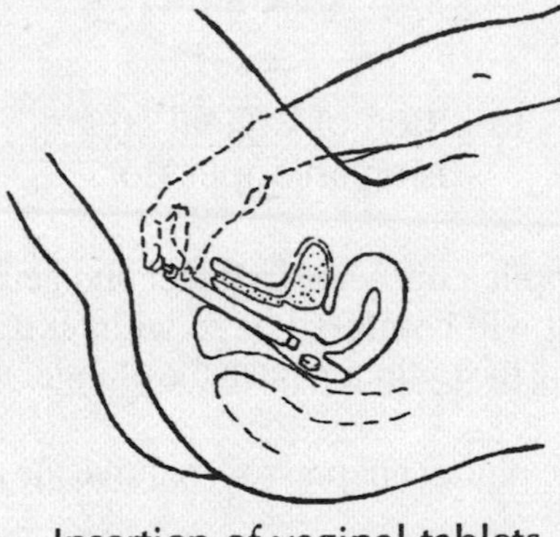

Insertion of vaginal tablets using an applicator

CLEANING THE APPLICATOR

- After each use, clean the applicator according to the instructions that came with your medicine. Extremely hot water should not be used on plastic applicators since it could soften them.
- Dry the applicator.

VAGINAL SUPPOSITORIES

- Remove the wrapper from the suppository.
- Lie on your back with your knees drawn up and spread apart.
- Insert the wide end of the suppository into the vagina.
- Remain lying down for a few minutes so that the suppository will melt.

Suppositories should generally be stored in a cool place. Do not store them in the refrigerator, however, unless directed by your pharmacist. If, for some reason, the suppositories become too soft to insert because of accidental storage in a warm place, they can be chilled in the refrigerator for a few minutes before use. Another method is to run cold water over the foil package *before* removing the suppository.

PRESCRIPTION DRUG INSTRUCTIONS

Disclaimer

These instructions are selective and do not cover all possible uses, actions, precautions, side effects or interactions of the medications included in this book. The information has been based on the official Canadian product labelling, the 1988 *Compendium of Pharmaceuticals and Specialties* and the recommendations of the distinguished physicians and pharmacists who reviewed the manuscript. The instructions may be altered by your doctor or pharmacist because of your medical condition or other drugs you may be taking.

The reader should not consult this book for decisions regarding the practice of medicine. This publication should be used for reference and information only. It should never take the place of your physician. You should not use this book to make medical decisions; rather, you should promptly consult your doctor whenever a medical question arises.

Allergic Reactions

Call your doctor immediately if you think you may be allergic to a medicine or if you develop a skin rash, hives, itching, swelling of the face, or difficulty in breathing. If you cannot reach your doctor, phone a hospital emergency department or the closest Emergency Medical Service.

ACETAMINOPHEN (ORAL)

ANACIN 3, ANACIN 3 EXTRA STRENGTH, APO-ACETAMINOPHEN, ATASOL, ATASOL FORTE, EXDOL, EXDOL STRONG, PANADOL, PANADOL CHEWABLE, ROBIGESIC, ROUNOX, TEMPRA, TEMPRA CHEWABLE, TEMPRA EXTRA STRENGTH, TEMPRA SYRUP, TYLENOL, TYLENOL CHEWABLE, TYLENOL EXTRA-STRENGTH, TYLENOL JUNIOR STRENGTH

ACETAMINOPHEN (RECTAL)

ABENOL SUPPOSITORIES, ACETAMINOPHEN SUPPOSITORIES

Purpose

This medicine is used to help reduce pain and/or fever.

Do not use for arthritic conditions without checking with your doctor because ACETAMINOPHEN does not treat the underlying cause (inflammation) of arthritic pain. ACETAMINOPHEN may relieve the pain but it will not relieve the inflammation (redness, swelling, stiffness) of arthritis.

Allergies/Warnings

If you have ever had an allergic reaction to acetaminophen or any other medicine, tell your doctor and pharmacist before you take any of this medicine.

How to Use This Medicine

How to Administer

This medicine may be taken with food or a full glass of water.

For drops:

- If a dropper is used to measure the dose and you do not fully understand how to use it, *see* How to Administer Medications (page 15). Caution: Some drops are very concentrated. Be sure you know how much to use.

For syrups and elixirs:

- If a spoon is used to measure the dose, it is recommended that you use a medicine spoon or an oral liquid syringe that you can obtain from your pharmacist. *See* How to Administer Medications (page 15).

For chewable tablets (PANADOL CHEWABLE, TEMPRA CHEWABLE, TYLENOL CHEWABLE):

- This medicine must be chewed completely before swallowing.

For suppositories: see How to Administer Medications (page 15).

Special Instructions

Length of Therapy

Children under 2 years of age should only be given this medicine with the approval of the doctor. Children under 12 years of age should not be given this medicine for more than 5 days in a row.

Pregnancy/Breastfeeding

Women who are pregnant, breastfeeding or planning to become pregnant should tell their doctor before taking this medicine.

Drug Interactions

Do not take any other medicine containing ACETAMINOPHEN without consulting your doctor or pharmacist while you are taking this medicine because you could take too much of this drug. Since many non-prescription drugs contain ACETAMINOPHEN, check the labels of any nonprescription drugs you may have and call your pharmacist if you have any questions about the contents.

Alcohol

Do not drink alcoholic beverages while taking this drug without the approval of your doctor. High doses of the drug taken for a long period in combination with large amounts of alcohol may cause liver damage.

When to Call Your Doctor

Call your doctor if the medicine does not relieve your symptoms or if they get worse. If you are using the medicine to lower a fever and if the fever does not go away (for example, within 2 or 3 days), call your doctor.

Most people experience few or no side effects from this drug. However, any medicine can sometimes cause unwanted effects. Call your doctor if you develop nausea or vomiting, stomach pain, diarrhea, unexplained sore throat or fever, unusual weakness or tiredness, unusual bruising or bleeding or a yellow color to the skin or eyes.

Get emergency help at once if you think that anyone has taken an overdose of this medicine. Overdoses can be very serious and treatment may need to be started even before the symptoms of an overdose appear because the symptoms of liver damage may not appear until 4 to 6 days after the overdose has been taken. Overdose symptoms include nausea, vomiting, diarrhea, stomach cramps, swelling of abdomen, increased sweating, fever, loss of appetite, or a yellow color to the skin or eyes.

Allergic Reactions

Call your doctor immediately if you think you may be allergic to the medicine or if you develop a skin rash, hives, itching, fever, swelling of the face, or difficulty in breathing. If you cannot reach your doctor, phone a hospital emergency department.

Storage

For tablets and capsules:

- Store the medicine in a cool, dark place.

For suppositories: *see* How to Administer Medications (page 15).

Did You Know That?

Whenever you receive a medicine from a pharmacist, you should know the answer to these questions:

- What is the name of the medicine?
- Why has the medicine been prescribed for me?
- How will I know if the medicine is working correctly?
- How long will it take to have an effect?
- How should I administer the medicine?
- How much of the medicine should I take?
- At what exact time(s) during the day and night should I administer the drug?
- Does the drug have to be taken before, during or after eating some food?
- What does it mean to take a drug on an empty stomach?
- Are there any foods that should be avoided?
- Should alcoholic beverages be avoided while taking this medicine?
- Are there any nonprescription medicines that can interact with this prescription drug and should not be taken at the same time?
- What are the side effects that most commonly occur with this medicine? What should I do if I experience one of these side effects?
- What adverse effects should prompt me to call the doctor?
- For how long should the medicine be taken?
- Can the prescription be refilled and how?
- How should the medicine be stored?

ACETAMINOPHEN-CODEINE (ORAL)

EMPRACET-30, EMPRACET-60, EMTEC-30, LENOLTEC WITH CODEINE NO. 4, ROUNOX + CODEINE, TYLENOL WITH CODEINE NO. 4, TYLENOL WITH CODEINE ELIXIR

ACETAMINOPHEN—CAFFEINE—CODEINE

ATASOL-8, ATASOL-15, ATASOL-30, EXDOL-8, EXDOL-15, EXDOL-30, LENOLTEC WITH CODEINE NO. 1, NO.2 AND NO. 3, TYLENOL NO. 1, TYLENOL NO. 1 FORTE, TYLENOL WITH CODEINE NO. 2, TYLENOL WITH CODEINE NO.3, VEGANIN

ACETAMINOPHEN-OXYCODONE

ENDOCET, OXYCOCET, PERCOCET, PERCOCET-DEMI

Purpose

This medicine is used to help relieve pain. Some products may also be used to reduce fever and coughing in some conditions.

Allergies/Warnings

If you have ever had an allergic reaction to ACETAMINOPHEN, CODEINE or any other medicine, tell your doctor and pharmacist before you take any of this medicine.

How to Use This Medicine

Time of Administration

If you are taking this medicine to help relieve pain, do not wait until the pain becomes severe. This medicine works best if you take it when the pain first occurs. If your doctor has prescribed this medicine on a regular schedule, take it as recommended and not on an "as needed" basis.

How to Administer

This medicine may be taken with food or a full glass of water.

For liquid medicines:

- If a spoon is used to measure the dose, it is recommended that you use a medicine spoon or an oral liquid syringe that you can obtain from your pharmacist. *See* How to Administer Medications (page 15).

Special Instructions

Length of Therapy

Do not take any more of this medicine than your doctor has prescribed. When used in large doses for a long period of time, these medicines can become habit forming and less effective.

Call your doctor if you feel you need the medicine more often than was prescribed. Do not take a larger dose without your doctor's approval.

Do not stop taking this medicine suddenly without the approval of your doctor. It may be necessary for your doctor to reduce your dose slowly. This will depend on the dose, length of therapy and the specific medicine you have been taking.

Pregnancy/Breastfeeding

Women who are pregnant, breastfeeding or planning to become pregnant should tell their doctor before taking this medicine.

Drug Interactions

It is important that you obtain the advice of your doctor or pharmacist before taking any other prescription or nonprescription medicines, including pain relievers, sleeping pills, tranquilizers or medicines for depression, cough, cold or allergy medicines. Some of these drugs may cause increased drowsiness if taken with this medicine.

Do not take any other medicine containing ACETAMINOPHEN without consulting your doctor or pharmacist while you are taking this medicine because you could take too much of this drug. Since many nonprescription drugs contain ACETAMINOPHEN, check the labels of any nonprescription drugs you may have and call your pharmacist if you have any questions about the contents.

There are other drug interactions that can occur. If you are taking any other medicines, be sure to check with your pharmacist or doctor.

Alcohol

Do not drink alcoholic beverages while taking this drug without the approval of your doctor because the combination could cause drowsiness. One drink may have the same effect that 2 or 3 drinks normally would have.

In addition, high doses of ACETAMINOPHEN taken for a long time in combination with large amounts of alcohol may cause liver damage.

Special Precautions

If you feel nauseated when you first start taking the medicine, it may help if you lie down for a few minutes.

In some people, this drug may cause dizziness or drowsiness. Do not drive a car, pilot an airplane, operate dangerous machinery or do jobs that require you to be alert if you are dizzy or drowsy. You should also be careful going up and down stairs. Get up slowly after you have been sitting or lying down. Sit or lie down at the first sign of dizziness. Tell your doctor if dizziness or drowsiness continues.

This medicine may cause some people to become constipated. To prevent constipation, try increasing the amount of bulk in your diet (for example, bran, fresh fruits and salads), exercising more often or drinking more fluids (unless otherwise directed). Call your doctor if the constipation continues.

When to Call Your Doctor

Call your doctor if the medicine does not relieve your symptoms or if they get worse.

Most people experience few or no side effects from this drug. However, any medicine can sometimes cause unwanted effects. Call your doctor if you develop nausea or vomiting, stomach pain, diarrhea, unexplained sore throat or fever, unusual weakness or tiredness, unusual bruising or bleeding, a yellow color to the skin or eyes, confusion, depression, severe nervousness, severe drowsiness or trembling.

Get emergency help at once if you think that anyone has taken an overdose of this medicine. Overdoses can be very serious and treatment may need to be started even before the symptoms of an overdose appear because the symptoms of liver damage may not appear until 4 to 6 days after the overdose has been taken. Overdose symptoms include nausea, vomiting, loss of appetite, diarrhea, stomach cramps, swelling of abdomen, increased sweating, fever, or a yellow color to the skin or eyes.

Did You Know That?

Medicines should not be stored in the traditional bathroom medicine cabinet. The bathroom often becomes hot and steamy and the heat and humidity can destroy some drugs.

Some medicines must be stored in the refrigerator. If this is the case, there will be a "Keep Refrigerated" label on the prescription container. Do not store any medicines in the refrigerator unless specified by your pharmacist. The cold temperature and high humidity can destroy some drugs.

In general, a cool dry place is the best storage place for most medications. Always keep your medicines in a place which is away from the reach or sight of children.

Allergic Reactions

Call your doctor immediately if you think you may be allergic to the medicine or if you develop a skin rash, hives, itching, fever, swelling of the face, or difficulty in breathing. If you cannot reach your doctor, phone a hospital emergency department.

Storage

Store the medicine in a cool, dark place.

ACETOHEXAMIDE (ORAL)

DIMELOR

CHLORPROPAMIDE

APO-CHLORPROPAMIDE, DIABINESE, NOVOPROPAMIDE

GLYBURIDE

DIABETA, EUGLUCON

METFORMIN

GLUCOPHAGE

TOLBUTAMIDE

APO-TOLBUTAMIDE, MOBENOL, NOVOBUTAMIDE, ORINASE

Purpose

This medicine is used in the treatment of diabetes. When you have diabetes, the body either is not producing enough insulin or is not able to use what is produced. Insulin is needed for the body's proper use of food, especially sugar. In a person with diabetes, the sugar in the blood can build up to dangerous levels and is passed out in the urine. Your doctor has prescribed this medicine to help keep your blood sugar at nearly normal levels.

Allergies/Warnings

If you have ever had an allergic reaction to any medicine or if you have a heart, liver or kidney condition, tell your doctor and pharmacist before you take any of this medicine.

How to Use This Medicine

Time of Administration

Do not take this medicine at bedtime unless your doctor tells you to.

It is very important that you take this medicine exactly as your doctor has prescribed. Do not miss any doses and take the medicine even if you feel well. Try to take this medicine at the same time(s) every day so that you have a constant level of medicine in your body. Do not take extra doses without your doctor's approval.

How to Administer

If you were prescribed ACETOHEXAMIDE, CHLORPROPAMIDE *or* TOLBUTAMIDE:

- This medicine may be taken with food if it upsets your stomach. Call your doctor if you continue to have stomach upset.

If you were prescribed GLYBURIDE *or* METFORMIN:

- It is best to take this medicine with food or immediately after meals.

Special Instructions

Length of Therapy

This medicine will not cure your diabetes but will help to control it. In order to receive the full benefit of the drug, you must take it as long as your doctor feels you need it. It may be necessary for you to take medicine for your diabetes the rest of your life.

Pregnancy/Breastfeeding

Women who are pregnant or planning to become pregnant should not take this medicine.

Women who are breastfeeding should tell their doctor before taking this medicine.

Drug Interactions

Before you purchase any nonprescription medicine (for example, cough and cold medicines), ask your pharmacist if the medicine is safe for diabetic patients to use. Some liquid nonprescription medicines contain a lot of sugar that could interfere with the control of your diabetes.

It is recommended that patients do not take products containing ASA, salicylates or large doses of vitamin C because the combination could cause hypoglycemia (low blood sugar). It is recommended that patients avoid the use of sodium bicarbonate (baking soda).

Alcohol

It is recommended that you avoid the use of alcoholic beverages until you have discussed this with your doctor. Some people who drink alcohol while taking this medicine react and develop low blood sugar early after ingestion and then high blood sugar several hours later. A pounding headache, flushing or upset stomach can also occur.

Patients taking METFORMIN could also develop high lactic acid levels.

Special Precautions

Follow the special diet your doctor has prescribed for you.

Test your urine or blood regularly for sugar and if your doctor recommends, test it for acetone. This is especially important during the first few weeks of treatment. Give the results of these tests to your doctor at every office visit unless he or she wants them more often.

See *General Instructions for Patients with Diabetes* (Appendix B) for signs of low blood sugar, high blood sugar, and proper foot care.

When to Call Your Doctor

Call your doctor if you become sick and have a fever, an infection, nausea or vomiting.

The Glove Compartment is not a Medicine Cabinet

Medications should not be stored in automobile glove compartments because the solar heating effect causes excessively high temperatures which can destroy the drug.

According to the *Journal of the American Medical Association,* temperatures in glove compartments between April and October in the northern hemisphere are up to 28 degrees C (50 degrees F) *higher* than outdoor temperatures. This means that medicines stored inside the glove compartment could be exposed to temperatures reaching 66 degrees C (150 degrees F). The temperature of floor areas shielded from direct sunlight was approximately 11 degrees C (20 degrees F) less. The study was conducted in California.

In general, medications should not be stored in the glove compartments of automobiles during the summer months because of the heat. If you are traveling during the summer, the best way to store medications in a car is in an insulated container on the floor of the car and shielded from direct sunlight. In addition, medications should not be stored in automobiles during the winter months in Canada because the extreme cold could freeze the medications.

Most people experience few or no side effects from this drug. However, any medicine can sometimes cause unwanted effects. Call your doctor if you develop a skin rash, sore throat, fever, mouth sores, dark-colored urine, increased sensitivity to sunlight or if you get a sunburn, a yellow color to the skin or eyes, unusual bruising or bleeding, unusual tiredness, diarrhea, light-colored stools or stomach pain.

If you are taking CHLOROROPAMIDE, also call your doctor if you develop any of the additional side effects: headache, swelling of the face, hands or legs, muscle cramps, or weakness.

If you are taking METFORMIN, also call your doctor if you develop vomiting, metallic taste in the mouth, stomach upset, diarrhea or loss of appetite.

When Insulin-Dependent Diabetics Travel Through Time Zones

When a diabetic patient who takes insulin travels by airplane through time zones, the dosage of insulin will have to be adjusted to allow for the rapid time changes.

A simple rule is:

When flying east, the insulin dose should be decreased.

When flying west, the insulin dose should be increased.

For example, if a man is flying from Ottawa to London, he will lose 6 hours of time, which is equivalent to one-fourth of a day. When he arrives in London, the first injection of insulin should be decreased by one-fourth. On the second day in London, he should return to his normal insulin dose.

When he flies back to Ottawa from London, he should increase the insulin dosage by one-fourth, since he will be gaining six hours. He should return to his normal dosage on the following day.

These guidelines will have to be tailored by the doctor in order to consider any factors, such as time of departure and meals served on the plane, that require additional adjustments. Therefore, if you have diabetes and take insulin, check with your doctor about your insulin dose before you travel through several time zones.

Reference: *Diabetes in the News* and *American Pharmacy*

Allergic Reactions

Call your doctor immediately if you think you may be allergic to the medicine or if you develop a skin rash, hives, itching, swelling of the face or difficulty in breathing. If you cannot reach your doctor, phone a hospital emergency department or emergency medical service.

Refills

Do not stop taking this medicine without your doctor's approval and do not go without medicine between prescription refills. Call your pharmacist for a refill 2 or 3 days before you will run out of the medicine.

Discuss with your pharmacist the implications of dispensing all your refills for this medicine with the same manufacturer's product. (*See* Generic Drugs, page 12.)

Miscellaneous

Carry an identification card (*See* Medicine Card) or wear a medical alert bracelet indicating that you are a diabetic and that you are taking this medicine. Always tell your pharmacist, dentist and other doctors who are treating you that you are taking this medicine.

ACYCLOVIR (ORAL)

ZOVIRAX

Purpose

This medicine is used to help shorten the duration and relieve the symptoms of initial episodes of herpes infections due to genital herpes. The drug attacks the herpes virus-infected cells and prevents spread of the virus to other cells. The drug does not act on normal cells that are not infected.

The drug is also used to manage recurrent herpes infections of the genitals. When given continuously to help prevent recurrences, the drug "stands by" in the cells and may stop the virus from spreading.

ACYCLOVIR will not cure genital herpes but it can help to reduce some of the pain and itching and help speed the healing of any sores. It can also help to reduce the number of attacks.

Allergies/Warnings

If you have ever had an allergic reaction to ACYCLOVIR, tell your doctor and pharmacist before you take any of this medicine.

How to Use This Medicine

Time of Administration

The medicine must be taken at regularly spaced intervals in order to be effective. Do not miss any doses.

In the treatment of recurrent herpes infections using 5-day treatments, start taking the medicine at the first sign of a recurrence, e.g. tingling, itching or pain. This helps prevent the virus from multiplying and destroying the skin cells.

If you were prescribed this medicine on a daily basis for long-term therapy, try not to miss any doses so that you have enough drug in the body at all times to prevent the virus from growing and multiplying.

How to Administer

Take the tablets with a full glass of water. The drug may also be taken at the same time as food.

Special Instructions

Length of Therapy

The length of treatment will depend on the severity of the infection and whether it is the first episode (10 days treatment) or a recurrent episode.

If you have recurrent genital herpes, your doctor will decide whether short-term (5 days) or long-term treatment (up to 12 months) is best for you.

The safety and effectiveness of continuous use of this drug has been established only for up to 12 months.

Pregnancy/Breastfeeding

Women who are pregnant, breastfeeding or planning to become pregnant should tell their doctor before taking this medicine.

Special Precautions

The herpes virus is contained in the blisters. When the blisters break, the infection will spread very easily. If you touch your skin sores, wash your hands immediately and do not touch other parts of your body until your hands are cleaned.

Genital herpes is a sexually transmitted disease and patients should avoid having sex when lesions (blisters) are present because there is a possibility of infecting the other person. The use of a condom will help prevent the spread of genital herpes. *The drug will NOT help prevent you from spreading the disease to others.*

Women with genital herpes should have yearly Pap smears because there appears to be a higher incidence of cancer of the cervix in women with genital herpes.

Do not share the medication with others.

Do not take a higher dose or take the medicine for longer periods of time than prescribed by your doctor.

Some patients may have worsening of symptoms after the first treatment has been completed. If this happens, call your doctor.

If you become dizzy, sit or lie down at the first sign of dizziness. Do not drive a car, pilot an airplane, operate dangerous machinery or do jobs that require you to be alert until you know how you are going to react to the drug. Tell your doctor if the dizziness continues.

It is important to drink adequate amounts of fluids while taking this medicine.

When to Call Your Doctor

Most people experience few or no side effects from this drug. However, any medicine can sometimes cause unwanted effects.

If you are taking the medicine for a *short time* (5 to 10 days), call your doctor if you develop severe nausea or vomiting, unusual headaches, diarrhea, painful urination, skin rash or leg pain.

If you are taking the medicine for a *long time*, call your doctor if you develop any of the previously listed symptoms or joint pain, muscle cramps, rapid heartbeats, insomnia, acne, back pain, swollen glands, hair loss, menstrual abnormalities or depression.

Allergic Reactions

Call your doctor immediately if you think you may be allergic to the medicine or if you develop a skin rash, hives, itching, swelling of the face or difficulty in breathing. If you cannot reach your doctor, phone a hospital emergency department.

Refills

Because of the importance of starting the drug at the first sign of a recurrence, it is a good idea to have at least one or two extra days' supply on hand. If you do not have at least one extra day's supply on hand, ask your doctor to prescribe it for you.

ACYCLOVIR (TOPICAL)

ZOVIRAX

Purpose

This ointment is used to treat initial herpes infections in the genital area. ACYCLOVIR will not cure herpes infections but it can help to reduce some of the pain and help speed the healing of the sores.

This ointment is NOT effective in the treatment of recurrent genital herpes infections.

Allergies/Warnings

If you have ever had an allergic reaction to ACYCLOVIR, or polyethylene glycol which is an inactive ingredient in the ointment, tell your doctor and pharmacist before you take any of this medicine.

How to Use This Medicine

Time of Administration

Start applying the ointment at the first sign of an attack (e.g. tingling, itching or pain).

The ointment is usually applied 4 to 6 times daily for up to 10 days. It is important not to miss any doses or the medication may be less effective.

How to Administer

Use a disposable rubber glove or finger cot to apply the ointment. Throw the glove or finger cot away after use. This will help prevent spreading of the infection to other parts of the body or to other people.

Cover all the sores (blisters) with a sufficient quantity of ointment.

Special Instructions

Length of Therapy

The usual length of treatment is 10 days.

Pregnancy/Breastfeeding

Women who are pregnant, breastfeeding or planning to become pregnant should tell their doctor before using this medicine.

Special Precautions

The herpes virus is contained in the blisters. When the blisters break,

Drugs That Cause Sexual Problems

More than 100 medications can interfere with sexual function in both men and women. They can cause decreased sex drive, interfere with erection or ejaculation in men and delay or prevent orgasm in women. Some of the drugs that may cause sexual problems include:

- Antihypertensives/Heart Drugs such as PROPRANOLOL, GUANETHIDINE, HYDRALAZINE, CAPTOPRIL, METHYLDOPA, PHENOXYBENZAMINE and RESERPINE
- Tranquilizers such as DIAZEPAM, CHLORDIAZEPOXIDE and MEPROBAMATE
- Antidepressants such as AMITRIPTYLINE, IMIPRAMINE and DESIPRAMINE
- Antipsychotic Drugs such as THIORIDAZINE and CHLORPROMAZINE
- Stomach Drugs such as CIMETIDINE, ATROPINE, BELLADONNA and PROPANTHELINE
- Cancer Drugs
- Diuretics such as SPIRONOLACTONE, CHLORTHALIDONE, THIAZIDES
- Clofibrate
- Alcohol

When a doctor prescribes a medication that may cause sexual problems, it has been suggested that he should question patients about possible sexual difficulties during the drug treatment. It is also wise advice for patients to discuss any sexual problems they are having with their doctor rather than blaming themselves or their partners. These problems can often be solved simply by reducing the dosage or switching to another drug.

In some cases, the sexual problems may be due to illnesses such as diabetes, heart disease, alcoholism, depression, fatigue, etc. which will require medical treatment.

the infection will spread very easily. If you touch your skin sores, wash your hands immediately and do not touch other parts of your body until your hands are clean.

Genital herpes is a sexually transmitted disease and you should avoid having sex when lesions (blisters) are present because there is a possibility of infecting the other person. The use of a condom will help prevent the spread of genital herpes. *The drug will NOT help prevent you from spreading the disease to others.*

Women with genital herpes should have yearly Pap smears because there appears to be a higher incidence of cancer of the cervix in women with genital herpes.

Do not share the medication with others.

Do not use this ointment in the eyes. It is meant only for application to the skin and mucous membranes.

The ointment normally causes a mild discomfort (e.g. tingling, itching or burning) when it is applied because the herpes lesions are very sensitive and tender.

When to Call Your Doctor

Most people experience few or no side effects from this drug. However, any medicine can sometimes cause unwanted effects. Call your doctor if you develop skin rash, redness or itching of the affected area.

Also call your doctor if your condition does not improve in 10 days.

Allergic Reactions

Call your doctor immediately if you think you may be allergic to the medicine or if you develop a skin rash, hives, itching, swelling of the face, or difficulty in breathing. If you cannot reach your doctor, phone a hospital emergency department.

ALLOPURINOL (ORAL)

ALLOPRIN, APO-ALLOPURINOL, NOVOPUROL, PURINOL, ZYLOPRIM

Purpose

This medicine is used in the treatment and prevention of gout. It will not be effective in relieving an attack that has already started. It is useful in treating certain types of kidney stones. It is also used in other conditions in which the body has high levels of uric acid.

Allergies/Warnings

If you have ever had an allergic reaction to ALLOPURINOL or if you have kidney or liver problems, tell your doctor and pharmacist before you take any of this medicine.

How to Use This Medicine

Time of Administration

It is very important that you take this medicine exactly as your doctor has prescribed. Do not miss any doses and take the medicine even if you feel well. Try to take this medicine at the same time(s) every day so that you will have a constant level of medicine in your body. Do not take extra tablets without your doctor's approval.

How to Administer

Take this medicine with food or a glass of milk or after meals to help prevent stomach upset. Call your doctor if you continue to have stomach upset.

Special Instructions

Length of Therapy

It may be necessary to take this medicine up to 2 to 6 weeks before you feel its full benefits.

Do not stop taking the medicine without your doctor's approval.

Pregnancy/Breastfeeding

Women who are pregnant or planning to become pregnant should tell their doctor before taking this medicine.

Women who are breastfeeding should tell their doctor before taking this medicine. This medicine may pass into the breast milk and cause side effects in the baby.

Drug Interactions

Do not take vitamin C supplements without the approval of your doctor while you are taking this medicine. Vitamin C (ascorbic acid) may make the urine more acidic and promote the development of kidney stones in people taking this medicine.

Special Precautions

Be sure to keep your regular doctor's appointments so that he or she can make sure that the medicine is working correctly and that your gout is under control.

To help prevent the formation of new kidney stones, drink at least 10 to 12 full 8-ounce glasses of water or other fluids every day while you are taking this medicine unless directed otherwise by your doctor. If the medicine is for a child, ask your doctor how much water the child should drink each day.

In some people, this drug may cause drowsiness. Do not drive a car, pilot an airplane, operate dangerous machinery or do jobs that require you to be alert until you know how you are going to react to the drug.

When to Call Your Doctor

Stop taking the drug and call your doctor immediately if you develop pain when you urinate (pass your water), blood in the urine, irritation of the eyes, swelling of the lips or mouth, a skin rash or red-purple spots that look like bruises. The skin rash has been reported to appear as late as 3 months after the medicine has been stopped.

Also call your doctor if you develop a sore throat, fever, chills, unusual bruising or bleeding, unusual tiredness or weakness, muscle aching, stomach pain, numbness, tingling or pain in the hands or feet, a yellow color to the skin or eyes, changes in vision or blurred vision, low back pain.

Allergic Reactions

Call your doctor immediately if you think you may be allergic to the medicine or if you develop a skin rash, hives or itching.

Did You Know That?

There are several look-alike and/or sound-alike drugs in Canada.

Pharmacists are especially careful when dispensing medications that either look alike on written prescriptions or sound alike when the prescription is received over the telephone.

Examples of such drugs are:

CORTONE .... CORDARONE
DONNATAL .... DONNAGEL
KAO-CON .... KAON
KEMADRIN .... COUMADIN
K-LOR .... CECLOR
KOFFEX .... KEFLEX
NORPRAMIN .... NORIPRAMINE
SELDANE .... FELDENE
THYROLAR .... THYTROPAR
ZANTAC .... XANAX

ALPRAZOLAM (ORAL)
XANAX

CHLORDIAZEPOXIDE HCl
APO-CHLORDIAZEPOXIDE, LIBRIUM, MEDILIUM, NOVOPOXIDE, SOLIUM

CLONAZEPAM
RIVOTRIL

CLORAZEPATE DIPOTASSIUM
NOVOCLOPATE, TRANXENE

DIAZEPAM
APO-DIAZEPAM, E-PAM, MEVAL, NOVODIPAM, RIVAL, VALIUM, VIVOL

BROMAZEPAM
LECTOPAM

LORAZEPAM (ORAL and SUBLINGUAL)
APO-LORAZEPAM, ATIVAN, NOVOLORAZEM

OXAZEPAM
APO-OXAZEPAM, NOVOXAPAM, OX-PAM, SERAX, ZAPEX

Purpose
This medicine (except CLONAZEPAM) is used to help relieve moderate to severe anxiety and tension and to treat some nervous conditions. It should not be used to treat nervousness or tension from the normal pressures of day-to-day living. DIAZEPAM is also used in some conditions to help relieve muscle cramps.

CLONAZEPAM is used in some patients to help prevent seizures. Some are used to treat the symptoms of alcohol withdrawal.

Allergies/Warnings
If you have ever had an allergic reaction to any medicine or if you have any medical problem, tell your doctor and pharmacist before you take any of this medicine.

How to Use This Medicine

How to Administer

This medicine may be taken without regard to meals. Take it either with food or on an empty stomach.

For ATIVAN *sublingual tablets, see* How to Administer Medications (page 15).

Special Instructions

Length of Therapy

Do not take this medicine more often or longer than recommended by your doctor. If large doses are taken for long periods of time (months), the drug can become habit-forming.

Do not stop taking this medicine suddenly without the approval of your doctor. It may be necessary for your doctor to reduce your dose slowly since your body may need time to adjust.

Check with your doctor if you develop any of the following symptoms while you are slowly stopping or after you have stopped the medicine: nausea or vomiting, trembling, seizures, muscle cramps, stomach cramps, unusual sweating, trouble sleeping. Also call your doctor if you become confused, irritable or nervous.

Pregnancy/Breastfeeding

Women who are pregnant, breastfeeding or planning to become pregnant should tell their doctor before taking this medicine. Generally, this medicine should not be used during pregnancy and is not generally recommended during breastfeeding.

Drug Interactions

It is important that you obtain the advice of your doctor or pharmacist before taking any other prescription or nonprescription medicines, including pain relievers, antacids, sleeping pills, tranquilizers or medicines for depression, cough, cold or allergy medicines.

There are other drug interactions that can occur. If you are taking any other medicines, be sure to check first with your pharmacist or doctor.

Alcohol

Do not drink alcoholic beverages while taking this drug or for a few days after you have stopped taking the drug without the approval of your doctor. The combination could cause drowsiness. One drink may have the same effect that 2 or 3 drinks normally would have.

Special Precautions

In some people, this drug may cause dizziness or drowsiness. Do not drive a car, pilot an airplane, operate dangerous machinery or do jobs that require you to be alert if you are dizzy or drowsy. You should also be careful going up and down stairs. Sit or lie down at the first sign of dizziness. Tell your doctor if the dizziness or drowsiness continues.

When to Call Your Doctor

Most people experience few or no side effects from this drug. However, any medicine can sometimes cause unwanted effects. Call your doctor if you develop a sore throat, fever, mouth sores, a staggering walk, a yellow color to the skin or eyes, slow heartbeats or shortness of breath, unusual tiredness or nervousness, stomach pain, unusual bruising or bleeding, confusion or depression, hallucinations, trouble sleeping, slurred speech or severe drowsiness.

If you are taking this medicine to treat epilepsy, call your doctor if you have an increase in the frequency of seizures.

Allergic Reactions

Call your doctor immediately if you think you may be allergic to the medicine or if you develop a skin rash, hives, itching, swelling of the face or difficulty in breathing. If you cannot reach your doctor, phone a hospital emergency department.

Did You Know That?

Two tablets with identical ingredients may perform differently in the body.

The manufacturing process has an important effect on the performance of the tablet in the body. Something as simple as the compression pressure used to shape the tablet powder into a tablet will influence the hardness of the tablet and how quickly it will break apart after being swallowed.

Tablets which are too hard may not break down, and may be excreted whole! All tablets manufactured in Canada must pass strict tests before they can be used in patients.

AMCINONIDE (TOPICAL)

CYCLOCORT

BECLOMETHASONE

PROPADERM

BETAMETHASONE
Beben, Betacort Scalp Lotion, Betaderm, Betaderm Scalp Lotion, Betnovate, Celestoderm-V, Celestoderm-V/2, Diprolene, Diprosone, Ectosone Mild, Ectosone Regular, Ectosone Scalp Lotion, Metaderm, Novobetamet, Valisone Scalp Lotion

CLOBETASOL PROPIONATE
Dermovate

CLOBETASONE
Eumovate

DESONIDE
Tridesilon

DESOXIMETASONE
Topicort

DIFLORASONE
Florone, Flutone

DIFLUCORTOLONE
Nerisone

FLUMETHASONE PIVALATE
Locacorten

FLUOCINOLONE ACETONIDE
Fluoderm, Fluolar, Fluonide, Synalar, Synamol

FLUOCINONIDE
Lidemol, Lidex, Lyderm, Topsyn Gel

FLURANDRENOLIDE
Drenison, Drenison Tape

HALCINONIDE
Halog

HYDROCORTISONE
Barriere-HC, Cortacet, Cortate, Cortef, Corticreme, Cortoderm, Emo-Cort, Hyderm, Novohydrocort, Sarna HC 1.0%, Unicort, Westcort

HYDROCORTISONE-NEOMYCIN
Neo-Cortef

METHYLPREDNISOLONE
MEDROL TOPICAL

METHYLPREDNISOLONE-NEOMYCIN
NEO-MEDROL TOPICAL

TRIAMCINOLONE
ARISTOCORT C, ARISTOCORT D, ARISTOCORT R, KENALOG, KENALOG SPRAY, TRIADERM, TRIANIDE MILD, TRIANIDE REGULAR

Purpose

This medicine is used to help relieve pain, itching, redness and swelling of certain types of skin conditions. NEO-CORTEF and NEO-MEDROL TOPICAL contain NEOMYCIN (an antibiotic) and are used to help prevent and treat skin infections.

Do not use this medicine for any other skin problems without checking with your doctor.

Allergies/Warnings

Be sure to tell your doctor and pharmacist if you are allergic to any medicine or have any other medical condition.

Children may absorb larger amounts of this medicine and should have frequent checkups by their doctors while using this medicine.

How to Use This Medicine

How to Administer

For cream, ointment, gel and lotion: see How to Administer Medications (page 15).

If you were prescribed HALOG *or* SYNALAR SOLUTION:

- Each time you apply the medicine, wash your hands with water unless otherwise directed by your doctor. Do not allow the skin to dry completely. Pat with a clean towel until slightly damp.
- Apply a small amount of the drug, drop by drop, to the affected area and spread lightly. Do not bandage unless otherwise directed by your doctor.
- In hairy areas, the hair should be parted before applying in order to get the medicine on the affected skin area.

For KENALOG SPRAY:

- *See* aerosol sprays in section How to Administer Medications

(page 15), except hold the container 7 to 15 cm away from the skin.
- To cover an area about the size of a hand, spray the area for only about 2 seconds.

For DRENISON TAPE:
- Each time you apply the tape, wash your hands and gently cleanse the skin area well with mild soap and water unless otherwise directed by your doctor. Allow the skin to dry 1 hour. The skin should be *clean and completely dry* before the tape is applied. If showers or tub baths are to be taken, they should be completed before applying the tape.
- In hairy areas, shave or clip the hair to allow good contact with the skin and easy removal of the tape.
- Remove the tape from the package and cut a piece slightly larger than the area to be covered. Round off the corners.
- The tape should always be cut— never tear it.
- Remove the paper liner from the back of the transparent tape. Be careful that the tape does not bend and stick to itself.
- Apply the tape and press it into place so that the surface is smooth.
- Unless otherwise directed by your doctor, replace the tape every 12 hours. Cleanse the skin and allow it to dry 1 hour before applying a new tape. If the tape loosens before the 12 hour period, cut and replace it.
- If an irritation or infection develops, remove the tape and call your doctor.

Did You Know That?

You should always keep your medicines in the containers in which they were dispensed by the pharmacist.

Do not remove the label until all the medication is taken.

The information on the label is necessary to properly identify the patient, the physician, the drug, the instructions for use and the date the prescription was dispensed.

This information is important when you need a refill of the prescription or in the event of an emergency.

Special Instructions

Length of Therapy

Do not use the drug more frequently or in larger quantities than prescribed by your doctor. Overuse of this medicine may cause you to absorb too much of the drug and increase the risk of side effects.

If the problem does not clear up within 10 to 14 days or if it reappears soon after treatment, see your doctor.

Pregnancy/Breastfeeding

Women who are pregnant, breastfeeding or planning to become pregnant should tell their doctor before using this medicine.

Drug Interactions

Do not apply cosmetics or lotions on top of the drug unless your doctor approves.

Do not use nonprescription creams or ointments (including those containing hydrocortisone) while using this medicine without first consulting with your doctor.

Special Precautions

Do not use this medicine for any other skin conditions that arise or on any other parts of your body without consulting your doctor or pharmacist.

This medicine is for external use only. Do not swallow it.

Some of the medicines may cause a temporary stinging sensation after they are applied. This will usually disappear within a few minutes.

Do not bandage the treated area unless your doctor has told you to do so. Do not apply this medicine to open wounds.

Keep the medicine away from the eyes, nose and mouth because it could cause serious side effects (e.g. cataracts or glaucoma).

When to Call Your Doctor

Call your doctor if the condition for which this drug is being used continues or becomes worse or if you have a constant irritation such as itching or burning that was not present before you started using this medicine or signs of a skin infection. Also call your doctor if you are using the medicine on the face, under the arms or between the legs and if you develop abnormal red-purple lines, easy bruising or thinning of the skin in these areas, increased facial hair or loss of scalp hair.

Storage

For KENLOG SPRAY: *see* How to Use Aerosol Sprays in How to Administer Medications (page 15).

Miscellaneous

Tell any other doctors you are seeing that you are using this medicine.

Did You Know That?

Taking prescription drugs at the correct times is like staying on a diet. You must motivate yourself and decide that you want to take the medications as they were prescribed.

AMILORIDE (ORAL)

MIDAMOR

AMILORIDE-HYDROCHLOROTHIAZIDE

MODURET

Purpose

This medicine is used to help the body get rid of excess fluids and to decrease swelling. The medicine does this by increasing the amount of urine and is commonly called a "water pill" or "fluid pill." It is used to treat high blood pressure and other medical conditions.

Allergies/Warnings

Be sure to tell your doctor or pharmacist if you are allergic to any medicine.

How to Use This Medicine

Time of Administration

Try to take this medicine at the same time(s) every day so that you have a constant level of the medicine in your body.

When you first start taking this medicine, you will probably urinate (pass your water) more often and in larger amounts than usual. Therefore, if you are to take 1 dose each day, take it in the morning after breakfast. Do not initially take a dose at bedtime or you may have to get up during the night to go to the bathroom.

If you are to take more than 1 dose each day, take the last dose approximately 6 hours before bedtime so that you will not have to get up during the night to go to the bathroom. This effect will usually lessen after you have taken the drug for a while.

How to Administer

Take this medicine with food, meals or milk.

Special Instructions

Length of Therapy

For patients with high blood pressure:

- High blood pressure (hypertension) is a long-term condition and it will probably be necessary for you to take the drug for a long time even if you feel better. If high blood pressure is not treated, it can lead to serious problems such as heart failure, strokes, blood vessel problems or kidney problems.

It is very important that you take this medicine as your doctor has directed and that you do not miss any doses. Otherwise, you cannot expect the drug to keep your blood pressure down or remove excess fluid.

Pregnancy/Breastfeeding

Women who are pregnant, breastfeeding or planning to become pregnant should tell their doctor before taking this medicine.

Drug Interactions

Some nonprescription drugs can aggravate high blood pressure. Do not take any of the following without the approval of your doctor or pharmacist: cough, cold or sinus products; asthma or allergy products since they may increase your blood pressure.

Read the label of the nonprescription drug product to see if there is a warning. If there is, check with your doctor or pharmacist before using the product.

Alcohol

Be careful drinking alcoholic beverages while taking this medicine because it could make the possible side effect of dizziness worse.

Special Precautions

If this medicine causes dizziness or lightheadedness, you should be careful going up or down stairs and you should not change positions too rapidly. Lightheadedness is more likely to occur if you stand up suddenly—this is due to blood collecting in the legs and lasts for a few seconds. Therefore, get up from a sitting or lying position more slowly and tighten and relax your leg muscles or wiggle your toes to help promote circulation. In the morning, get out of bed slowly and dangle your feet over the edge of the bed for a few minutes before standing up. Sit or lie down at the first sign of dizziness. Do not drive a car, pilot an airplane, operate dangerous machinery or do jobs that require you to be alert if you are dizzy. Tell your doctor if you have been dizzy.

In order to help prevent dizziness or fainting, your doctor may also recommend that you avoid strenuous exercise, standing for long periods of time (especially in hot weather), hot showers, hot baths or saunas.

People more than 65 years of age may be more sensitive to the side effect of dizziness.

This medicine may make some people more sensitive to sunlight and various tanning lamps. When you begin taking this medicine, try to avoid too much sun until you see how you are going to react. If your skin does become more sensitive to sunlight, tell your doctor and try not to stay in direct sunlight for extended periods of time. While in the sun, wear protective clothing and sunglasses. You may wish to ask your pharmacist about suitable sunscreen products. Call your doctor if you become sunburned.

This medicine does not cause your body to lose potassium as some other types of water pills do. Therefore, it is not usually necessary for you to eat foods rich in potassium. In fact, too much potassium while you are taking this medicine could be harmful. Call your doctor if you develop any of the warning signs of too much potassium: irregular heartbeats; numbness or tingling in the hands, feet or lips; confusion; difficulty breathing; unusual tiredness or weakness; unexplained nervousness; weakness or a feeling of heaviness in the legs. Since not all patients develop these symptoms, your doctor may want to check your blood occasionally to see if the potassium level is normal.

Do not use salt substitutes, low-salt milk or low-salt soups without the approval of your doctor. They may contain large amounts of potassium, which could affect the way you respond to this medicine.

If you are a diabetic and were prescribed MODURET:

- This medicine may cause your blood sugar to rise. Carefully test your blood or urine for sugar while you are taking this medicine. Call your doctor if you think your blood sugar is higher than normal or harder to control.

When to Call Your Doctor

Most people experience few or no side effects from this drug. However, any medicine can sometimes cause unwanted effects. Call your doctor if you develop nausea, vomiting, a skin rash, headaches, diarrhea, weakness, tiredness, muscle cramps, numbness or tingling of the hands, feet or lips, a yellow color to the skin or eyes or dark yellow-colored urine.

Also call your doctor if you become sick or develop persistent vomiting or diarrhea.

If you were prescribed MODURET:

- Also call your doctor if you develop sharp joint pain or unusual bruising or bleeding.

DID YOU KNOW THAT?

You should tell your doctor if you did not have a prescription filled or if you did not take your medicine exactly as prescribed.

Otherwise, your doctor will think that the medicine was not effective and prescribe another medicine that is used to treat the same condition but could have more side effects or be less effective.

Allergic Reactions

Call your doctor immediately if you think you may be allergic to the medicine or if you develop a skin rash, hives, itching, swelling of the face or difficulty in breathing. If you cannot reach your doctor, phone a hospital emergency department.

Refills

Do not stop taking this medicine without your doctor's approval and do not go without medicine between prescription refills. Call your pharmacist for a refill 2 or 3 days before you will run out of the medicine.

AMITRIPTYLINE HCl (ORAL)
APO-AMITRIPTYLINE, ELAVIL, LEVATE, NOVOTRIPTYN

AMOXAPINE
ASENDIN

CLOMIPRAMINE
ANAFRANIL

DESIPRAMINE
NORPRAMIN, PERTOFRANE

DOXEPIN
SINEQUAN, TRIADAPIN

IMIPRAMINE
APO-IMIPRAMINE, IMPRIL, NOVOPRAMINE, TOFRANIL

MAPROTILINE
LUDIOMIL

NORTRIPTYLINE
AVENTYL

PROTRIPTYLINE
TRIPTIL

TRAZODONE
DESYREL

TRIMIPRAMINE
APO-TRIMIP, SURMONTIL

Purpose

This medicine is used to help relieve the symptoms of depression and may be used to treat other nervous conditions.

IMIPRAMINE and AMITRIPTYLINE are also used to treat bed-wetting in children.

Allergies/Warnings

If you have ever had an allergic reaction to any medicine or if you have high blood pressure, seizures, heart problems, enlarged prostate, difficulty urinating (passing your water), Parkinson's disease, thyroid problems or glaucoma, tell your doctor and pharmacist before you take any of this medicine.

How to Use This Medicine

How to Administer

If you develop stomach upset while taking this medicine, take it with food or immediately after a snack, unless otherwise directed.

For ELAVIL SYRUP:

- Shake the bottle well each time before pouring so that you will measure an accurate dose.
- If a spoon is used to measure the dose, it is recommended that you use a medicine spoon or an oral liquid syringe that you can obtain from

your pharmacist. *See* How to Administer Medications (page 15).

Special Instructions

Length of Therapy

It is important that you take the medicine regularly and that you do not miss any doses. The full effect of the medicine may not be noticed immediately, but usually takes 10 days or up to several weeks. Early signs of improvement are increased appetite, better sleep, increased energy and improved mood. *Do not stop taking* the medicine when you first feel better or you may feel worse in 3 or 4 days.

Since the medicine does not have an immediate effect on your mood, do not attempt to adjust the dose according to your moods but continue to take the dose prescribed for you. Do NOT take an extra dose if you are having a bad day.

Do not stop taking this medicine suddenly without the approval of your doctor. It will be necessary for your doctor to reduce your dose slowly since your body will need time to adjust. It could make your condition worse if you suddenly stopped taking the medicine. After you have stopped taking this medicine, you must continue to observe the following precautions (*see* Alcohol below) for 1 to 2 weeks since some of the medicine will still be in your body.

If you take this medicine only at bedtime and miss a dose, do not take the missed dose the next morning until you check with your doctor. Depending on your dose, the drug may cause some unwanted effects during the day if you took the whole dose the next morning.

Pregnancy/Breastfeeding

Women who are pregnant, breastfeeding or planning to become pregnant should not use this medicine without their doctor's approval.

Drug Interactions

It is important that you obtain the advice of your doctor or pharmacist before taking any prescription or nonprescription medicines, including pain relievers, sleeping pills, tranquilizers or other medicines for depression, cough, cold or allergy medicines.

There are other drug interactions that can occur. If you are taking any other medicines, be sure to check first with your pharmacist or doctor.

Alcohol

Do not drink alcoholic beverages while taking this drug without the approval of your doctor. The combination could irritate your stomach and could cause drowsiness or dizziness. One drink may have the same effect that 2 or 3 drinks normally would have.

If you have been taking this medicine regularly for several days or weeks, it is recommended not to drink alcohol for 2 weeks *after* you have stopped taking the medicine. Depending on your dose, it may take this long for the drug to be eliminated from your body.

Special Precautions

Any medicine has a few unwanted side effects. Many of these side effects are annoying but you should try to keep taking the medicine unless your doctor tells you to stop it. Because this medicine takes a few weeks to work, the side effects show the doctor that the drug is starting to work. Most of these side effects will go away as your body adjusts to the medicine but some may not.

If this medicine causes dizziness or lightheadedness, you should be careful going up and down stairs and you should not change positions too rapidly. Lightheadedness is more likely to occur if you stand up suddenly—this is due to blood collecting in the legs and lasts for a few seconds. Therefore, get up from a sitting or lying position more slowly and tighten and relax your leg muscles or wiggle your toes to help promote circulation. In the morning, get out of bed slowly and dangle your feet over the edge of the bed for a few minutes before standing up. Sit or lie down at the first sign of dizziness. Tell your doctor if you have been dizzy. In order to help prevent dizziness or fainting, your doctor may also recommend that you avoid strenuous exercise, standing for long periods of time (especially in hot weather), hot showers, hot baths, saunas, or Jacuzzis.

Make sure you know how you are going to react to this medicine and whether it will make you dizzy or drowsy. Do not drive a car, pilot an airplane, operate dangerous machinery or do jobs that require you to be alert if you are dizzy or drowsy. The drowsiness may decrease over time.

An urge to urinate (pass your water) with an inability to do so sometimes occurs with this drug. Urinating before taking the drug each time may help relieve this problem. Tell your doctor if you are having this problem.

If your mouth becomes dry, drink water, suck ice chips or a hard, sour candy (sugarless) or chew gum (sugarless). Sugarless products are recommended in order to avoid dental problems. You may wish to ask your pharmacist about special solutions, called artificial saliva, that can also be used to help restore moisture in the mouth. Call your doctor if your mouth becomes extremely dry.

It is especially important to brush and floss your teeth regularly if you develop a dry mouth to help prevent gum problems.

This medicine may cause some people to become constipated. To help prevent constipation, try increasing the amount of bulk in your diet (for example, bran, fresh fruits and salads), exercising more often or drinking more fluids (unless otherwise directed). Call your doctor if the constipation continues.

This medicine (except TRAZODONE) may make some people more sensitive to sunlight and sunlamps. When you begin taking this medicine, try to avoid too much sun until you see how you are going to react. If your skin does become more sensitive to sunlight, tell your doctor and try to stay out of direct sunlight for extended periods of time. While in the sun, wear protective clothing and sunglasses. You may wish to ask your pharmacist about suitable sunscreen products. Call your doctor if you become sunburned.

There have been some reports that smoking may decrease the effect of this drug.

This medicine may cause nasal congestion (stuffy nose). Do not try to treat this yourself with cold or allergy medicines. Check with your doctor.

When to Call Your Doctor

Any medicine can cause unwanted side effects. Call your doctor if you develop a sore throat, fever, mouth sores, eye pain or blurred vision, difficulty in urinating (passing your water), dizziness or drowsiness, difficulty speaking, unexplained nervousness, unusually high energy or irritability, a yellow color in the skin or eyes, fast heartbeats, difficulty breathing, a skin rash, nausea or vomiting, confusion, fainting spells, seizures or shakiness, or convulsions.

For patients prescribed AMOXAPINE:

- Also call your doctor if you develop tremors, drooling, unusual muscle stiffness, shuffling walk, inability to sit still or sleep, unexplained fever, shakiness or unusual movements of the face, tongue or hands, stiffness of the face or body, irregular menstrual periods (in women), pain or discharge from the breasts, numbness or tingling of the hands or feet.

For patients prescribed TRAZODONE:

- Call your doctor if you develop a skin rash, confusion, chest pain, nausea and vomiting, shortness of breath, blood in the urine, dizziness, fainting, trembling or severe drowsiness, changes in sexual ability, fast or slow heartbeats or confusion.

For men:

- Stop taking the drug and call your doctor *immediately* if you develop a painful, long-lasting erection. Immediate treatment is necessary to help avoid serious problems.

What if My Drug Causes a Dry Mouth?

Some helpful hints to help prevent dental problems if you have a dry mouth are:

- Suck bitter or lemon-flavored sugarless candies. This will help to stimulate the flow of saliva.
- Avoid gums and candies that contain sugar because they can promote dental cavities.
- Brush your teeth after each meal and floss your teeth daily to remove the plaque on your teeth. Remember the plaque can build up more quickly if you have a dry mouth and plaque is responsible for many gum problems.
- Small sips of water and ice chips will help to moisturize a dry mouth.
- Bland mouth rinses such as salt and sodium bicarbonate may soothe, lubricate and moisturize dry, irritated mouths.
- Spraying the mouth with warm water from a small atomizer can be very soothing.
- Ask your doctor or dentist about the use of lubricating products that can be purchased in a pharmacy. Though they lack the infection-fighting substances and digestive enzymes of natural saliva, they do help to lubricate the mouth.

Refills

Do not stop taking this medicine without your doctor's approval and do not go without medicine between prescription refills. Call your pharmacist for a refill 2 or 3 days before you will run out of the medicine.

Discuss with your pharmacist the implications of dispensing all your refills for this medicine with the same manufacturer's product. (*See* Generic Drugs, page 12.)

Miscellaneous

Carry an identification card in your wallet or wear a medical alert bracelet indicating that you are taking this medicine as well as the names and phone numbers of your doctors. If you do not already carry such a card, complete the Medicine Card in this book. Always tell your dentist, pharmacist and other doctors who are treating you that you are taking this medicine.

AMITRIPTYLINE-PERPHENAZINE (ORAL)

ELAVIL PLUS, ETRAFON 2-10, ETRAFON-A, ETRAFON-D, ETRAFON-F, PMS LEVAZINE, PROAVIL, TRIAMED, TRIAVIL

Purpose

This medicine is used to help relieve the symptoms of anxiety and depression and certain other types of emotional conditions.

Allergies/Warnings

If you have ever had an allergic reaction to any medicine or if you have high blood pressure, seizures, heart problems, enlarged prostate, difficulty urinating (passing your water), Parkinson's disease, thyroid problems, glaucoma or any other medical condition, tell your doctor and pharmacist before you take any of this medicine.

How to Use This Medicine

How to Administer

If you develop stomach upset while taking this medicine, take it with food or immediately after a snack, unless otherwise directed.

Special Instructions

Length of Therapy

It is important that you take the medicine regularly and that you do not miss any doses. The full effect of the medicine may not be noticed immediately, but may take from a few days to several weeks. Early signs of improvement are increased appetite, better sleep, increased energy and improved mood. *Do not stop taking the medicine* when you first feel better or you may feel worse in 3 or 4 days.

Since the medicine does not have an immediate effect on your mood, do not attempt to adjust the dose according to your moods but continue to take the dose prescribed for you. Do NOT take an extra dose if you are having a bad day.

Do not stop taking this medicine suddenly without the approval of your doctor. It will be necessary for your doctor to reduce your dose slowly since your body will need time to adjust. It could make your condition worse if you suddenly stopped taking the medicine. After you have stopped taking this medicine, you must continue to observe the following precautions for 1 to 2 weeks since some of the medicine will still be in your body.

Pregnancy/Breastfeeding

Women who are pregnant, breastfeeding or planning to become pregnant should not use this medicine without their doctor's approval.

Drug Interactions

It is best not to take this medicine at the same time as an antacid or an anti-diarrhea medicine containing aluminum. Try to space them 2 hours apart if you must take them while you are on this medicine.

It is important that you obtain the advice of your doctor or pharmacist before taking any prescription or nonprescription medicines, including pain relievers, sleeping pills, tranquilizers or medicines for depression, cough, cold or allergy medicines.

There are other drug interactions that can occur. If you are taking any other medicines, be sure to check with your pharmacist or doctor.

Alcohol

Do not drink alcoholic beverages while taking this drug without the approval of your doctor. The combination could irritate your stomach and could cause drowsiness or dizziness. One drink may have the same effect that 2 or 3 drinks normally would have.

If you have been taking this medicine regularly for several days or weeks, it is recommended not to drink alcohol for 2 weeks *after* you have stopped taking the medicine. Depending on your dose, it may take this long for the drug to be eliminated from your body.

Special Precautions

Any medicine has a few unwanted side effects. Many of these side effects are annoying but you should try to keep taking the medicine unless your doctor tells you to stop it. Because this medicine takes a few weeks to work, the side effects show the doctor that the drug is starting to work. Most of these side effects will go away as your body adjusts to the medicine but some may not.

If this medicine causes dizziness or lightheadedness, you should be careful going up and down stairs and you should not change positions too rapidly. Lightheadedness is more likely to occur if you stand up suddenly—this is due to blood collecting in the legs and lasts for a few seconds. Therefore, get up from a sitting or lying position more slowly and tighten and relax your leg muscles or wiggle your toes to help promote circulation. In the morning, get out of bed slowly and dangle your feet over the edge of the bed for a few minutes before standing up. Sit or lie down at the first sign of dizziness. Tell your doctor if you have been dizzy.

You may become more sensitive to heat because your body may perspire less while you are taking this drug. Be careful not to become overheated during exercise or in hot weather. Try to avoid strenuous exercise, standing for long periods of time (especially in hot weather), hot showers, hot baths, saunas or Jacuzzis while taking this medicine.

Some patients may also become more sensitive to cold and should dress warmly during cold weather and limit exposure to cold temperatures.

This medicine commonly causes drowsiness. Do not drive a car, pilot an airplane, operate dangerous machinery or do jobs that require you to be alert if you are dizzy or drowsy.

If your mouth becomes dry, drink water, suck ice chips or a hard, sour candy (sugarless) or chew gum (sugarless). Sugarless products are recommended in order to avoid dental problems. You may wish to ask your pharmacist about special solutions, called artificial saliva, that can also be used to help restore moisture in the mouth.

It is especially important to brush and floss your teeth regularly if you develop a dry mouth to help prevent gum problems.

This medicine may cause some people to become constipated. To help prevent constipation, try increasing the amount of bulk in your diet (for example, bran, fresh fruits and salads), exercising more often or drinking more fluids (unless otherwise directed). Call your doctor if the constipation continues.

This medicine may make some people more sensitive to sunlight and sunlamps. When you begin taking this medicine, try to avoid too much sun until you see how you are going to react. If your skin does become more sensitive to sunlight, tell your doctor and try to stay out of direct sunlight for extended periods of time. While in the sun, wear protective clothing and sunglasses. You may wish to ask your pharmacist about suitable sunscreen products. Call your doctor if you become sunburned.

There have been some reports that this medicine may cause the urine to turn pink or red. This is only temporary and will go away after you have finished taking the medicine.

This medicine may cause nasal congestion (stuffy nose). Do not try to treat this yourself with cold or allergy medicines. Check with your doctor.

An urge to urinate (pass your water) with an inability to do so sometimes occurs with this drug. Urinating before taking the drug each time may help relieve this problem. Tell your doctor you are having this problem.

When to Call Your Doctor

Stop taking the medicine and call your doctor if you become restless or unable to sit still or sleep or if you develop unusually high energy or irritability.

Also call your doctor immediately if you develop a sore throat, fever, mouth sores, eye pain or blurred vision, difficulty in urinating (passing your water), difficulty in breathing, speaking or swallowing, increased sweating, a yellow color in the skin or eyes, dark, yellow-colored urine, irregular heartbeats, a skin rash, unusual bruising or bleeding, nausea or vomiting, unusual tiredness, confusion, nightmares, fainting spells, unusual muscle stiffness, and drooling, seizures or shakiness or unusual movements of the face, tongue or hands.

If you develop painful muscle spasms, call your doctor or go to the hospital emergency room since treatment can be given to provide rapid relief of this problem.

Refills

Do not stop taking this medicine without your doctor's approval and do not go without medicine between prescription refills. Call your pharmacist for a refill 2 or 3 days before you will run out of the medicine.

Discuss with your pharmacist the implications of dispensing all your refills for this medicine with the same manufacturer's product. (*See* Generic Drugs, page 12.)

Miscellaneous

Carry an identification card in your wallet or wear a medical alert

bracelet indicating that you are taking this medicine as well as the names and phone numbers of your doctors. If you do not already carry such a card, complete the Medicine Card in this book. Always tell your dentist, pharmacist and other doctors who are treating you that you are taking this medicine.

Did You Know That?

Smoking cigarettes can alter the way some people respond to some medications.

Cigarette smoke contains substances that can alter enzymes in the liver to cause some drugs to be less effective. People who smoke more than 20 cigarettes a day tend to experience these drug interactions more often than those who smoke fewer cigarettes per day. Little is known about drug interactions that may occur with pipe or cigar smoking.

Smoking has been shown to interfere with the effects of the following drugs:

- Pain Relievers such as PENTAZOCINE and PROPOXYPHENE
- Oral Contraceptives
- Tricyclic Antidepressants such as AMITRIPTYLINE, DESIPRAMINE, IMIPRAMINE and NORTRIPTYLINE
- Antianxiety Drugs such as CHLORDIAZEPOXIDE and DIAZEPAM
- HEPARIN (a "blood thinner")
- Phenothiazines such as CHLORPROMAZINE
- PROPRANOLOL, especially if used to treat angina
- THEOPHYLLINE

If you smoke cigarettes, be sure to tell your doctor and pharmacist so that they can watch for any signs that smoking is adversely affecting your response to the medications.

The Canadian Pharmaceutical Association was the first pharmacy association to join Health and Welfare Canada in the fight for a "Generation of Non-Smokers." Over the past two years, almost

3,500 pharmacists have participated in the program and have information available to help people stop smoking.

Because of the success of this program and the dangers of smoking, the Canadian Pharmaceutical Association has started a new program called "Pharmacists Against Cigarette and Tobacco Sales." Many Canadian pharmacists are refusing to sell cigarette and tobacco products because they feel it is time to take an even harder line against the leading cause of preventable death in the developed world.

AMOBARBITAL (ORAL AND RECTAL)

AMYTAL

AMOBARBITAL-SECOBARBITAL

TUINAL

BUTABARBITAL

BUTISOL SODIUM, DAY-BARB

PENTOBARBITAL

NEMBUTAL, NOVA-RECTAL

PHENOBARBITAL

GARDENAL

SECOBARBITAL

SECONAL SODIUM

Purpose

This medicine is used in the treatment of some sleep disorders and some nervous problems.

PHENOBARBITAL is also used in the long-term treatment of certain types of seizures.

Allergies/Warnings

If you have ever had an allergic reaction to any medicine or have liver or lung problems, tell your doctor and pharmacist before you take any of this medicine.

How to Use This Medicine

Time of Administration

If you are taking this medicine to help you sleep:

- Take the medicine about 20 minutes before you want to fall asleep. Go

to bed after you have taken the medicine.
- If you do not fall asleep after taking the prescribed amount, do *not* take another dose unless advised by your physician.
- Do not smoke in bed after you have taken this medicine because you could fall asleep and cause a fire.

If you are taking this medicine to treat seizures or nervous problems:
- Take the medicine at the times prescribed by your doctor.

How to Administer
For tablets and capsules:
- This medicine may be taken either with food or on an empty stomach.

For liquid medicines:
- If a spoon is used to measure the dose, it is recommended that you use a medicine spoon or an oral liquid syringe that you can obtain from your pharmacist. *See* How to Administer Medications (page 15).

For suppositories: *see* How to Administer Medications (page 15).

Special Instructions

Length of Therapy
Sleeping medicines are only useful for a short time. If too much is used, they could become habit forming. Do not take any more of this medicine than your doctor has prescribed.

Do not stop taking this medicine suddenly without the approval of your doctor. It may be necessary for your doctor to slowly reduce your dose since your body may need time to adjust.

If you are taking PHENOBARBITAL to control seizures, suddenly stopping the medicine could cause seizures.

Check with your doctor if you develop any of the following while you are slowly stopping the medicine: nausea or vomiting, feeling faint, trembling, seizures, changes in vision or trouble sleeping. You may have a sleep problem on the first night or two after stopping the drug. This is not a reason for restarting the drug.

Pregnancy/Breastfeeding
Women who are pregnant, breastfeeding or planning to become pregnant should not take this medicine without their doctor's permission.

Drug Interactions
It is important that you obtain the advice of your doctor or pharmacist before taking any other prescription or nonprescription medicines,

including pain relievers, anticoagulants (blood thinners), drugs used to treat epilepsy, sleeping pills, other tranquilizers or medicines for depression, cough, cold or allergy medicines.

If you have problems sleeping, you should avoid caffeinated beverages, certain cold decongestants and strenuous exercise in the evenings as they make it more difficult to fall asleep. There are other drug interactions that can occur. If you are taking any other medicines, be sure to check with your pharmacist or doctor.

There have been some reports that oral contraceptives (birth control pills) may not work as well while taking this medicine. Unplanned pregnancies may occur. Ask your doctor about using another form of birth control or adjusting the dose of your birth control pill while you are taking this medicine. Also call your doctor if you develop spotting or breakthrough bleeding since these can be signs of decreased birth control effect.

Do You Know the Warning Signs of Drug Dependence?

Call your doctor immediately if you suspect you are becoming dependent on a medication. The warning signs are:

- You need a larger dose to produce the desired effect.
- You start taking the medication automatically without considering whether it is needed.

Drug dependence most commonly occurs with pain relievers, sleeping pills, tranquilizers and diet pills.

Alcohol

Do not drink alcoholic beverages while taking this drug or for a few days after you have stopped taking the drug without the approval of your doctor. The combination could cause drowsiness. One drink (even during the day) may have the same effect that 2 or 3 drinks normally would have.

If you are taking PHENOBARBITAL on a long-term basis to control epilepsy, check with your doctor to see what amount of alcohol (if any) you can drink safely. Be careful because the combination can cause severe drowsiness and increase the frequency of seizures.

Special Precautions

If this medicine causes dizziness or drowsiness the day after you take it, do not drive a car, pilot an airplane, use a sewing machine, operate dangerous machinery or do jobs that require you to be alert if you are dizzy or drowsy. You should also be careful going up and down stairs. Sit or lie down at the first sign of dizziness.

If this hangover drowsiness becomes bothersome, call your doctor.

When to Call Your Doctor

Call your doctor if you do not feel that the drug is working. Do not increase your dose without your doctor's approval.

Most people experience few or no side effects from this drug. However, any medicine can sometimes cause unwanted effects. Call your doctor if you develop a sore throat, fever, mouth sores, a staggering walk, a yellow color to the skin or eyes, unusual bruising or bleeding, muscle or joint pain, slow heartbeats or shortness of breath, bothersome sleepiness or tiredness during the day, unusual nervousness, confusion or depression, hallucinations, trouble sleeping, nightmares or slurred speech.

Caffeine and Insomnia

Does the caffeine in coffee, tea and cola beverages cause you to stay awake at night? If so, you should be aware that caffeine is contained in more than 100 nonprescription drugs and more than 65 commonly prescribed drugs. A cup of drip coffee contains approximately 146 mg caffeine. Some nonprescription drugs contain up to 200 mg per tablet or capsule. Always read the label of the nonprescription products before you purchase them.

If you are sensitive to caffeine, tell your doctor and pharmacist so that they can make sure you are not prescribed a medicine that contains caffeine.

Anyone who suffers from insomnia due to caffeine should not take any beverage or medicine containing caffeine within 6 hours of bedtime.

Allergic Reactions

Call your doctor immediately if you think you may be allergic to the medicine or if you develop a skin rash, hives, itching, swelling of the face

or difficulty in breathing. If you cannot reach your doctor, phone a hospital emergency department.

Storage

Do not store this medicine by the bedside. Keep it out of the reach of children.

For suppositories see How to Administer Medications (page 15).

AMOXICILLIN TRIHYDRATE (ORAL)

AMOXIL, APO-AMOXI, NOVAMOXIN

AMOXICILLIN-POTASSIUM CLAVULANATE

CLAVULIN

Purpose

This medicine is an antibiotic used to treat certain types of infections.

Your doctor has prescribed this antibiotic for your present infection only. Do not use it for other infections or give it to other people.

Allergies/Warnings

If you have ever had an allergic reaction to penicillin, a cephalosporin, or any other medicine or if you have any allergies (for example, asthma or hay fever), tell your doctor and pharmacist before you take any of this medicine.

How to Use This Medicine

Time of Administration

This medicine may be taken with meals or on an empty stomach.

It has been suggested that when CLAVULIN is taken with food, nausea occurs less often.

Space your doses of the medicine around the clock (throughout the entire day of 24 hours). For example, if you are to take 3 doses each day, space the doses 8 hours apart. This will keep a constant level of the medicine in your body.

How to Administer

For tablets or capsules:

- If you were prescribed AMOXIL CHEWABLE TABLETS, chew or crush the tablets well before swallowing. Do not swallow them whole. *After* you have chewed and swallowed the small pieces of the tablet, you

may wish to drink some water.
- Take the other brands of tablets or capsules with a full glass of water (8 ounces) unless otherwise directed. Swallow them whole.

For liquid medicines:
- If you were prescribed a SUSPENSION, shake the bottle well each time before pouring so that you can measure an accurate dose.
- If a dropper is used to measure the dose and you do not fully understand how to use it, *see* How to Administer Medications (page 15).
- If a spoon is used to measure the dose, it is recommended that you use a medicine spoon or an oral liquid syringe that you can obtain from your pharmacist. For instructions on their use *see* How to Administer Medications (page 15).

Special Instructions

Length of Therapy

It is important to take all of this medicine plus any refills that your doctor told you to take. Do not stop taking this medicine earlier than your doctor has recommended even if you begin to feel better. If you stop taking the medicine too soon, the infection may return.

This is especially important if you are taking the medicine to cure a strep infection because if the infection is not completely cleared up, serious heart problems could develop later. After treatment for a strep infection, your doctor may want to do a test to make sure that the infection is gone.

Pregnancy/Breastfeeding

Women who are pregnant or planning to become pregnant should tell their doctor before taking this medicine.

Women who are breastfeeding should tell their doctor before taking this medicine. This medicine can pass into the breast milk and may cause unwanted side effects in the baby.

Drug Interactions

There have been some reports that oral contraceptives (birth control pills) may not work as well while taking this medicine. Unplanned pregnancies may occur. Ask your doctor about using another form of birth control while you are taking this medicine. Also call your doctor if you develop spotting or breakthrough bleeding since these can be signs of decreased birth control effect.

Special Precautions

If you develop diarrhea, do not treat it yourself without first checking with your doctor or pharmacist.

When to Call Your Doctor

Call your doctor if your symptoms do not improve within a few days or if they become worse.

Most people experience few or no side effects from this drug. However, any medicine can sometimes cause unwanted effects. Call your doctor if you develop fever, chills, severe watery diarrhea, yellow-green stools, nausea or vomiting, abdominal or stomach cramps, bloating, unusual thirst, unusual weakness or unusual weight loss. These effects are rare and may occur even after the medicine has been stopped. Also call your doctor if you develop rectal itching or, in women, vaginal itching or a vaginal discharge that was not present before you started taking the medicine.

Did You Know That?

Bacterial infections can be transmitted to people by their pets.

If a family has repeated episodes of *streptococcal pharyngitis* and if they have a pet, they should have a veterinarian test the pet for *streptococcal* infection. According to the *American Family Physician*, it is possible that the animal has a "strep" infection and is reinfecting the family members.

Animals often develop infections in skin lesions after prolonged scratching. A child with atopic eczema can also develp a *staphylococcal* or *streptococcal* infection from a pet with an infected eczemoid condition.

If the pet does have a *streptococcal* infection, it should be treated with an antibiotic such as penicillin.

Allergic Reactions

Call your doctor immediately if you think you may be allergic to the medicine or if you develop a skin rash, hives, itching, swelling of the face or difficulty in breathing. If you cannot reach your doctor, phone a hospital emergency department.

Storage

For liquid medicines:

- Store the bottle of medicine in a refrigerator unless otherwise directed. Do not freeze.

If for some reason you cannot take all of the medicine, discard the unused portion by flushing it down the toilet. Throw away any unused medicine after the discard (expiration) date on the bottle. Do not take or save old medicine.

Refills

Do not go without medicine between prescription refills. Call your pharmacist for a refill 2 or 3 days before you will run out of the medicine.

AMPICILLIN (ORAL)
APO-AMPI, NOVO-AMPICILLIN, PENBRITIN

BACAMPICILLIN
PENGLOBE

CLOXACILLIN
APO-CLOXI, NOVOCLOXIN, ORBENIN

DICLOXACILLIN
DYNAPEN

FLUCLOXACILLIN
FLUCLOX

PIVAMPICILLIN
PONDOCILLIN

Purpose
This medicine is an antibiotic used to treat certain types of infections.

Your doctor has prescribed this antibiotic for your present infection only. Do not use it for other infections or give it to other people.

Allergies/Warnings
If you have ever had an allergic reaction to penicillin, or cephalosporin, or any other medicine or if you have any allergies (for example, asthma or hay fever), tell your doctor and pharmacist before you take any of this medicine.

How to Use This Medicine

Time of Administration

For Apo-Ampi, Apo-Cloxi, Dynapen, Fluclox, Novo-Ampicillin, Novocloxin, Orbenin, Penbritin:

- It is best to take this medicine on an empty stomach 1 hour before (or 2 hours after) meals or food unless otherwise directed by your doctor. Take it at the proper time even if you skip a meal.
- Space your doses of the medicine around the clock (throughout the entire day of 24 hours). For example, if you are to take 4 doses each day, space the doses 6 hours apart. This will keep a constant level of the medicine in your body.

For Penglobe *and* Pondocillin *only:*

- This medicine may be taken without regard to meals. Take with food or on an empty stomach.

How to Administer

For tablets or capsules:

- Take the tablets or capsules with a full glass of water (8 ounces) unless otherwise directed.

For liquid medicines:

- If you were prescribed a *suspension*, shake the bottle well each time before pouring so that you can measure an accurate dose.
- If a spoon is used to measure the dose, it is recommended that you use a medicine spoon or an oral liquid syringe that you can obtain from your pharmacist. *See* How to Administer Medications (page 15).

Special Instructions

Length of Therapy

It is important to take all of this medicine plus any refills that your doctor told you to take. Do not stop taking this medicine earlier than your doctor has recommended even if you begin to feel better.

If you stop taking the medicine too soon, the infection may return. This is especially important if you are taking the medicine to cure a strep infection because if the infection is not completely cleared up, serious heart problems could develop later. After treatment for a strep infection, your doctor may want to do a test to make sure that the infection is gone.

Pregnancy/Breastfeeding

Women who are pregnant or planning to become pregnant should tell their doctor before taking this medicine.

Women who are breastfeeding should tell their doctor before taking this medicine. This medicine can pass into the breast milk and may cause unwanted side effects in the baby.

Drug Interactions

There have been some reports that oral contraceptives (birth control pills) may not work as well while taking this medicine. Unplanned pregnancies may occur. Ask your doctor about using another form of birth control while you are taking these antibiotics. Also call your doctor if you develop spotting or breakthrough bleeding since these can be signs of decreased birth control effect.

When to Call Your Doctor

Call your doctor if your symptoms do not improve within a few days or if they become worse.

This medicine sometimes causes diarrhea. Call your doctor if the diarrhea becomes severe or lasts for more than two days. Do not try to treat the diarrhea yourself without first checking with your doctor or pharmacist.

Most people experience few or no side effects from this drug. However, any medicine can sometimes cause unwanted effects. Call your doctor if you develop fever, chills, nausea or vomiting, yellow-green stools, abdominal or stomach cramps, bloating, unusual thirst, unusual weakness or unusual weight loss. These effects are rare and may occur even after the medicine has been stopped. Also call your doctor if you develop rectal itching or, in women, vaginal itching or a vaginal discharge that was not present before you started taking the medicine.

Allergic Reactions

Call your doctor immediately if you think you may be allergic to the medicine or if you develop a skin rash, hives, itching, swelling of the face or difficulty in breathing. If you cannot reach your doctor, phone a hospital emergency department.

Storage

For APO-AMPI, FLUCLOX, NOVO-AMPICILLIN *and* PENBRITIN liquid medicines:

- Store the bottle of medicine in a refrigerator unless otherwise directed. Do not freeze.

If for some reason you cannot take all of the medicine, discard the unused portion by flushing it down the toilet. Throw away any unused medicine after the discard (expiration) date on the bottle. Do not take or save old medicine.

Refills

Do not go without medicine between prescription refills. Call your pharmacist for a refill 2 or 3 days before you will run out of the medicine.

Does the Medicine Taste Bad?

Some helpful hints to make bad-tasting medicines taste better:

- If the medicine is a liquid, it may help to chill the medicine in the refrigerator for a few minutes before it is taken.
- If the medicine is a tablet, place the tablet closer to the front of the tongue. The taste buds on the tongue that detect bitter tastes are located near the back of the tongue. By placing the tablet near the front of the tongue, you are placing it on the sweet taste buds and there is less perception of the bitter taste.
- Suck some ice chips before taking a bitter medication. This will help numb the taste buds.
- It may help to hold your nose as you swallow the medicine. The sense of smell is involved in the sensation of taste and by decreasing your ability to smell the medicine, it may not taste as bad.
- Ask your pharmacist if it is safe to dilute your liquid medicine with juice or some other liquid. Some medicines interact with some liquids and it is important not to dilute your medicine with one that interacts with your drug.
- Drink some water after taking the medicine to help get rid of the aftertaste—unless you are taking a cough syrup which acts by coating the throat to soothe it.
- It may also help to gargle or rinse your mouth or suck a hard candy after taking the medicine.

ASA-BARBITURATE (ORAL)
PHENAPHEN

ASA-BARBITURATE-CODEINE
PHENAPHEN NO. 2, PHENAPHEN NO. 3, PHENAPHEN NO. 4

ASA-BARBITURATE-CAFFEINE
FIORINAL, TECNAL

ASA-BARBITURATE-CAFFEINE-CODEINE
FIORINAL-C 1/4, FIORINAL-C 1/2, TECNAL C 1/4, TECNAL C 1/2

Purpose
This medicine is used to help relieve pain associated with muscle tension (e.g. tension headache).

Allergies/Warnings
If you have a stomach ulcer, hay fever, asthma, nasal polyps or have ever had an allergic reaction to ASA (acetylsalicylic acid), codeine, caffeine, a barbiturate or any other medicine, tell your doctor and pharmacist before you take any of this medicine.

Check with your doctor before giving any medicine containing ASA or salicylates to children, teenagers and young adults with chicken pox, flu or other viral infections. Studies have shown a possible link between ASA/salicylate products and Reye's Syndrome, a rare but serious disease. The first symptoms of Reye's Syndrome are usually vomiting, tiredness, and loss of concentration that may lead to delirium and coma.

How to Use This Medicine

Time of Administration

Do not wait until the pain becomes severe. This medicine works best if you take it at the beginning of the pain.

How to Administer

This medicine should be taken with food or a full glass of water to help prevent stomach upset.

Do not take this medicine if it smells strongly like vinegar since this may mean the ASA is not fresh and may be losing strength.

Special Instructions

Length of Therapy

If your doctor has prescribed this medicine to be taken on a regular schedule, take it as recommended and not on an "as needed" basis.

Do not take any more of this medicine than your doctor has prescribed. When used for a long period of time, the drug can become less effective. These products contain codeine and/or a barbiturate and when used in large doses for a long period of time, these drugs can become habit forming. Call your doctor if you feel you need the medicine more often than was prescribed. Do not take a larger dose without your doctor's approval.

If you have been taking this medicine in large doses or for several weeks, do not stop taking this medicine suddenly without the approval of your doctor. It may be necessary for your doctor to reduce your dose slowly. This will depend on the dose and thc specific medicine you have been taking.

Pregnancy/Breastfeeding

Women who are pregnant, breastfeeding or planning to become pregnant should tell their doctor before taking this medicine.

Drug Interactions

It is important that you obtain the advice of your doctor or pharmacist before taking any other prescription or nonprescription medicines, including other pain relievers, sleeping pills, tranquilizers or medicines for depression, cough, cold or allergy medicines or blood thinners.

There are other drug interactions which can occur. If you are taking any other medicines, be sure to check first with your pharmacist or doctor.

Alcohol

Do not drink alcoholic beverages while taking this drug because the combination could cause dizziness or drowsiness. One drink may have the same effect that 2 or 3 drinks normally would have. The combination could also cause stomach problems.

Special Precautions

If you feel nauseated when you first start taking the medicine, it may help if you lie down for a few minutes.

In some people, this drug may cause dizziness or drowsiness. Do not drive a car, pilot an airplane, operate dangerous machinery or do jobs that require you to be alert if you are dizzy or drowsy. You should also be careful going up and down stairs. Get up slowly after you have been sitting or lying down. Sit or lie down at the first sign of dizziness. Tell your doctor if the dizziness or drowsiness continues.

This medicine may cause some people to become constipated. To help prevent constipation, try increasing the amount of bulk in your diet (for example, bran, fresh fruits and salads), exercising more often or drinking more fluids (unless otherwise directed). Call your doctor if the constipation continues.

ASA can thin the blood and prolong the bleeding time; therefore, you may have to stop taking it before surgery or dental work. Check with your doctor or dentist at least one week before you have any surgery or dental work.

When to Call Your Doctor

Call your doctor if the medicine does not relieve your symptoms or if they get worse.

Most people experience few or no side effects from this drug. However, any medicine can sometimes cause unwanted effects. Call your doctor if you develop stomach pain, vomiting, vomiting of blood or material that looks like coffee grounds, bloody or black stools, blood in the urine, ringing or buzzing in the ears or difficulty hearing, a feeling of fullness in the ears, severe drowsiness or dizziness, bothersome sleepiness or laziness during the day, nightmares, staggering walk, a slow heartbeat, unusual nervousness, confusion, unusual bruising or bleeding, a yellow color to the skin or eyes or severe diarrhea.

Allergic Reactions

Call your doctor immediately if you think you may be allergic to the medicine or if you develop a skin rash, hives, itching, unexplained fever, swelling of the face or difficulty in breathing. If you cannot reach your doctor, phone a hospital emergency department.

Storage

Store the medicine in a cool, dark place.

Miscellaneous

Carry an identification card in your wallet or wear a medical alert bracelet indicating that you are taking this medicine as well as the names and phone numbers of your doctors. If you do not already carry such a card, complete the Medicine Card in this book. Always tell your dentist, pharmacist and other doctors who are treating you that you are taking this medicine.

ASA Hypersensitivity

Thousands of people in Canada are hypersensitive to ASA. There are two major types of symptoms that can result. One type consists of shortness of breath or asthma-like symptoms. The other type consists of skin reactions such as edema (swelling), rash or hives. ASA hypersensitivity occurs more commonly (up to 20%) in people who have asthma or chronic urticaria (hives). The incidence of ASA hypersensitivity in the general population is much lower (0.3%).

According to the *Journal of the American Geriatrics Society*, a person who is hypersensitive to ASA may also be hypersensitive to other drugs that have a similar chemical structure. This is called cross-sensitivity. Many ASA-sensitive patients are also allergic to nonsteroidal anti-inflammatory drugs (IBUPROFEN, FENOPROFEN, INDOMETHACIN, KETOPROFEN, MEFENAMIC ACID, NAPROXEN, PIROXICAM, SULINDAC, TOLMETIN).

The ASA-sensitive patient may also react to a number of foods that naturally contain salicylate such as:

Almonds
Apples
Apricots
Blackberries
Cherries
Currants
Gooseberries
Grapes
Nectarines
Oranges
Raisins
Raspberries
Strawberries

ASA-CAFFEINE-CODEINE (ORAL)

AC&C, ANACIN WITH CODEINE, ANCASAL 8, ANCASAL 15, ANCASAL 30, 222, 222 FORTE, 282, 292, 293, C2 WITH CODEINE, C2 BUFFERED WITH CODEINE

ASA-CODEINE

CORYPHEN-CODEINE

ASA-OXYCODONE

ENDODAN, OXYCODAN, PERCODAN, PERCODAN-DEMI

Purpose

This medicine is used to help relieve pain and fever.

Allergies/Warnings

If you have a stomach ulcer, asthma, hay fever, nasal polyps or have ever had an allergic reaction to ASA (acetylsalicylic acid), codeine, caffeine or any other medicine, tell your doctor and pharmacist before you take any of this medicine.

Check with your doctor before giving any medicine containing ASA or salicylates to children, teenagers and young adults with chicken pox, flu or other viral infections. Studies have shown a possible link between ASA/salicylate products and Reye's Syndrome, a rare but serious disease. The first symptoms of Reye's Syndrome are usually vomiting and tiredness that may lead to delirium and coma.

How to Use This Medicine

Time of Administration

Do not wait until the pain becomes severe. This medicine works best if you take it at the beginning of the pain.

How to Administer

This medicine should be taken with food or a full glass of water to help prevent stomach upset.

Do not take this medicine if it smells strongly like vinegar since this may mean the ASA in it is not fresh and may be losing strength.

If you were prescribed 293 TABLETS:

- These tablets are long-acting and must be swallowed whole. Do not crush, chew or break them into pieces.

Special Instructions

Length of Therapy

Do not take any more of this medicine than your doctor has prescribed. When used for a long period of time, the drug can become less effective. These products contain codeine and/or a barbiturate and when used in large doses for a long period of time, the drug can become habit forming. Call your doctor if you feel you need the medicine more often than was prescribed. Do not take a larger dose without your doctor's approval.

If you have been taking this medicine in large doses or for several weeks, do not stop taking this medicine suddenly without the approval of your doctor. It may be necessary for your doctor to reduce your dose slowly. This will depend on the dose and the specific medicine you have been taking.

Pregnancy/Breastfeeding

Women who are pregnant, breastfeeding or planning to become pregnant should tell their doctor before taking this medicine.

Do Not Place ASA Tablets Directly on a Sore Tooth or Gum

ASA tablets should not be sucked or placed directly on a canker sore, sore gum or sensitive tooth and allowed to dissolve.

ASA is an acidic drug, and if left in one spot and allowed to dissolve, there is a good chance that it will irritate the sore area even more. With continued use, the ASA could even cause a severe chemical burn and destroy that area of the skin. When this happens, the skin will turn white and slough off leaving a painful ulceration. When this happens, it is known as *aspirin burn*.

Drug Interactions

It is important that you obtain the advice of your doctor or pharmacist before taking any other prescription and nonprescription medicines, including other pain relievers, sleeping pills, tranquilizers or medicines for depression, or cough, cold or allergy medicines.

There are other drug interactions which can occur. If you are taking any other medicines, be sure to check first with your pharmacist or doctor.

Alcohol

Do not drink alcoholic beverages while taking this drug without the approval of your doctor because the combination could cause dizziness or drowsiness. One drink may have the same effect that 2 or 3 drinks normally would have. The combination could also cause stomach problems.

Special Precautions

If you feel nauseated when you first start taking the medicine, it may help if you lie down for a few minutes.

In some people, this drug may cause dizziness or drowsiness. Do not drive a car, pilot an airplane, operate dangerous machinery or do jobs that require you to be alert if you are dizzy or drowsy. You should also be careful going up and down stairs. Get up slowly after you have been sitting or lying down. Sit or lie down at the first sign of dizziness. Tell your doctor if the dizziness and drowsiness continue.

This medicine may cause some people to become constipated. To help prevent constipation, try increasing the amount of bulk in your diet (for example, bran, fresh fruits and salads), exercising more often or drinking more fluids (unless otherwise directed). Call your doctor if the constipation continues.

ASA can thin the blood and prolong the bleeding time; therefore, you may have to stop taking it before surgery or dental work. Check with your doctor or dentist at least one week before you have any surgery or dental work.

Did You Know That?

ASA and alcohol should not be taken together.

Both ASA and alcohol are capable of irritating the lining of the stomach and, when taken together, there is a chance that the double irritation could cause bleeding. ASA can also thin the blood and prolong the bleeding time. This unwanted effect will not happen in everyone but it is especially important in people who have or have had peptic ulcers.

Whenever possible, avoid ASA use within 8 to 10 hours of heavy alcohol use. Taking ASA the morning after alcoholic overindulgence would seem less likely to cause difficulty than taking ASA before retiring since the gastric irritation caused by the alcohol would have been at least partially relieved by the next morning.

When to Call Your Doctor

Call your doctor if the medicine does not relieve your symptoms or if they get worse.

Most people experience few or no side effects from this drug. However, any medicine can sometimes cause unwanted effects. Call your doctor if you develop stomach pain, vomiting, vomiting of blood or

Did You Know That?

Any medicine that causes blurred vision, drowsiness, dizziness, hearing problems, decreased reflexes, inability to concentrate, or muscle incoordination has the potential to impair your ability to drive a car safely.

In the past few years, increased attention has been focused on the dangers of drinking and driving. Governments have set strict limits on blood alcohol concentrations at which a driver's performance could be considered to be "impaired". Until recently, little attention has been given to the effect of medications on driving. There are some medications that are capable of decreasing a person's mental alertness and physical coordination, thereby damaging or lessening that person's ability to drive a car safely.

The Canadian Pharmaceutical Association with the support of interested consumer groups has undertaken "A Drugs and Driving Program: Take Care". This is a project designed to help make consumers more aware of medicines that can adversely affect driving skills. A booklet, "Drugs and Driving", is available by writing: The Canadian Pharmaceutical Association, 1785 Alta Vista Drive, Ottawa, Ontario K1G 3Y6.

Other sources of information are also available. The Drug Caution Code, a program developed by pharmacists in Manitoba and available in Saskatchewan, Newfoundland, and Alberta, informs consumers on the hazards of over-the-counter medicines and driving. The individual prescription drug monographs in *Understanding Canadian Prescription Drugs* contain information on prescription drugs that may impair a person's ability to drive a car or do tasks that require mental alertness.

The best advice is to ask your doctor or pharmacist about possible side effects that could affect your driving performance whenever you are prescribed a medication. Not everyone will respond the same way to a medication. Until you know how you are going to respond to the medication, your doctor or pharmacist may advise you to refrain from, or minimize, driving for a few days after starting the medication. In this way, you can assess whether it will be safe for you to drive while undergoing the treatment.

material that looks like coffee grounds, bloody or black stools, blood in the urine, ringing or buzzing in the ears or difficulty hearing, a feeling of fullness in the ears, severe drowsiness or dizziness, bothersome sleepiness or laziness during the day, sweating, unusual nervousness, severe constipation, diarrhea, confusion or depression.

Allergic Reactions

Call your doctor immediately if you think you may be allergic to the medicine or if you develop a skin rash, hives, itching, unexplained fever, swelling of the face or difficulty in breathing. If you cannot reach your doctor, phone a hospital emergency department.

Storage

Store the medicine in a cool, dark place.

Miscellaneous

Carry an identification card in your wallet or wear a medical alert bracelet indicating that you are taking this medicine as well as the names and phone numbers of your doctors. If you do not already carry such a card, complete the Medicine Card in this book. Always tell your dentist, pharmacist and other doctors who are treating you that you are taking this medicine.

ATROPINE-SCOPOLAMINE-HYOSCYAMINE-PHENOBARBITAL (ORAL)

DONNATAL

Purpose

This medicine is used to help relieve cramps and spasms of the bowels and as an aid to treating some cases of duodenal ulcers by lowering the stomach acid secretions.

Allergies/Warnings

If you have ever had an allergic reaction to atropine, bromides, barbiturates or any other drug, or if you have glaucoma, enlarged prostate, difficulty urinating (passing your water) or any other medical condition, tell your doctor and pharmacist before you take any of this medicine.

How to Use This Medicine

Time of Administration

Take this medicine approximately 30 minutes to 1 hour before a meal unless otherwise directed.

The DONNATAL EXTENTABS are usually taken in the morning and at night since they are long-acting.

How to Administer

If you were prescribed DONNATAL EXTENTABS:

- These tablets are long-acting and must be swallowed whole. Do not crush, chew or break them into pieces.

For liquid medicines:

- If a spoon is used to measure the dose, it is recommended that you use a medicine spoon or an oral liquid syringe that you can obtain from your pharmacist. These are more accurate than the average household teaspoon. *See* How to Administer Medications (page 15).

Special Instructions

Length of Therapy

Do not take this medicine more often or longer than recommended by your doctor. To do so may increase your chance of developing side effects.

Do not stop taking this medicine suddenly without the approval of your doctor.

Pregnancy/Breastfeeding

Women who are pregnant, breastfeeding or planning to become pregnant should tell their doctor before taking this medicine.

Drug Interactions

It is important that you obtain the advice of your doctor or pharmacist before taking any other prescription or nonprescription medicines, including pain relievers, sleeping pills, tranquilizers or medicines for depression, or cough, cold or allergy medicines.

Do not take antacids or medicines for diarrhea within 1 hour of taking this medicine because they could make this medicine less effective.

There are other drug interactions that can occur. If you are taking any other medicines, be sure to check first with your pharmacist or doctor.

Alcohol

Do not drink alcoholic beverages while taking this drug without the approval of your doctor because the combination could cause severe drowsiness. One drink may have the same effect that 2 or 3 drinks normally would have.

Special Precautions

If your mouth becomes dry, drink water, suck ice chips or a hard, sour candy (sugarless) or chew gum (sugarless). Sugarless products are recommended in order to avoid dental problems. You may wish to ask your pharmacist about special solutions, called artificial saliva, that can also be used to help restore moisture in the mouth.

It is especially important to brush and floss your teeth regularly if you develop a dry mouth to help prevent gum problems.

In some people, this drug may cause dizziness, drowsiness or blurred vision. Do not drive a car, pilot an airplane, operate dangerous machinery or do jobs that require you to be alert until you know how you are going to react to this drug. You should also be careful going up and down stairs. Sit or lie down at the first sign of dizziness. Tell your doctor if these problems continue.

If your eyes become more sensitive to sunlight, it may help to wear sunglasses.

An urge to urinate (pass your water) with an inability to do so sometimes occurs with this drug. Urinating before taking the drug each time may help relieve this problem. Tell your doctor if you are having this problem.

This medicine will often cause you to sweat less and you may become more sensitive to heat. Be careful not to become overheated during exercise or to stand for long periods of time, especially if the weather is hot. Avoid hot showers, hot baths, Jacuzzis or saunas while taking this medicine.

This medicine may cause some people to become constipated. This side effect occurs more often in people over 65 years of age. To help prevent constipation, try increasing the amount of bulk in your diet (for example, bran, fresh fruits and salads), exercising more often or drinking more fluids (unless otherwise directed). Call your doctor if the constipation continues.

When to Call Your Doctor

Most people experience few or no side effects from this drug. However, any medicine can sometimes cause unwanted effects. Call your doctor if you develop a skin rash, difficulty in breathing, diarrhea, unusual restlessness, flushing, eye pain or changes in vision, a sore throat, fever, headache, nausea or vomiting, bothersome constipation, a yellow color to the skin or eyes, easy bruising or bleeding, unusual tiredness, a change in the heart rate, difficulty in urinating (passing your water), confusion or slurred speech.

Allergic Reactions

Call your doctor immediately if you think you may be allergic to the medicine or if you develop a skin rash, hives, itching, swelling of the face or difficulty in breathing. If you cannot reach your doctor, phone a hospital emergency department.

Miscellaneous

Carry an identification card in your wallet or wear a medical alert bracelet indicating that you are taking this medicine as well as the names and phone numbers of your doctors. If you do not already carry such a card, complete the Medicine Card in this book. Always tell your dentist, pharmacist and other doctors who are treating you that you are taking this medicine.

BECLOMETHASONE (INHALATION)

BECLOVENT INHALER, BECLOVENT ROTACAPS, VANCERIL ORAL INHALER

FLUNISOLIDE

BRONALIDE AEROSOL

Purpose

This medicine is a steroid (cortisone) and is used to help prevent asthmatic attacks. It is not effective in treating an asthma attack that has already begun and should not be used during an attack.

Allergies/Warnings

If you have ever had an allergic reaction to any steroid (cortisone) medicines or inhalation spray medicines, tell your doctor and pharmacist before you use any of this medicine.

How to Use This Medicine

How to Administer

BECLOVENT ROTACAPS must *not* be swallowed. The capsules are to be used with the BECLOVENT ROTAHALER.

For aerosol inhaler:

- *See* How to Administer Medications (page 15) for general instructions.
- Follow the specific instructions for your brand of inhaler on the sheet that comes with the medicine.
- The VANCERIL ORAL INHALER has a "dosage reminder" at the top of the

canister to help you remember to take each dose. Each time you take a dose, set the number of your dose opposite the arrow on the plastic shell.

- If your doctor has prescribed a second dose, wait about 1 minute before shaking the container again and repeating this procedure.
- Rinse your mouth and gargle with lukewarm water after you have used the inhaler. This will help prevent your throat from becoming dry or sore, your voice from becoming hoarse, and an infection.

Special Instructions

Length of Therapy

Patients vary in the dose they require, and your doctor will determine the dosage that is best for you. Take the medicine regularly. It may take 1 to 4 weeks before you feel the full benefit of this medicine. If you develop difficulty in breathing, contact your doctor immediately.

Do not take any more of this medicine than your doctor has prescribed and do not stop taking this medicine suddenly without the approval of your doctor. If you should suddenly stop taking it or reduce the dose, you may experience a worsening of your asthma.

Since this drug is used to help prevent asthma attacks, you may need to take it for a prolonged period of time. Discuss the length of therapy with your doctor.

Pregnancy/Breastfeeding

Women who are pregnant, breastfeeding or planning to become pregnant should tell their doctor before taking this medicine.

Drug Interactions

Some nonprescription drugs can aggravate your condition. Do not take any of the following without the approval of your doctor or pharmacist: cough, cold or sinus products; asthma or allergy products; or ASA-containing products. Read the label of the product to see if there is a warning. If there is, check first with your doctor or pharmacist before using the product.

Do not take other inhaled medicines that have not been prescribed by your doctor while you are using this medicine.

Special Precautions

Do not change the dose of your regular asthma or bronchitis medicines except on the advice of your doctor.

If you are also using another inhaler medicine (bronchodilator) that opens up the air passages in the lungs, use it several minutes before using this medicine as directed by your doctor. The bronchodilator will help open up the air passages in the lungs and increase the amount of this steroid medicine that can get into the lungs.

When to Call Your Doctor

Call your doctor if you develop difficulty breathing or coughing when you use the medicine, if your sputum turns yellow or green in color or if you develop an infection of the mouth, throat or lungs, fever, congestion, skin rash, hives, fast heartbeats, or white curdlike patches inside the mouth.

Also call your doctor if you develop a soreness in the mouth or throat, a bad taste in the mouth that will not go away, insomnia, hoarseness, or if your asthma gets worse.

Storage

For inhalers: see How to Administer Medications (page 15).

Refills

To determine the amount of medicine left in the inhaler and when a refill will be needed, *see* How to Administer Medications (page 15).

Miscellaneous

Carry an identification card in your wallet or wear a medical alert bracelet indicating that you are taking this medicine as well as the names and phone numbers of your doctors. If you do not already carry such a card, complete the Medicine Card in this book. Always tell your dentist, pharmacist and doctors treating you that you are taking this medicine.

BECLOMETHASONE (NASAL)

BECONASE, BECONASE AQUEOUS NASAL SPRAY, VANCENASE NASAL INHALER

FLUNISOLIDE

RHINALAR

Purpose

This medicine is used in the treatment of hay fever and to help prevent or relieve the symptoms of nasal stuffiness and runny nose associated with allergic conditions.

Allergies/Warnings

If you have ever had an allergic reaction to any cortisone medicines or inhalation spray medicines, tell your doctor and pharmacist before you take any of this medicine.

How to Use This Medicine

How to Administer

Follow the special instructions for your specific brand on the sheet that comes with the medicine.

It is very important that you use this medicine regularly as your doctor has prescribed. It will not relieve your symptoms immediately. It is not like ordinary nasal decongestants that you take only when you feel it is necessary.

Children should use the nasal medicine under the supervision of an adult who is aware of its proper use.

Special Instructions

Length of Therapy

Do not take any more of this medicine than your doctor has prescribed and do not stop taking this medicine suddenly without the approval of your doctor. If you should suddenly stop taking it or reduce the dose, you may experience a worsening of your symptoms.

If this medicine is going to work in your condition, you should notice an improvement in your symptoms, usually in a few days to two weeks when used regularly.

Pregnancy/Breastfeeding

Women who are pregnant, breastfeeding or planning to become pregnant should tell their doctor before taking this medicine.

When to Call Your Doctor

Call your doctor if you develop an infection of the nose, sinuses, mouth, throat or lungs. It may be necessary to stop this medicine until you have recovered.

Most people experience few or no side effects from this drug. However, any medicine can sometimes cause unwanted effects. Call your doctor if you develop unexplained nosebleeds, blood in the mucus, sore throat, sneezing attacks, headaches, burning or soreness in the nose or if your condition does not improve within 2 or 3 weeks.

Storage

For BECONASE *and* VANCENASE:

- Store the nasal inhaler at room temperature. Do not place it in hot water or near radiators, stoves or other sources of heat. Do not puncture, burn or incinerate the container (even when it is empty).

For BECONASE AQUEOUS NASAL SPRAY:
- Discard 3 months after first using the spray.

Miscellaneous

Carry an identification card in your wallet or wear a medical alert bracelet indicating that you are taking this medicine as well as the names and phone numbers of your doctors. If you do not already carry such a card, complete the Medicine Card in this book. Always tell your dentist, pharmacist and other doctors who are treating you that you are taking this medicine.

BENZTROPINE MESYLATE (ORAL)

APO-BENZTROPINE, BENSYLATE, COGENTIN, PMS BENZTROPINE

Purpose

This medicine is used to improve various symptoms of Parkinson's disease such as tremors, uncontrolled shaking movements, muscle rigidity, or problems in walking.

Allergies/Warnings

If you have ever had an allergic reaction to any medicine or if you have glaucoma, enlarged prostate, difficulty urinating (passing your water), high blood pressure or any other medical condition, tell your doctor and pharmacist before you take any of this medicine.

This medicine should not be used in children less than 3 years of age and with caution in older children.

How to Use This Medicine

Time of Administration

Take this medicine with food or immediately after meals to help prevent stomach upset unless otherwise directed.

Your doctor may prescribe the medicine at bedtime to help prevent drowsiness during the day.

Special Instructions

Length of Therapy

Do not take this medicine more often or longer than recommended by your doctor. To do so may increase your chance of developing side effects.

Do not stop taking this medicine suddenly without the approval of your doctor. It may be necessary for your doctor to reduce your dose slowly since your body may need time to adjust. It could be harmful and make your condition worse if you suddenly did not receive the medicine.

Pregnancy/Breastfeeding

Women who are pregnant, breastfeeding or planning to become pregnant should tell their doctor before taking this medicine.

Drug Interactions

It is important that you obtain the advice of your doctor or pharmacist before taking any other prescription or nonprescription medicines including pain relievers, sleeping pills, tranquilizers, medicine for seizures, muscle relaxants, anesthetics, medicines for depression or medicines for allergies, colds or sinus conditions. Combining this medication with some of these drugs could cause drowsiness or dizziness.

Do not take antacids or diarrhea medicines within 1 hour of taking this medicine as it could make this medicine less effective.

There are other drug interactions that can occur. If you are taking any other medicines, be sure to check first with your pharmacist or doctor.

Alcohol

Do not drink alcoholic beverages while taking this drug without the approval of your doctor because the combination could cause severe drowsiness or dizziness. One drink may have the same effect that 2 or 3 drinks normally would have.

Special Precautions

People over 60 years of age may be more sensitive to some of these side effects.

If your mouth becomes dry, drink water, suck ice chips or a hard, sour candy (sugarless) or chew gum (sugarless). Sugarless products are recommended in order to avoid dental problems. You may wish to ask your pharmacist about special solutions, called artificial saliva, that can also be used to help restore moisture in the mouth.

It is especially important to brush and floss your teeth regularly if you develop a dry mouth to help prevent gum problems.

If your mouth becomes extremely dry and you have difficulty swallowing or speaking or if you lose your appetite, call your doctor. It may be necessary to lower your dose.

In some people, this drug may cause dizziness, drowsiness or blurred vision, particularly during the first 2 weeks of use. This will usually go away as your body adjusts to the medicine. Do not drive a car, pilot an airplane, operate dangerous machinery or do jobs that require you to be alert until you know how you are going to react to the drug.

If this medicine causes dizziness or lightheadedness, you should be careful going up and down stairs and you should not change positions too rapidly. Lightheadedness is more likely to occur if you stand up suddenly—this is due to blood collecting in the legs and lasts for a few seconds. Therefore, get up from a sitting or lying position more slowly and tighten and relax your leg muscles or wiggle your toes to help promote circulation. In the morning, get out of bed slowly and dangle your feet over the edge of the bed for a few minutes before standing up. Sit or lie down at the first sign of dizziness. Tell your doctor if you have been dizzy.

You may become more sensitive to heat because your body may perspire less while you are taking this drug. Be careful not to become overheated during exercise or in hot weather. Try to avoid strenuous exercise, standing for long periods of time (especially in hot weather), hot showers, hot baths, saunas or Jacuzzis while taking this medicine.

This medicine may cause some people to become constipated. To help prevent constipation, try increasing the amount of bulk in your diet (for example, bran, fresh fruits and salads), exercising more often or drinking more fluids (unless otherwise directed). Call your doctor if the constipation continues.

If your eyes become more sensitive to sunlight, it may help to wear sunglasses.

An urge to urinate (pass your water) with an inability to do so sometimes occurs with this drug. Urinating before taking the drug each time may help relieve this problem. Tell your doctor if you are having this problem.

When to Call Your Doctor

Most people experience few or no side effects from this drug. However, any medicine can sometimes cause unwanted effects. Call your doctor if you develop a skin rash, eye pain, difficulty reading, fainting spells, fast heartbeats, shortness of breath or difficulty breathing, confusion, unusual restlessness, seizures, abdominal pain, muscle weakness, severe constipation or continued difficulty urinating.

Allergic Reactions

Call your doctor immediately if you think you may be allergic to the medicine or if you develop a skin rash, hives, itching, swelling of the face or difficulty in breathing. If you cannot reach your doctor, phone a hospital emergency department.

Refills

Do not stop taking this medicine without your doctor's approval and do not go without medicine between prescription refills. Call your pharmacist for a refill 2 or 3 days before you will run out of the medicine.

BETAMETHASONE (ORAL)
BETNELAN, BETNESOL, CELESTONE

CORTISONE
CORTONE

DEXAMETHASONE
DECADRON, DERONIL, DEXASONE, HEXADROL, ORADEXON

HYDROCORTISONE
CORTEF

METHYLPREDNISOLONE
MEDROL

PREDNISONE
APO-PREDNISONE, DELTASONE, WINPRED

TRIAMCINOLONE
ARISTOCORT, KENACORT

Purpose
This medicine is a hormone (corticosteroid) used to help decrease inflammation. This then relieves pain, redness and swelling. It is used to treat certain kinds of arthritis, severe allergies or skin conditions as well as a variety of other medical conditions. If you do not know why you were prescribed this medicine, ask your doctor.

Allergies
If you have ever had an allergic reaction to any medicine or if you have or have had tuberculosis (TB), a positive skin test for TB, an infection,

ulcers, high blood pressure or any other medical condition, tell your doctor and pharmacist before you take any of this medicine.

How to Use This Medicine

Time of Administration

If your doctor has prescribed only *one* dose of this medicine every day or every other day, it is best to take it before 9 A.M. or with breakfast.

Try to take this medicine at the same time(s) every day so that you will have a constant level of medicine in your body. The time of day affects the way your body responds to this medicine. It is important to follow your doctor's directions as closely as possible.

How to Administer

Take this medicine after meals or with a snack in order to help prevent stomach upset. Call your doctor if you develop stomach upset, stomach pain, heartburn (especially if it awakens you during the night) or if your stools become black and tarry. Do not try to treat these problems yourself.

If you were prescribed CELESTONE REPETABS:

- These tablets are long-acting and must be swallowed whole. Do not crush, chew or break them into pieces.

If you were prescribed BETNESOL TABLETS:

- These are effervescent tablets and must be dissolved in a full glass of water before taking. Let the bubbles disappear before drinking the solution.

If you were prescribed BETNESOL PELLETS:

- These tablets should be placed close to the ulcer in the mouth and allowed to dissolve.

For liquid medicines:

- If a spoon is used to measure the dose, it is recommended that you use a medicine spoon or an oral liquid syringe that you can obtain from your pharmacist. *See* How to Administer Medications (page 15).

Special Instructions

Length of Therapy

Do not take this medicine more often or longer than recommended by your doctor. To do so may increase your chance of developing side effects. Your doctor will want you to take the lowest dose possible.

Do not stop taking this medicine suddenly without the approval of your doctor. It may be necessary for your doctor to reduce your dose slowly since your body will need time to adjust. It could be harmful and make your condition worse if you suddenly stopped taking the medicine. You might then experience symptoms of too rapid withdrawal including nausea, tiredness, loss of appetite, difficulty breathing, fainting, joint and muscle pains.

Pregnancy/Breastfeeding

Women who are pregnant, breastfeeding or planning to become pregnant should tell their doctor before taking this medicine.

Drug Interactions

It is best not to take ASA or medicines containing salicylates while you are taking this medicine without the approval of your doctor or pharmacist. The combination could cause stomach problems.

Alcohol

It is best not to drink alcoholic beverages while you are taking this medicine because the combination could cause stomach problems.

Special Precautions

While you are taking this medicine you may gain some weight. This could be due to an increase in your appetite or to increased water in your body. Your doctor may prescribe a special diet to decrease the number of calories you eat, and/or to lower the amount of sodium or to increase the amount of potassium in your diet. Follow any diet that your doctor may order.

Bruising may occur more easily. Try to protect yourself from all injuries to prevent bruising.

Diabetic patients should regularly check the sugar in their urine or blood and report any unusual levels to their doctor.

It is generally not recommended that patients taking this medicine (especially high doses) receive vaccinations against infectious diseases. The body is not usually able to respond in the normal manner.

When to Call Your Doctor

Call your doctor if you are taking this medicine or have recently stopped taking it and you experience severe stress.

Most people experience few or no side effects from this drug. However, any medicine can sometimes cause unwanted effects. Call your doctor if you develop stomach pain, sore throat, fever, swelling of the legs or ankles, eye pain or changes in vision, frequent urination (passing your water), nightmares or a change in your mood, depression, unusual bruising, changes in the skin, increased facial hair (in women), muscle cramps, stomach or back pain, bloody or black stools, puffy face, irregular heartbeats, dizziness, weakness, unusual thirst, menstrual problems (women) or an infection that does not clear up as quickly as usual.

Helpful Hint for Relief of Dry Mouth

The husband of a semiconscious woman discovered an ingenious way to relieve her dry mouth. He filled a small perfume atomizer with fresh water and misted his wife's mouth frequently. According to the *American Journal of Nursing,* the condition of the woman's throat and mouth improved. After the wife recovered, she commented that the misting had been very comforting.

If you decide to use this technique, use fresh water and change the water at least once daily to help prevent bacterial contamination of the water.

Allergic Reactions

Call your doctor immediately if you think you may be allergic to this medicine or if you develop a skin rash, hives, itching, swelling of the face or difficulty in breathing. If you cannot reach your doctor, phone a hospital emergency department.

Refills

Do not stop taking this medicine without your doctor's approval and do not go without medicine between prescription refills. Call your pharmacist for a refill 2 or 3 days before you will run out of the medicine.

Miscellaneous

Carry an identification card in your wallet or wear a medical alert bracelet indicating that you are taking this medicine as well as the names and phone numbers of your doctors. If you do not already carry such a card, complete the Medicine Card in this book. Always tell your dentist, pharmacist and other doctors who are treating you that you are taking this medicine. This is especially important if you have an infection or injury or if you plan to have an operation, vaccination, skin tests or dental surgery. This medicine can affect the way your body responds to stress, such as surgery. Your doctor may need to adjust your dose.

If you were taking the medicine for a long time, your body's response to stress may take several months to return to normal. It is important to tell your future doctors and dentists this even after you have stopped the medicine for 1 year.

Did You Know That?

Prescription drugs available in Canada are frequently different from those available in the United States even though they may be manufactured by the same pharmaceutical company and sold under the same brand name.

During the preparation of the manuscript for this book, it became evident that more than one-third of the medication instructions differed between the two countries. There are many cases of a Canadian product requiring different administration instructions from the American product because of differences in formulation of the product between the two countries. Even the types of medical problems that the federal governments have approved for the drug to be safe and effective often differ between the two countries. There are some Canadian medications that have exactly the same name as the American product but have different ingredients or different strengths of the medicine. As a result, the contraindications, warnings and side effects can vary between the two products.

It is very important for Canadians to follow the medication instructions for Canadian products and not to use American reference sources.

BROMPHENIRAMINE (ORAL)

DIMETANE

BROMPHENIRAMINE MALEATE-PHENYLEPHRINE-PHENYLPROPANOLAMINE

DIMETAPP, DIMETAPP ORAL INFANT DROPS

BROMPHENIRAMINE-PHENYLEPHRINE-PHENYLPROPANOLAMINE-GUAIFENESIN

DIMETANE EXPECTORANT

BROMPHENIRAMINE-PHENYLEPHRINE-PHENYLPROPANOLAMINE-ACETAMINOPHEN
DIMETAPP-A, DIMETAPP-A PEDIATRIC

BROMPHENIRAMINE-PHENYLEPHRINE-PHENYLPROPANOLAMINE-DEXTROMETHORPHAN
DIMETAPP-DM

BROMPHENIRAMINE-PHENYLEPHRINE-PHENYLPROPANOLAMINE-GUAIFENESIN-CODEINE
DIMETANE EXPECTORANT-C

BROMPHENIRAMINE-PHENYLEPHRINE-PHENYLPROPANOLAMINE-GUAIFENESIN-HYDROCODONE
DIMETANE EXPECTORANT-DC

BROMPHENIRAMINE-PHENYLEPHRINE-PHENYLPROPANOLAMINE-CODEINE
DIMETAPP-C, DIMETAPP WITH CODEINE

Purpose

This medicine is used to help relieve or prevent the symptoms of certain types of allergic conditions (such as hay fever), coughs and colds and certain allergic skin conditions.

Allergies/Warnings

If you have ever had an allergic reaction to any medicine or if you have asthma, glaucoma, an enlarged prostate, urinary retention (a type of bladder problem), high blood pressure or diabetes, tell your doctor and pharmacist before you take any of this medicine.

How to Use This Medicine

Time of Administration

This medicine may be taken without regard to meals. Take it either with food or on an empty stomach. If stomach upset occurs, take it with some food or a glass of milk.

How to Administer

If you were prescribed DIMETANE EXTENTABS, DIMETAPP EXTENTABS:

- These tablets must be swallowed whole. Do not crush, chew or break them into pieces. Do not take chipped tablets.

If your child was prescribed DIMETAPP ORAL INFANT DROPS:
- Use the special dropper that comes with the medicine.
- If you do not understand how to use the dropper to measure an accurate dose, *see* How to Administer Medications (page 15).

If you were prescribed DIMETANE ELIXIR, DIMETAPP ELIXIR, DIMETANE EXPECTORANTS, DIMETAPP-C, DIMETAPP-DM ELIXIR:
- Use a medicine spoon to measure each dose. Household teaspoons are not accurate.

Special Instructions

Length of Therapy

Do not take this medicine more often or longer than recommended by your doctor. To do so may increase your chance of developing side effects.

Prolonged use of DIMETANE EXPECTORANT-C, DIMETANE EXPECTORANT-DC, DIMETAPP-C, and DIMETAPP WITH CODEINE should be avoided. Do not use more often than recommended by your physician.

Pregnancy/Breastfeeding

Women who are pregnant, breastfeeding or planning to become pregnant should tell their doctor before taking this medicine. Some of the products should not be taken during pregnancy or while breastfeeding.

Drug Interactions

It is important that you obtain the advice of your doctor or pharmacist before taking any other prescription or nonprescription medicines including pain relievers, sleeping pills, tranquilizers, medicine for seizures, muscle relaxants, anesthetics, medicines for depression or other medicines for allergies. Combining this medicine with some of these drugs could cause drowsiness or dizziness.

There are other drug interactions that can occur. If you are taking any other medicines, be sure to check first with your pharmacist or doctor.

Alcohol

Do not drink alcoholic beverages while taking this drug without the approval of your doctor because the combination could cause drowsiness. One drink may have the same effect that 2 or 3 drinks normally would have.

Special Precautions

In some people, this drug may initially cause dizziness or drowsiness. Do not drive a car, pilot an airplane, operate dangerous machinery or do jobs that require you to be alert until you know how you are going to react to the drug. If you become dizzy or drowsy, you should be careful going up and down stairs. Sit or lie down at the first sign of dizziness. Tell your doctor if the dizziness continues.

People over 65 years of age may be more sensitive to these side effects.

If your mouth becomes dry, drink water, suck ice chips or a hard, sour candy (sugarless) or chew gum (sugarless). Sugarless products are recommended in order to avoid dental problems. You may wish to ask your pharmacist about special solutions, called artificial saliva, that can also be used to help restore moisture in the mouth. It is especially important to brush and floss your teeth regularly if you develop a dry mouth to help prevent gum problems.

When to Call Your Doctor

Most people experience few or no side effects from these drugs. However, any medicine can sometimes cause unwanted effects. Call your doctor if you develop a skin rash, fast or irregular heartbeats, blurred vision, stomach pain, unexplained weakness or tiredness, unexplained sore throat or fever, unusual bruising or bleeding, unexplained nervousness, restlessness or irritability (especially in children), trouble sleeping or difficulty in urinating (passing your water), severe constipation or if mucus (lung secretions) becomes thicker than normal.

How to Break Tablets in Half

Most tablets that are intended to be broken in half have an indented line (score line) down the middle. In addition, the tablet surfaces are frequently convexly curved. These two properties allow the tablet to be split fairly easily by using the following procedure:

- Hold the tablet so the indented line is facing you.
- Place a thumb on each side of the indented line.
- Press down firmly until the tablet breaks.

The tablet will usually break along the indented line with very little loss of the drug.

CAPTOPRIL (ORAL)
CAPOTEN

ENALAPRIL
VASOTEC

Purpose
This medicine is used to treat high blood pressure and may also be used to treat heart failure.

Allergies/Warnings
Be sure to tell your doctor and pharmacist if you are allergic to any medicine.

How to Use This Medicine

Time of Administration

Try to take this medicine at the same time every day so that you have a constant level of the medicine in your body.

How To Administer

For CAPOTEN:
- Take this medicine with a glass of water on an empty stomach at least 1 hour before or 2 hours after eating food.

For VASOTEC:
- This medicine is not affected by food and may be taken with food or on an empty stomach.

Special Instructions

Length of Therapy

For patients with high blood pressure:
- High blood pressure (hypertension) is a long-term condition, and it will probably be necessary for you to take the drug for a long time in spite of the fact that you feel better. If high blood pressure is not treated, it can lead to serious problems such as heart failure, strokes, blood vessel problems or kidney problems. It is very important that you take this medicine as your doctor has directed and that you do not miss any doses. Otherwise, you cannot expect the drug to keep your blood pressure down.

Do not take any more of this medicine than your doctor has prescribed and do not stop taking this medicine suddenly without the approval of your doctor. It will be necessary for your doctor to reduce your dose slowly since your body will need time to adjust. It could be harmful and make your condition worse if you suddenly stopped taking the medicine.

Pregnancy/Breastfeeding

Women who are pregnant, breastfeeding or planning to become pregnant should tell their doctor before taking this medicine.

Drug Interactions

Some nonprescription drugs can aggravate your condition. Do not take any of the following without the approval of your doctor or pharmacist: cough, cold, or sinus products; products containing ASA; asthma or allergy products since they may increase your blood pressure. Read the label of the product to see if there is a warning. If there is, check with your doctor or pharmacist before using the product.

Special Precautions

In order to prevent dizziness or fainting, you should avoid strenuous exercise, standing for long periods of time (especially in hot weathcr), how showers, hot baths, Jacuzzis or saunas. If this medicine causes dizziness or lightheadedness, you should be careful going up and down stairs and you should not change positions too rapidly. Sit or lie down at the first sign of dizziness. Do not drive a car, pilot an airplane, operate dangerous machinery or do jobs that require you to be alert if you are dizzy. Tell your doctor if you have been dizzy.

Do not use salt substitutes, low-salt milk or low-salt soups without the approval of your doctor. They may contain large amounts of potassium, which could affect the way you respond to this medicine. Do not start any special diets without first consulting your physician.

This medicine may cause a temporary loss of taste or change in taste. This is not harmful and disappears after 2 or 3 months of treatment.

When to Call Your Doctor

Most people experience few or no side effects from this drug. However, any medicine can sometimes cause unwanted effects. Call your doctor if you develop a skin rash, sore throat, fever or mouth sores, chills, insomnia, increased or decreased amount of urine, chest pain, fast or irregular heartbeats, fainting, or swelling of the face, mouth, hands or feet.

Call your doctor if you develop any of the warning signs of too much potassium: irregular heartbeats, numbness or tingling in the hands, feet or lips, confusion, difficulty breathing, unusual tiredness or weakness, unexplained nervousness, weakness or a feeling of heaviness in the legs. Since not all patients develop these symptoms, your doctor may want to check your blood occasionally to see if the potassium level is normal.

Call your doctor if you become sick or develop persistent nausea, vomiting or diarrhea or excessive perspiration. These conditions could cause the blood pressure to fall more than desired.

Chewable Tablets — How Much Chewing Is Necessary

Chewable tablets should be completely chewed and broken into very small pieces before swallowed.

Since the pieces of the tablet must still dissolve in the stomach fluids in order to be absorbed into the bloodstream, the smaller the pieces, the quicker the tablet will dissolve and then be absorbed. Always drink some water after you have chewed and swallowed the small tablet pieces unless otherwise directed.

Allergic Reactions

Call your doctor immediately if you think you may be allergic to the medicine or if you develop a skin rash, hives, itching, swelling of the face or difficulty in breathing. If you cannot reach your doctor, phone a hospital emergency department.

Refills

Do not stop taking this medicine without your doctor's approval and do not go without medicine between prescription refills. Call your pharmacist for a refill 2 or 3 days before you will run out of the medicine.

Miscellaneous

Carry an identification card in your wallet or wear a medical alert bracelet indicating that you are taking this medicine as well as the names and phone numbers of your doctors. If you do not already carry such a card, complete the Medicine Card in this book. Always tell your dentist, pharmacist and other doctors who are treating you that you are taking this medicine.

Did You Know That?

Most people with high blood pressure do not have any symptoms.

The only way to determine if your blood pressure is higher than normal is to have it measured.

CARBAMAZEPINE (ORAL)

APO-CARBAMAZEPINE, MAZEPINE, TEGRETOL, TEGRETOL-CR

Purpose

This medicine is used to help control convulsions and seizures. It is commonly used in the treatment of epilepsy. It is also used to help relieve a certain type of face pain called trigeminal neuralgia, glossopharyngeal neuralgia, and other types of "nerve pain."

Do not take this medicine for ordinary aches and pains. It is *not* an ordinary pain reliever.

Allergies/Warnings

If you have ever had an allergic reaction to an anticonvulsant (seizure medicine) or a medicine for depression or if you have glaucoma, heart disease, anemia or other blood problems, tell your doctor and pharmacist before you take any of this medicine.

How to Use This Medicine

Time of Administration

It is very important that you take this medicine exactly as your doctor has prescribed. Do not miss any doses and take the medicine even if you feel well. Try to take this medicine at the same time(s) every day so that you will have a constant level of medicine in your body. This is the only way that you can receive the full benefit of the medicine.

How to Administer

Take this medicine after food to help prevent stomach upset and to improve absorption of the drug into the body. Call your doctor if you continue to have stomach upset.

For TEGRETOL-CR:

- This medicine is long-acting and must not be crushed or chewed.

Swallow the medicine whole.

If you were prescribed Tegretol Chewtabs:

- These tablets should be swallowed whole or chewed well before swallowing. Always take them the same way so that you receive the same amount of medicine each time.

Special Instructions

Length of Therapy

If you are taking this medicine to treat epilepsy, do not stop taking it suddenly without the approval of your doctor. It will usually be necessary for your doctor to reduce your dose slowly, since your body will need time to adjust. You could develop seizures if you suddenly stopped taking the medicine. The only time this medicine should be stopped quickly is if certain serious side effects develop.

Pregnancy/Breastfeeding

Women who are pregnant, planning to become pregnant or breastfeeding should tell their doctor before taking this medicine.

Drug Interactions

It is important that you obtain the advice of your doctor or pharmacist before taking any other prescription or nonprescription medicines including pain relievers, sleeping pills, birth control pills, erythromycin antibiotics, tranquilizers, medicine for seizures, muscle relaxants, anesthetics, medicines for depression or medicines for allergies. Combining this medicine with some of these drugs could cause drowsiness or dizziness.

There are other drug interactions that can occur. If you are taking any other medicines, be sure to check first with your pharmacist or doctor.

There have been some reports that oral contraceptives (birth control pills) may not work as well while taking this medicine. Unplanned pregnancies may occur. Ask your doctor about using another form of birth control or adjusting your dose of birth control pills while you are taking this medicine. Also call your doctor if you develop spotting or breakthrough bleeding since these can be signs of decreased birth control effect.

Alcohol

Do not drink alcoholic beverages while taking this drug without a doctor's approval because the combination could cause drowsiness.

Special Precautions

Be sure to keep your doctor's appointments so that your doctor can check your progress. This is especially important during the first few months of therapy when the doctor will decide the best dose of this medicine for your condition. To make sure that your dose is correct, your doctor may wish to take a blood sample periodically to measure the amount of medicine in it.

This medicine may cause dizziness, drowsiness or blurred vision in some people. Do not drive a car, operate dangerous machinery or do jobs that require you to be alert until you know how you are going to react to the drug. If you become dizzy, you should be careful going up and down stairs. Sit or lie down at the first sign of dizziness. Tell your doctor if you are dizzy, drowsy or have blurred vision.

If this medicine is for a child, do not let him or her ride a bike, climb trees, etc. until you can determine how he or she is going to react to this medicine. Children could hurt themselves if they participated in these activities when they were dizzy.

This medicine may make some people more sensitive to sunlight and various tanning lamps. When you begin taking this medicine, try to avoid too much sun until you see how you are going to react. If your skin does become more sensitive to sunlight, tell your doctor and try not to stay in direct sunlight for extended periods of time. While in the sun, wear protective clothing and sunglasses. You may wish to ask your pharmacist about suitable sunscreen products. Call your doctor if you become sunburned.

When to Call Your Doctor

Most people experience few or no side effects from this drug. However, any medicine can sometimes cause unwanted effects. Call your doctor immediately if you develop a sore throat, fever or mouth sores, chills, swollen glands, fainting, muscle weakness, unexplained coughing, difficulty breathing, unusual bruising or bleeding, dark-colored urine, a yellow color to the skin or eyes, unusual tiredness or weakness, continuous back-and-forth or rolling eye movements, numbness or tingling in the hands or feet, fast or slow heartbeats, chest pain, trembling, abdominal pain, light-colored stools, ringing or buzzing in the ears, confusion, hallucinations, nightmares or depression, swelling of the legs or ankles or if you urinate (pass your water) in smaller amounts than usual.

Call your doctor if you are taking this medicine for seizures and you have an increase in the frequency of seizures.

Allergic Reactions

Call your doctor immediately if you think you may be allergic to the medicine or if you develop a skin rash, hives, itching, swelling of the face or difficulty in breathing. If you cannot reach your doctor, phone a hospital emergency department.

Storage

Protect the medicine from heat and humidity.

Refills

Do not stop taking this medicine without your doctor's approval and do not go without medicine between prescription refills. Call your pharmacist for a refill 2 or 3 days before you will run out of the medicine.

Miscellaneous

Carry an identification card in your wallet or wear a medical alert bracelet indicating that you are taking this medicine as well as the names and phone numbers of your doctors. If you do not already carry such a card, complete the Medicine Card in this book. Always tell your dentist, pharmacist and other doctors who are treating you that you are taking this medicine.

Did You Know That?

When a medicine is prescribed, you should ask the doctor what you should expect to feel and what you can do if a common side effect occurs. Then if the effect occurs, you will know whether it is a sign that the drug is working or whether you should contact your doctor.

CEFACLOR (ORAL)
CECLOR

CEFADROXIL
DURICEF

CEPHALEXIN MONOHYDRATE
CEPOREX, KEFLEX, NOVOLEXIN

CEPHRADINE
VELOSEF

Purpose

This medicine is an antibiotic used to treat certain types of infections. Your doctor has prescribed this antibiotic for your present infection only. Do not use it for other infections or give it to other people.

Allergies/Warnings

If you have ever had an allergic reaction to penicillin, a cephalosporin or any other medicine or if you have any allergies (for example, asthma or hay fever), tell your doctor and pharmacist before you take any of this medicine.

How to Use This Medicine

Time of Administration

This medicine may be taken with meals or on an empty stomach. However, if you develop an upset stomach after taking the drug, take it with some food. Call your doctor if you continue to have stomach upset.

Space your doses of the medicine around the clock (throughout the entire day of 24 hours). For example, if you are to take 4 doses each day, space the doses 6 hours apart. This will keep a constant level of the medicine in your body.

How to Administer

For tablets and capsules:

- Take the medicine with a full glass of water unless otherwise directed.

For liquid medicines:

- If you were prescribed a *suspension*, shake the bottle well each time before pouring so that you can measure an accurate dose.
- If a spoon is used to measure the dose, it is recommended that you use a medicine spoon or an oral liquid syringe that you can obtain from your pharmacist. *See* How to Administer Medications (page 15).

Special Instructions

Length of Therapy

It is important to take all of this medicine plus any refills that your doctor told you to take. Do not stop taking this medicine earlier than your doctor has recommended even if you begin to feel better. If you stop taking the medicine too soon, the infection may return.

This is especially important if you are taking the medicine to cure a strep infection because if the infection is not completely cleared up, serious heart problems could develop later. After treatment for a strep infection, your doctor may want to do a test to make sure that the infection is gone.

Pregnancy/Breastfeeding

Women who are pregnant, breastfeeding or planning to become pregnant should tell their doctor before taking this medicine.

Special Precautions

For patients with diabetes:

- If you have diabetes, this medicine may interfere with some of the tests for sugar in the urine. Check with your doctor or pharmacist for advice on which test you should use for detecting sugar in the urine while you are taking this antibiotic.

When to Call Your Doctor

Call your doctor if your symptoms do not improve within a few days or if they become worse.

Most people experience few or no side effects from this drug. However, any medicine can sometimes cause unwanted effects. Call your doctor if you develop nausea, vomiting, fever, chills, sore mouth or sore tongue, severe or persistent watery or bloody diarrhea, severe stomach cramps and bloating, unusual weight loss, rectal or genital itching or, in women, a vaginal discharge that was not present before you started taking the medicine.

Allergic Reactions

Call your doctor immediately if you think you may be allergic to the medicine or if you develop a skin rash, hives, itching, swelling of the face or difficulty in breathing. If you cannot reach your doctor, phone a hospital emergency department.

Storage

For liquid medicines:

- Store the bottle of medicine in a refrigerator unless otherwise directed. Do not freeze.

If for some reason you cannot take all of the medicine, discard the unused portion by flushing it down the toilet. Throw away any unused medicine after the discard (expiration) date on the bottle. Do not take or save old medicine.

Did You Know That?

You should not mix pediatric medicines with infant formulas or foods.

If the child detects a strange taste in the food due to the medicine, he or she may refuse that particular food in the future.

Also, if the infant does not drink all the formula, he or she will not receive the full dose of the medicine.

CHLORDIAZEPOXIDE-CLIDINIUM (ORAL)

APO-CHLORAX, CORIUM, LIBRAX

Purpose

This medicine is used to decrease the amount of acid in the stomach and help relax the muscles of the stomach and bowels.

Allergies/Warnings

If you have ever had an allergic reaction to any medicine or if you have glaucoma, depression, an enlarged prostate, difficulty in urinating (passing your water) or any medical problem, tell your doctor and pharmacist before you take any of this medicine.

How to Use This Medicine

Time of Administration

Take this medicine 1/2 hour to 1 hour before meals unless otherwise directed by your doctor.

Special Instructions

Length of Therapy

Do not take this medicine more often or longer than recommended by your doctor. If large doses are taken for long periods of time (months), the drug can become habit forming.

If you are taking the medicine regularly, do not stop taking it suddenly without the approval of your doctor. It may be necessary for your doctor to reduce your dose slowly since your body may need time to adjust.

Check with your doctor if you develop any of the following while you are slowly stopping the medicine: nausea or vomiting, trembling, seizures, muscle cramps, stomach cramps, unusual sweating or trouble sleeping or if you become confused, irritable or nervous.

Pregnancy/Breastfeeding

Women who are pregnant, breastfeeding or planning to become pregnant should tell their doctor before taking this medicine. This medicine should generally not be used during pregnancy and is not generally recommended during breastfeeding.

Drug Interactions

It is important that you obtain the advice of your doctor or pharmacist before taking any other prescription or nonprescription medicines, including pain relievers, sleeping pills, tranquilizers or medicines for depression, cough, cold or allergy medicines because the combination could cause drowsiness or confusion.

There are other drug interactions that can occur. If you are taking any other medicines, be sure to check first with your pharmacist or doctor.

Alcohol

Do not drink alcoholic beverages while taking this drug or for a few days after you have stopped taking the drug without the approval of your doctor. The combination could cause drowsiness. One drink may have the same effect that 2 or 3 drinks normally would have.

Special Precautions

In some people, this drug may cause dizziness or drowsiness. Do not drive a car, pilot an airplane, operate dangerous machinery or do jobs that require you to be alert if you are dizzy or drowsy. You should also be careful going up and down stairs. Sit or lie down at the first sign of dizziness. Tell your doctor if the dizziness or drowsiness continues.

If your mouth becomes dry, drink water, suck ice chips or a hard, sour candy (sugarless) or chew gum (sugarless). Sugarless products are recommended in order to avoid dental problems. You may wish to ask your pharmacist about special solutions, called artificial saliva, that can also be used to help restore moisture in the mouth. It is especially important to brush and floss your teeth regularly if you develop a dry mouth to help prevent gum problems.

You may become more sensitive to heat because your body may perspire less while you are taking this drug. Be careful not to become overheated during exercise or in hot weather. Try to avoid strenuous exercise, standing for long periods of time (especially in hot weather), hot showers, hot baths, saunas or Jacuzzis while taking this medicine.

When to Call Your Doctor

If you develop constipation, do not try to treat it yourself with nonprescription drugs. Call your doctor.

Most people experience few or no side effects from this drug. However, any medicine can sometimes cause unwanted effects. Call your doctor if you develop a sore throat, fever, mouth sores, a staggering walk, a yellow color to the skin or eyes, slow heartbeats or shortness of breath, unusual tiredness or nervousness, stomach pain, confusion or depression, hallucinations, trouble sleeping, seizures, slurred speech or severe drowsiness. Also call your doctor if you develop constipation, difficulty urinating (passing your water), eye pain or fast heartbeats.

Allergic Reactions

Call your doctor immediately if you think you may be allergic to the medicine or if you develop a skin rash, hives, itching, swelling of the face or difficulty in breathing. If you cannot reach your doctor, phone a hospital emergency department.

CHLOROTRIANISENE (ORAL)
TACE

CONJUGATED ESTROGENS
C.E.S., PREMARIN

ESTRADIOL
ESTRACE

ESTROPIPATE
OGEN

ETHINYL ESTRADIOL
ESTINYL

ESTRADIOL (TRANSDERMAL)
ESTRADERM PATCH

ESTROGENS (VAGINAL)
OESTRILIN VAGINAL, ORTHO DIENESTROL CREAM, PREMARIN VAGINAL CREAM

Purpose

This medicine is a hormone commonly used to relieve hot flashes, sleep problems, and sweating that may occur during menopause. The medicine has many other uses and the reason it was prescribed depends on your condition. If you do not understand why you are taking it, check with your doctor.

Allergies/Warnings

If you have ever had an allergic reaction to any medicine, tell your doctor and pharmacist before you take any of this medicine.

Also tell your doctor if you have had cancer or problems of the breast or uterus, changes in vaginal bleeding, endometriosis, blood clotting problems, migraine headaches, strokes or liver disease. The medicines should not be used in these conditions.

Also tell your doctor if you have had high blood pressure, heart or kidney disease, asthma, epilepsy, diabetes or depression. This will help your doctor decide whether estrogen therapy should be prescribed.

How to Use This Medicine

How to Administer

For tablets:

- Take the tablets after meals or with a snack if they upset your stomach. Call your doctor if the stomach upset continues.

For vaginal creams and suppositories: see How to Administer Medications (page 15).

For ESTRADERM PATCHES:

- Apply the patch on the same 2 days of the week. If you forget to change the patch on the correct day, change it as soon as you remember and continue to follow your ORIGINAL schedule. The patch is worn continuously for 3 to 4 days and is changed twice weekly.
- Apply the patch to a non-hairy area of the body that is not oily, damaged, irritated or exposed to the sun. Do not apply the patch over skin folds (for example, waistline or under tight clothing) since the patch may fall off. Suggested areas to apply the patch include on the side of the torso, lower back or buttocks. Do not apply ESTRADERM to the breasts or to skin that is exposed to the sun. The skin should be clean and dry so that the patch will stick to the skin.

- Tear open the foil pouch and remove the ESTRADERM PATCH. Do not use scissors to open the pouch since you may accidentally cut the patch.
- Loosen the protective liner on the back of the pouch by sliding the patch sideways between your thumb and index finger. Then remove the protective liner by holding at the edge with one hand and peeling back the liner with the other hand. Do not touch the sticky surface of the pouch.
- Apply the patch immediately by pressing the sticky side onto the chosen area of the skin. Press the patch firmly in place with the palm of your hand for about 10 seconds.
- Water (bath, pool, shower) will not damage the patch; however, very hot water or steam may loosen it.
- When it is time to apply a new patch, select a different area of the skin. You can use the same spot more than once — but not twice in a row.
- When you remove the used patch, fold it in half (with the sticky side inside) and throw it away, safely out of the reach of children.
- If the patch falls off, reapply the SAME patch to a DIFFERENT area of skin that is clean and dry. Continue to follow your ORIGINAL schedule for changing patches. If this patch will not stick to the new area, apply a new patch but continue with your original dosing schedule.
- Be sure to read the booklet, "Estraderm and How to Use It," that comes with the medicine.

Special Instructions

Length of Therapy

Do not take this medicine more often or longer than recommended by your doctor. To do so may increase your chance of developing side effects.

Do not stop taking this medicine suddenly without the approval of your doctor.

Pregnancy/Breastfeeding

Women who are pregnant or planning to become pregnant should not take this medicine because it can cause birth defects.

Women who are breastfeeding should tell their doctor before taking this medicine.

Special Precautions

If you are taking the oral medicine for a long time, do not smoke while you are on this medicine because smoking can increase the incidence of heart attacks and slow down the circulation of the blood.

Diabetic patients should regularly check the sugar in their urine or blood while they are taking this medicine.

If you are taking this medicine for a long time, it is recommended that you visit your doctor every 6 or every 12 months for follow-up to make sure that you are not developing side effects.

Call your doctor if you develop brown, blotchy spots. These spots may disappear or fade after you have stopped taking the drug.

If you were prescribed a vaginal cream or suppository:

- You may wish to wear a sanitary napkin to protect your clothing from the medicine. Do not use tampons while you are using the vaginal cream or suppository.

For additional information, read the leaflet "Information for the Patient," which was given to you by your pharmacist.

When to Call Your Doctor

Most people experience few or no side effects from this drug. However, any medicine can sometimes cause unwanted effects. Call your doctor immediately or go to the nearest hospital emergency department if you develop:

- Sudden, severe headaches.
- Sudden loss of coordination.
- Blurred vision or slurred speech.
- Pain in the calves or numbness in an arm or leg.
- Chest pain, shortness of breath, or coughing of blood.

These side effects are rare but could be a sign that blood clots have formed.

Also call your doctor if you develop a skin rash, white vaginal discharge, abnormal vaginal bleeding, irregular or missed menstrual period, breast tenderness, lumps in the breast, dizziness, skin irritation with ESTRADERM PATCH, severe depression, a yellow color to the skin or eyes or dark-colored urine, severe abdominal pain, weight gain or swelling of the hands or ankles.

If you are using a vaginal cream or suppository:

- Call your doctor if the condition for which the drug is being used persists or becomes worse or if the medication causes a constant irritation such as itching or burning that was not present before you started using it.

If you are using ESTRADERM PATCHES:

- If you develop bothersome redness or irritation in the area where the patch has been applied, tell your doctor.

Did You Know That?

Medicines for estrogen replacement and motion sickness now come in the form of small adhesive bandages. They are called transdermal patches.

The medicine is contained in a thin membrane and is slowly released through the skin directly into the bloodstream. Because the medicine bypasses the stomach and liver, lower dosages can be used and fewer side effects occur. This new form of treatment makes it much easier to "take" medicines since the person does not have to take the medicine as often.

Not every medicine is suitable for this dosage form. The molecules of the medicine must be small enough to pass through the skin and must not cause skin irritation. The medicine must be released at a rate that will result in correct blood levels. Some medicines are absorbed too slowly and are unsuitable. Another important factor is the quality of the person's skin. A young person's skin absorbs medicines differently from an older person's skin. Oiliness of the skin can affect the absorption of the drug and this is why the skin area should be cleansed and dried before a patch is applied. Hair can also interfere with the ability of the patch to stick and with the absorption of the medicine. For this reason, patches should be applied to non-hairy areas of skin.

Allergic Reactions

Call your doctor immediately if you think you may be allergic to the medicine or if you develop a skin rash, hives, itching, swelling of the face

or difficulty in breathing. If you cannot reach your doctor, phone a hospital emergency department.

Storage
For suppositories: see How to Administer Medications (page 15).

For ESTRADERM PATCHES:
- Store the patch in its original pouch at room temperature.

Refills
Do not stop taking this medicine without your doctor's approval and do not go without medicine between prescription refills. Call your pharmacist for a refill 2 or 3 days before you will run out of the medicine.

CHLORPHENIRAMINE MALEATE (ORAL)
CHLOR-TRIPOLON, NOVOPHENIRAM

CHLORPHENIRAMINE MALEATE-PHENYLEPHRINE
HISTASPAN-P

CHLORPHENIRAMINE-PHENYLPROPANOLAMINE
CHLOR-TRIPOLON DECONGESTANT SYRUP, DRISTAN LONG LASTING CAPSULES, ORNADE, ORNADE-A.F.

CHLORPHENIRAMINE-PHENYLPROPANOLAMINE-GUAIFENESIN
ORNADE EXPECTORANT

CHLORPHENIRAMINE-PHENYLPROPANOLAMINE-DEXTROMETHORPHAN
ORNADE-DM 10 PEDIATRIC, ORNADE-DM 15, ORNADE DM 30

PHENIRAMINE-PHENYLPROPANOLAMINE-PYRILAMINE
TRIAMINIC, TRIAMINIC ORAL INFANT DROPS

PHENIRAMINE-PHENYLPROPANOLAMINE-PYRILAMINE-GUAIFENESIN
TRIAMINIC EXPECTORANT

PHENIRAMINE-PHENYLPROPANOLAMINE-PYRILAMINE-GUAIFENESIN-DEXTROMETHORPHAN
TRIAMINIC-DM

Purpose
This medicine is used to help relieve the symptoms of certain types of allergic conditions (such as hay fever), coughs and colds. Some of the

products are also used to treat certain types of allergic skin conditions.

Allergies/Warnings

If you have ever had an allergic reaction to any medicine or if you have asthma, glaucoma, an enlarged prostate, urinary retention (a type of bladder problem), high blood pressure or diabetes, tell your doctor and pharmacist before you take any of this medicine.

How to Use This Medicine

Time of Administration

This medicine may be taken without regard to meals. Take it either with food or on an empty stomach. If stomach upset occurs, take it with some food or a glass of milk.

How to Administer

If you were prescribed a long-acting form of this medicine (CHLOR-TRIPOLON REPETABS, DRISTAN LONG LASTING CAPSULES, HISTASPAN-P, ORNADE CAPSULES, ORNADE A.F. CAPSULES):

- This medicine lasts approximately 12 hours or longer and must be swallowed whole. Do not crush, chew or break it into pieces.

For liquid medicines:

- It is recommended that a medicine spoon be used to measure the dose. An average household teaspoon is not accurate.

Special Instructions

Length of Therapy

Do not take this medicine more often or longer than recommended by your doctor. To do so may increase your chance of developing side effects.

Pregnancy/Breastfeeding

Women who are pregnant, breastfeeding or planning to become pregnant should tell their doctor before taking this medicine. Some of the products should not be taken during pregnancy or while breastfeeding.

Drug Interactions

It is important that you obtain the advice of your doctor or pharmacist before taking any other prescription or nonprescription medicines including pain relievers, sleeping pills, tranquilizers, medicine for seizures, muscle relaxants, anesthetics, medicines for depression or other medicines for allergies. Combining this medicine with some of these drugs could cause drowsiness or dizziness.

Drug interactions can occur. If you are taking any other medicines, be sure to check first with your pharmacist or doctor.

Alcohol

Do not drink alcoholic beverages while taking this drug without the approval of your doctor because the combination could cause drowsiness. One drink may have the same effect that 2 or 3 drinks normally would have.

Special Precautions

In some people, this drug may initially cause dizziness or drowsiness. Do not drive a car, pilot an airplane, operate dangerous machinery or do jobs that require you to be alert until you know how you are going to react to the drug. If you become dizzy or drowsy, you should be careful going up and down stairs. Sit or lie down at the first sign of dizziness. Tell your doctor if the dizziness or drowsiness continues.

People over 65 years of age may be more sensitive to these side effects.

If your mouth becomes dry, drink water, suck ice chips or a hard, sour candy (sugarless) or chew gum (sugarless). Sugarless products are recommended in order to avoid dental problems. You may wish to ask your pharmacist about special solutions, called artificial saliva, that can also be used to help restore moisture in the mouth. It is especially important to brush and floss your teeth regularly if you develop a dry mouth to help prevent gum problems.

What Can You Do If?

You have a dry mouth and cannot swallow tablets.

This is a common problem in patients who sleep with their mouths open, in elderly patients who are dehydrated and in patients taking medicines that can cause a dry mouth. It is very difficult to swallow a tablet if the mouth and throat are dry.

It may be easier for these patients to swallow tablets if they have a drink of water before putting the medication in their mouths. This will moisten and lubricate the mucous membranes of the mouth and make it more slippery. Then they should put the tablet on the tongue and swallow the medicine with some more water.

When to Call Your Doctor

Most people experience few or no side effects from this drug. However, any medicine can sometimes cause unwanted effects. Call your doctor if you develop a skin rash, fast or irregular heartbeats, blurred vision, stomach pain, unexplained weakness or tiredness, unexplained sore throat or fever, unusual bruising or bleeding, unexplained nervousness, restlessness or irritability (especially in children), trouble sleeping, difficulty in urinating (passing your water) or if mucus (lung secretions) becomes thicker than usual.

CHLORPROMAZINE HCl (ORAL and RECTAL)

LARGACTIL, NOVOCHLORPROMAZINE

FLUPHENAZINE HCl

APO-FLUPHENAZINE, MODITEN, PERMITIL

MESORIDAZINE

SERENTIL

METHOTRIMEPRAZINE

NOZINAN

PERPHENAZINE

APO-PERPHENAZINE, PHENAZINE, TRILAFON

PROCHLORPERAZINE

STEMETIL

PROMAZINE

SPARINE

THIORIDAZINE HCl

APO-THIORIDAZINE, MELLARIL, NOVORIDAZINE, PMS THIORIDAZINE

TRIFLUOPERAZINE HCl

APO-TRIFLUOPERAZINE, NOVOFLURAZINE, SOLAZINE, STELAZINE, TERFLUZINE

Purpose

This medicine is used in the treatment of anxiety and tension and certain types of emotional problems such as severe anxiety, mood problems, confusion, and troubling thoughts and feelings. Some products are also used to treat severe nausea and vomiting and some are used to treat severe hiccups. Check with your doctor if you do not fully understand why you are taking it.

Allergies/Warnings

If you have ever had an allergic reaction to any medicine or if you have high blood pressure, seizures, heart problems, enlarged prostate, difficulty urinating (passing your water), Parkinson's disease, liver disease, glaucoma or any other medical condition, tell your doctor and pharmacist before you take any of this medicine.

How to Use This Medicine

How to Administer

For tablets and capsules:

- If you develop stomach upset while taking this medicine, take it with food or immediately after a snack, unless otherwise directed.

For liquid medicine:

- If a dropper is used to measure the dose and you do not fully understand how to use it, *see* How to Administer Medications (page 15).
- If a spoon is used to measure the dose, it is recommended that you use a medicine spoon or an oral liquid syringe that you can obtain from your pharmacist. These are more accurate than the average household teaspoon. *See* How to Administer Medications (page 15).
- *If you were prescribed* the LARGACTIL LIQUID or SERENTIL CONCENTRATE, the proper dose should be mixed with 2 or more ounces of fruit juice, milk, carbonated beverages or water just before taking. Do not let the solution stand. Drink it at once.
- *If you were prescribed* STELAZINE LIQUID CONCENTRATE, each dose of the medicine can be mixed with 2 or more ounces of fruit juice, milk, carbonated beverages or water just before taking.
- *For other liquid medicines*, check with your pharmacist to see if you can dilute it.
- *If you were prescribed* MELLARIL SUSPENSION, shake the bottle well each time before measuring a dose.

For suppositories: see How to Administer Medications (page 15).

Special Instructions

Length of Therapy

The full effect of this medicine may not be noticed immediately and may take several weeks. Be patient. Take the medicine regularly and try not to miss any doses.

Do not stop taking this medicine suddenly without the approval of your doctor. It may be necessary for your doctor to reduce your dose slowly since your body will need time to adjust. It could make your condition worse if you suddenly stopped taking the medicine. After you have stopped taking this medicine, you may have to continue to observe the following precautions for 1 to 2 weeks since some of the medicine may still be in your body.

Pregnancy/Breastfeeding

Women who are pregnant, breastfeeding or planning to become pregnant should not take this medicine without their doctor's approval.

Drug Interactions

It is best not to take this medicine at the same time as an antacid or an anti-diarrhea medicine containing aluminum. Try to space them 2 hours apart if you must take them while you are on this medicine.

It is important that you obtain the advice of your doctor or pharmacist before taking any other prescription or nonprescription medicines, including pain relievers, sleeping pills, other tranquilizers or medicines for depression, cough, cold or allergy medicines.

There have been some reports that caffeine (in coffee, tea, colas, and in some nonprescription drugs) may decrease the effect of this medicine.

There are other drug interactions that can occur. If you are taking any other medicines, be sure to check first with your pharmacist or doctor.

Alcohol

Do not drink alcoholic beverages while taking this drug without the approval of your doctor. The combination could irritate your stomach and could cause drowsiness or dizziness. One drink may have the same effect that 2 or 3 drinks normally would have.

If you have been taking this medicine regularly for several days or weeks, it is recommended not to drink alcohol for 2 weeks *after* you have stopped taking the medicine. Depending on your dose, it may take this long for the drug to be eliminated from your body.

Special Precautions

If this medicine causes dizziness or lightheadedness, you should be careful going up and down stairs and you should not change positions too rapidly. Lightheadedness is more likely to occur if you stand up suddenly—this is due to blood collecting in the legs and lasts for a few seconds. Therefore, get up from a sitting or lying position more slowly and tighten and relax your leg muscles or wiggle your toes to help promote circulation. In the morning, get out of bed slowly and dangle your feet over the edge of the bed for a few minutes before standing up. Sit or lie down at the first sign of dizziness. Tell your doctor if you have been dizzy.

You may become more sensitive to heat because your body may perspire less while you are taking this drug. Be careful not to become overheated during exercise or in hot weather. Try to avoid strenuous exercise, standing for long periods of time (especially in hot weather), hot showers, hot baths, saunas or Jacuzzis while taking this medicine.

Some patients may also become more sensitive to cold and should dress warmly during cold weather and limit exposure to cold temperatures.

This medicine commonly causes drowsiness, especially during the first week of treatment. Make sure you know how you are going to react to this medicine and whether it will make you dizzy or drowsy. Do not

Did You Know That?

Certain drugs may make a person more vulnerable to heat exhaustion and heatstroke.

Recent summer heat waves have caused thousands of cases of heat-related illness. The most important method of regulating the temperature of the body is sweating. As sweat evaporates on the skin, it has a cooling effect. Sweat must evaporate, however, and when the relative humidity increases, less sweat evaporates. The hotter the temperature, the higher the humidity and the brighter the sun's rays, the greater the risk.

Patients taking any of the following drugs are at greater risk because the medications may:

- impair their ability to sweat or regulate the body temperature
- increase fluid loss
- increase the rate of metabolism of the body which in turn increases the body temperature

Anticholineric Drugs such as ATROPINE, BENZTROPINE and SCOPOLAMINE

Diuretics ("Water Pills") such as
HYDROCHLOROTHIAZIDE and FUROSEMIDE
Phenothiazines such as CHLORPROMAZINE
Tricyclic Antidepressants such as AMITRIPTYLINE, IMIPRAMINE, NORTRIPTYLINE and PROTRIPTYLINE
Monoamine Oxidase Inhibitors such as ISOCARBOXAZID, PHENELZINE and TRANYLCYPROMINE
Beta-Blockers such as PROPRANOLOL
Alcohol
Excessive Laxative Use
Use of Sunscreens while exercising in hot weather
Other Drugs such as AMPHETAMINE, anesthetics, barbiturates and some cancer drugs

Patients taking any medicine that can increase their sensitivity to heat should take precautions to stay as cool as possible during heat waves. Unless fluids and salt are restricted because of a medical condition, they should be increased. Strenuous exercise should be avoided. Jacuzzis and hot showers should be avoided year-round. At the slightest sign of heat illness, contact a physician.

drive a car, pilot an airplane, operate dangerous machinery or do jobs that require you to be alert if you are dizzy or drowsy. The drowsiness may decrease over time.

If your mouth becomes dry, drink water, suck ice chips or a hard, sour candy (sugarless) or chew gum (sugarless). Sugarless products are recommended in order to avoid dental problems. You may wish to ask your pharmacist about special solutions, called artificial saliva, that can also be used to help restore moisture in the mouth. It is especially important to brush and floss your teeth regularly if you develop a dry mouth to help prevent gum problems.

This medicine often makes some people more sensitive to sunlight and various tanning lamps. When you begin taking this medicine, try to avoid too much sun until you see how you are going to react. If your skin does become more sensitive to sunlight, tell your doctor and try not to stay in direct sunlight for extended periods of time. While in the sun, wear protective clothing and sunglasses. You may wish to ask your pharmacist about suitable sunscreen products. Call your doctor if you become sunburned.

An urge to urinate (pass your water) with an inability to do so sometimes occurs with this drug. Urinating before taking the drug each time may help relieve this problem. Tell your doctor if you are having this problem.

There have been some reports that this medicine may cause the urine to turn pink, red or red-brown. This is only temporary and will go away after you have finished the medicine.

When to Call Your Doctor

Call your doctor if you become restless, unable to sit still or sleep, or if you develop unusual muscle stiffness, drooling, disturbed gait, shuffling walk, tremors, shakiness or unusual movements of the face, tongue or hands or stiffness of the face or body. If you develop painful muscle spasms, call your doctor or the hospital emergency room since treatment can be given to provide rapid relief of this problem.

Check with your doctor if you develop constipation.

Any medicine can sometimes cause unwanted effects. Call your doctor if you develop a sore throat, fever, mouth sores, eye pain or changes in vision, difficulty in urinating (passing your water), difficulty breathing, speaking or swallowing, a yellow color in the skin or eyes, dark yellow-colored urine, fast heartbeats, fever, seizures, a skin rash, fainting spells or decreased sexual ability.

Storage

For liquid medicine:

- Store the liquid medicine in a cool, dark place and do not get the liquid on your skin or clothing.

For LARGACTIL LIQUID *or* LARGACTIL ORAL DROPS:

- Throw away the medicine if it turns dark in color.

For suppositories: *see* How to Administer Medications (page 15).

Refills

Do not stop taking this medicine without your doctor's approval and do not go without medicine between prescription refills. Call your pharmacist for a refill 2 or 3 days before you will run out of the medicine.

Discuss with your pharmacist the implications of dispensing all your refills for this medicine with the same manufacturer's product. (*See* Generic Drugs, page 12.)

Miscellaneous

Carry an identification card in your wallet or wear a medical alert

bracelet indicating that you are taking this medicine as well as the names and phone numbers of your doctors. If you do not already carry such a card, complete the Medicine Card in this book. Always tell your dentist, pharmacist and other doctors who are treating you that you are taking this medicine.

CIMETIDINE
APO-CIMETIDINE, NOVOCIMETINE, PEPTOL, TAGAMET

FAMOTIDINE (ORAL)
PEPCID

NIZATIDINE
AXID

RANITIDINE
APO-RANITIDINE, ZANTAC

Purpose
This medicine is used in the treatment and prevention of certain types of stomach and duodenal ulcers and in conditions in which the stomach is producing too much acid. The medicine is also used to help relieve both day- and night-time symptoms (e.g. heartburn, sour taste, coughing, choking, etc.) of gastroesophageal reflux disease.

Allergies/Warnings
If you have ever had an allergic reaction to any medicine, tell your doctor and pharmacist before you take any of this medicine.

How to Use This Medicine

How to Administer

This medicine may be taken with or without food depending upon your condition.

If you develop stomach pain between doses of this medicine, ask your doctor if you may take an antacid between doses. The two medicines should not be taken at the same time. Ask your doctor or pharmacist how many hours you must wait before you take the other medicine.

For TAGAMET LIQUID:
- It is recommended that you use a medicine spoon to measure each

dose. A medicine spoon is more accurate than the average household teaspoon.

Special Instructions

Length of Therapy

It is very important that you take this medicine for the full length of treatment as your doctor has prescribed even if your symptoms have stopped. Try not to miss any doses because the medicine will not be as effective. It may take several days or a few weeks before you feel the full benefit of this medicine.

Do not stop taking the medicine suddenly without the approval of your doctor.

Pregnancy/Breastfeeding

Women who are pregnant, breastfeeding or planning to become pregnant should tell their doctor before taking this medicine.

Drug Interactions

There have been some reports that antacids may decrease the effect of this medicine. The interaction can probably be avoided by taking them at different times. Ask your doctor or pharmacist how many hours you must wait before you take the other medicine.

Smoking cigarettes appears to decrease the effect of this medicine and lengthen the time it takes an ulcer to heal. Do not smoke while taking this drug.

There are other interactions that can occur. If you are taking any other medicines, be sure to check with your doctor or pharmacist.

Alcohol

Do not drink alcoholic beverages while taking this drug because it may make the ulcer pain worse and interfere with healing of the ulcer.

Special Precautions

People with ulcers should generally avoid medicines that can upset the stomach, such as ASA or salicylates since they may interfere with healing of the ulcer. Always read the label and check with your pharmacist if you have any questions. Also avoid those foods and beverages that cause your ulcer symptoms to reappear.

Rarely, this drug may cause dizziness. Do not drive a car, pilot an airplane, operate dangerous machinery or do jobs that require you to be alert until you know how you are going to react to the drug. If you become dizzy, you should be careful going up and down stairs. Sit or lie down at the first sign of dizziness. Tell your doctor if the dizziness continues.

For AXID *and* TAGAMET:

- Rarely, some people taking this medicine may notice a slight increase in the size of their breasts or some breast soreness. This is temporary and will go away after the treatment has ended. Tell your doctor if you develop this problem.

When to Call Your Doctor

Call your doctor immediately if you are being treated for an ulcer and you develop fainting spells, unusual thirst, dizziness, sweating, vomiting of blood or bloody or black stools. This may mean your condition is getting worse.

Most people experience few or no side effects from this drug. However, any medicine can sometimes cause unwanted effects. Call your doctor if you develop a skin rash, unexplained sore throat, fever, muscle cramps or joint pain, unusual bruising or bleeding, severe diarrhea, changes in sexual ability, bothersome headaches, bothersome constipation, hallucinations or if you become confused or restless.

Allergic Reactions

Call your doctor immediately if you think you may be allergic to the medicine or if you develop a skin rash, hives, itching, swelling of the face or difficulty in breathing. If you cannot reach your doctor, phone a hospital emergency department.

CLONIDINE (ORAL)

CATAPRES

CLONIDINE-CHLORTHALIDONE (ORAL)

COMBIPRES

Purpose

This medicine is commonly used to treat high blood pressure as well as some other medical conditions.

Allergies/Warnings

Tell your doctor and pharmacist if you are allergic to any medicine.

If you were prescribed COMBIPRES:

- Be sure to tell your doctor and pharmacist if you are allergic to sulfa drugs, thiazide diuretics or any medicine.

How to Use This Medicine

Time of Administration

Try to take the medicine at the same time(s) each day so that you have a constant level of the medicine in your body.

If you were prescribed CATAPRES:

- The last daily dose of CATAPRES is usually taken immediately before going to bed. This helps to control your blood pressure during the night and also helps to reduce daytime drowsiness.

If you were prescribed COMBIPRES:

- When you first start taking this medicine, you will probably urinate (pass your water) more often and in larger amounts than usual. Therefore, if you are to take 1 dose each day, your doctor may want you to take it in the morning after breakfast. If you do take it in the morning, be alert for possible drowsiness and dizziness (*see* Special Precautions below).
- If you are to take more than 1 dose each day, ask your doctor if you can take the last dose approximately 6 hours before bedtime so that you will not have to get up during the night to go to the bathroom. This effect will usually lessen after you have taken the drug for a while.

How to Administer

Take the medicine with food or a glass of water.

Special Instructions

Length of Therapy

High blood pressure (hypertension) is a long-term condition and it will probably be necessary for you to take the drug for a long time in spite of the fact that you feel better. If high blood pressure is not treated, it can lead to serious problems such as heart failure, strokes, blood vessel problems or kidney problems.

It is very important that you take this medicine as your doctor has directed and that you do not miss any doses. Otherwise, you cannot expect the drug to keep your blood pressure down.

Do not take any more of this medicine than your doctor has prescribed and *do not stop taking this medicine suddenly without the approval of your doctor*. It will be necessary for your doctor to reduce your dose slowly over 2 to 4 days since your body will need time to adjust. It could be harmful and make your condition worse if you suddenly stopped taking the medicine. Call your doctor if you develop any of the following symptoms as you are stopping the medicine: fast heartbeats, chest pain, nausea, vomiting, unexplained nervousness, shaking, headache, flushing, or stomach pain.

Pregnancy/Breastfeeding

Women who are pregnant, breastfeeding or planning to become pregnant should tell their doctor before taking this medicine.

Drug Interactions

Do not take any nonprescription drugs without the approval of your doctor or pharmacist. Some of these products can aggravate your condition and some can combine with this medicine and make the drowsiness or dizziness worse. Read the label of the product to see if there is a warning. If there is, check with your doctor or pharmacist before using the product.

Alcohol

You may become more sensitive to alcohol while you are taking this medicine. Do not drink alcoholic beverages while you are on this drug because the combination could make the possible side effects of dizziness and drowsiness worse.

Special Precautions

If this medicine causes dizziness or lightheadedness, you should be careful going up and down stairs and you should not change positions too rapidly. Lightheadedness is more likely to occur if you stand up suddenly—this is due to blood collecting in the legs and lasts for a few seconds. Therefore, get up from a sitting or lying position more slowly and tighten and relax your leg muscles or wiggle your toes to help promote circulation. In the morning, get out of bed slowly and dangle your feet over the edge of the bed for a few minutes before standing up. Sit or lie down at the first sign of dizziness. Tell your doctor if you have been dizzy.

In order to help prevent dizziness or fainting, your doctor may also recommend that you avoid strenuous exercise, standing for long periods of time (especially in hot weather), hot showers, hot baths or saunas.

Do not drive a car, operate dangerous machinery, pilot an airplane or do jobs that require you to be alert if you are dizzy or drowsy.

If your mouth becomes dry, drink water, suck ice chips or a hard, sour candy (sugarless) or chew gum (sugarless). Sugarless products are recommended in order to avoid dental problems. You may wish to ask your pharmacist about special solutions, called artificial saliva, that can also be used to help restore moisture in the mouth. It is especially important to brush and floss your teeth regularly if you develop a dry mouth to help prevent gum problems.

This medicine may cause some people to become constipated. To help prevent constipation, try increasing the amount of bulk in your diet (for example, bran, fresh fruits and salads), exercising more often or drinking more fluids (unless otherwise directed). Call your doctor if the constipation continues.

The side effects of dizziness, constipation and tiredness usually decrease after you have taken the medicine for 4 to 6 weeks.

Follow any special diet your doctor may have prescribed. It may be necessary to limit the amount of salt in your diet.

Your doctor may want you to have regular eye checkups if you will be taking this medicine for a long period of time.

If your eyes become dry, ask your doctor or pharmacist to recommend artificial tears to wet the eyes. Call your doctor if you experience itching or burning of your eyes.

If you were prescribed COMBIPRES, *the following special instructions also apply:*

- This medicine normally causes your body to lose potassium. The body has warning signs to let you know if too much potassium is being lost. Call your doctor if you become unusually thirsty or if you develop leg cramps, unusual weakness, fatigue, vomiting, confusion or an irregular pulse. Since these symptoms may not be present in all patients, your doctor may wish to check your blood occasionally to see if it is low in potassium. Depending upon your dose, your doctor may prescribe some medicine to replace the potassium or he or she may recommend that you regularly eat foods that contain a lot of potassium (see Appendix A).

  Do not change your diet unless your doctor tells you to.

- This medicine may make some people more sensitive to sunlight and various tanning lamps. When you begin taking this medicine, try to avoid too much sun until you see how you are going to react. If your skin does become more sensitive to sunlight, tell your doctor and try not to stay in direct sunlight for extended periods of time. While in the sun, wear protective clothing and sunglasses. You may wish to ask your pharmacist about suitable sunscreen products. Call your doctor if you become sunburned.

- If you have diabetes, this medicine may cause your blood sugar to rise. Carefully test your blood or urine for sugar while you are taking this medicine. Call your doctor if you think your blood sugar is higher than normal or harder to control.

When to Call Your Doctor

Any medicine can sometimes cause unwanted effects. Call your doctor if you develop paleness or coldness in the fingertips or toes, nightmares, impotence, decreased sexual function, difficulty breathing, unusual tiredness or weakness, swelling of the feet or ankles or depression.

If you were prescribed COMBIPRES:

- In addition to the previous symptoms, also call your doctor if you develop an unexplained sore throat or fever, sharp stomach pain, sharp joint pain, unusual bruising or bleeding, a yellow color to the skin or eyes, or a sudden weight gain of 5 pounds (2.5 kg) or more.

Allergic Reactions

Call your doctor immediately if you think you may be allergic to the medicine or if you develop a skin rash, hives, itching, swelling of the face or difficulty in breathing. If you cannot reach your doctor, phone a hospital emergency department.

Refills

Do not stop taking this medicine without your doctor's approval and do not go without medicine between prescription refills. Call your pharmacist for a refill 2 or 3 days before you will run out of the medicine.

Miscellaneous

Carry an identification card in your wallet or wear a medical alert bracelet indicating that you are taking this medicine as well as the names and phone numbers of your doctors. If you do not already carry such a card, complete the Medicine Card in this book. Always tell your dentist, pharmacist and other doctors who are treating you that you are taking this medicine.

Did You Know That?

You should have all of your prescriptions filled at the same pharmacy so that the pharmacist can keep a complete record of your medicines.

This is especially important if you are being treated by more than one doctor. Some drugs can interact with each other. Just as your doctor keeps your medical record, many pharmacists keep "drug records" or "drug profiles" for their patients. These drug profiles make it possible for the pharmacist to review your drug therapy each time you have a prescription filled and to help prevent you from receiving any drugs which can interact with each other.

CLOTRIMAZOLE (TOPICAL)

CANESTEN, MYCLO

CLOTRIMAZOLE (VAGINAL)

CANESTEN, CANESTEN 3, CANESTEN 1, CANESTEN 1 COMBI-PAK, MYCLO

Purpose

This medicine is used to treat fungal and yeast infections.

Allergies/Warnings

Be sure to tell your doctor and pharmacist if you are allergic to any medicine.

How to Use This Medicine

Time of Administration

The vaginal medicine is usually used at bedtime when you are lying down so that the drug is less likely to drain out.

How to Administer

For skin cream and solution, vaginal creams, and vaginal tablets, see How to Administer Medications (page 15).

For CANESTEN SOLUTION with SPRAY:

- Cleanse the affected area well unless otherwise directed by your doctor. Dry the area.

- Spray the prescribed amount of solution and massage into the affected and surrounding areas. Do NOT spray the solution on the face.

Special Instructions

Length of Therapy

It is important to use all of this medicine, plus any refills that your doctor told you to use. Do not stop using it earlier than your doctor has recommended in spite of the fact that your symptoms seem to have improved. Otherwise, the infection may return.

Pregnancy/Breastfeeding

Women who are pregnant, breastfeeding or planning to become pregnant should tell their doctor before taking this medicine. The vaginal medicines should not be used during the first 3 months of pregnancy unless otherwise directed by your doctor.

If you are pregnant, check with your doctor before using the applicator to insert the vaginal cream or tablets.

Special Precautions

If you are using this medicine to treat a fungal infection of the feet, it is important to dry the feet (especially between the toes) well after washing.

If you are using this medicine to treat a vaginal infection, you may wish to wear a sanitary napkin to protect your clothing from any drainage of the drug. Do *not* use menstrual tampons without your doctor's approval while using this drug.

In the treatment of vaginal infections, the drug is usually used throughout the menstrual period. Check with your doctor if you can have sexual intercourse or if you can douche during treatment.

It is important to wash all towels, linens, bedding and clothing in hot water after they have been in contact with the affected skin area. If it is not possible to wash them in hot water, they should be dry-cleaned. This will help prevent reinfection.

Keep the affected skin areas as dry as possible. Do not bandage the affected skin area unless directed by your doctor.

When to Call Your Doctor

Call your doctor if the condition for which you are using this medicine has not improved after 1 or 2 weeks or becomes worse or if the medicine causes itching or burning of the skin or vagina for more than a few minutes after instillation.

Also call your doctor if you are using this medicine to treat a vaginal infection and if you develop increased frequency of urination (passing your water) or stomach cramps or pains.

Also call your doctor if you are applying the medicine to the skin and you develop stinging, blistering, swelling, peeling, hives or itching of the skin.

Miscellaneous

For creams, solutions and lotions:

- This medicine is for external use only. Do not swallow it and keep it away from the eyes.

Did You Know That?

Couples with infertility problems or couples wishing to conceive now have available a reliable test that can be used to help predict ovulation.

The new ovulation test kits can be purchased without a prescription and will predict ovulation 24 to 36 hours BEFORE it occurs. Older methods of measuring the basal body temperature indicated ovulation after it had occurred. The woman is most likely to become pregnant if she has sex within the 24 hours following a positive test result. The tests are very reliable and are based on testing the urine with a small plastic strip containing monoclonal antibodies. These are highly specific molecules that detect the presence of a sharp increase in luteinizing hormone (LH), which occurs just before ovulation.

CROMOGLYCATE SODIUM (ORAL)

NALCROM

Purpose

This medicine is used to help prevent food-related allergies and some types of bowel disease.

Allergies/Warnings

If you have ever had an allergic reaction to CROMOGLYCATE, tell your doctor and pharmacist before you take any of this medicine.

How to Use This Medicine

Time of Administration

It is very important that you take this medicine exactly as your doctor has prescribed. Do not miss any doses, and take the medicine even if you feel well. Try to take this medicine at the same time(s) every day so that you will have a constant level of medicine in your body.

Take this medicine 15-20 minutes before a meal.

How to Administer

There are 2 ways to take the NALCROM CAPSULES:

(1) The preferred method is to dissolve the contents of the capsule(s) in a teaspoonful of very hot water and then dilute with 4 teaspoonsful of cold water.

(2) Take the capsules by swallowing whole with a glass of water.

Special Instructions

Length of Therapy

After you have taken this medicine for a while, the number of times you will have to use this medicine may be slowly decreased by your doctor.

Do not take any more of this medicine than your doctor has prescribed and do not stop taking this medicine suddenly without the approval of your doctor. It may be necessary for your doctor to slowly reduce your dose since your body may need time to adjust. If you should suddenly stop taking it or reduce your dose, you may experience a worsening of your condition.

Pregnancy/Breastfeeding

Women who are pregnant, breastfeeding, or planning to become pregnant should tell their doctor before taking this medicine.

When to Call Your Doctor

Most people experience few or no side effects from this drug. However, any medicine can sometimes cause unwanted effects. Call your doctor if you develop fever, nausea, unusual headaches, difficulty sleeping, skin rashes or joint pains.

Allergic Reactions

Call your doctor immediately if you think you may be allergic to the medicine or if you develop a skin rash, hives, itching, swelling of the face or difficulty in breathing. If you cannot reach your doctor, phone a hospital emergency department.

Storage

Store the capsules in a cool, dry, dark place.

Senility Due to Medicines

If an older person becomes confused or forgetful, thinks more slowly, or cannot care for himself, don't jump to the conclusion that it is due to old age. *Emergency Medicine* reports that in a research study of 308 elderly patients, adverse reactions to medications were causing symptoms of forgetfulness, confusion, falling down, and slow thought processes in 35. The types of medicines causing the problem included sleeping pills, tranquilizers, high blood pressure medicines, aspirin, CIMETIDINE, and insulin. Do not stop taking any medicines without medical advice.

CROMOGLYCATE SODIUM (INHALATION)

FIVENT INHALER, INTAL SPINCAPS, INTAL NEBULIZER

Purpose

This medicine is used to help prevent asthma attacks. It is to be taken on a continuous basis to prevent symptoms from appearing. The medicine will not help an asthma attack that has already begun—and may even make the attack worse. If an asthma attack occurs, check with your doctor regarding treatment. In some cases, the medicine will have to be changed.

This medicine is also used to help prevent bronchospasm and wheezing caused by exercise and is taken shortly before physical exertion.

Allergies/Warnings

If you have ever had an allergic reaction to CROMOGLYCATE, tell your doctor and pharmacist before you take any of this medicine.

How to Use This Medicine

Time of Administration

It is very important that you take this medicine exactly as your doctor has prescribed. Do not miss any doses, and take the medicine even if you feel well. Try to take this medicine at the same time(s) every day so that you will have a constant level of medicine in your body.

How to Administer

For INTAL SPINCAPS (INHALATION):

- These capsules must be used in the special Spinhaler or Halermatic device designed for them. DO NOT SWALLOW THE CAPSULES. The medicine must be inhaled in order to work.
- It is important to get the powder as deep as possible into the lungs.
- Follow the special administration instructions that come with these capsules. Insert one end of the capsule down into the device. *See* How to Administer Medications (page 15) for general instructions on how to hold the head and when to inhale the powder.
- Repeat the inhalation procedure until the capsule is empty.
- Do not exhale into the Spinhaler or Halermatic device because moisture from the mouth can cause powder to plug up the inhaler.
- A little powder may stick to the Spinhaler or Halermatic device during use. This is normal but the inhalers should be cleaned and dried before reuse. If there are large amounts of powder sticking to the inhaler, you may not be using it correctly.
- Wash the inhalers at least once a week and dry thoroughly. It is recommended that the inhalers be replaced after six months of use. You may obtain a new one from your pharmacist.

Special note for parents: Your doctor or pharmacist can show you how to attach a whistle on the end of the Spinhaler. This could make taking the Intal more fun for your child and may help him or her learn to use the Spinhaler properly.

For INTAL NEBULIZER SOLUTION:

- A power-operated (not hand-operated) nebulizer must be used to administer this solution.
- Be sure you understand how to use the equipment, including the face mask or mouthpiece.

For FIVENT INHALER:

- *See* How to Administer Medications (page 15).
- To test the inhaler, press down on the canister once. The dose can be seen as a fine white mist. This mist should never be seen to escape from the mouth or nose during a treatment. If it is seen, you are not using the inhaler correctly.
- Keep the cap on the inhaler when it is not in use. This will keep dirt out of the inhaler.

- The inhaler should be cleaned approximately once a week. Remove the canister from the plastic mouthpiece. Wash the mouthpiece in warm water and dry thoroughly before replacing the canister.

Special Instructions

Length of Therapy

It may take 1 to 4 weeks before you feel the full benefit of this medicine.

If you are also using another inhaler containing a bronchodilator to open up the air passages in your lungs, use the bronchodilator several minutes before you use this CROMOGLYCATE inhaler.

After you have taken CROMOGLYCATE for a while and your asthma symptoms have decreased, the number of times you will have to use this medicine may be slowly reduced by your doctor.

Do not take any more of this medicine than your doctor has prescribed and do not stop taking this medicine suddenly without the approval of your doctor. It may be necessary for your doctor to slowly reduce your dose since your body may need time to adjust. If you should suddenly stop taking it or reduce your dose, you may experience a worsening of your asthma.

Pregnancy/Breastfeeding

Women who are pregnant, breastfeeding, or planning to become pregnant should tell their doctor before taking this medicine.

Special Precautions

Drinking a few sips of water or gargling after each inhalation may help decrease mild throat irritation, cough or hoarseness which may be caused by the powder.

If you develop coughing or wheezing after using this drug, check with your doctor. Use of a bronchodilator aerosol may be helpful prior to inhaling the CROMOGLYCATE.

When to Call Your Doctor

Most people experience few or no side effects from this drug. However, any medicine can sometimes cause unwanted effects. Call your doctor if you develop fever or coughing, difficulty in urinating (passing your water), dizziness or severe headaches, joint or muscle pain, nausea or vomiting, trouble in swallowing, swollen glands, severe nasal congestion, difficulty in breathing or increased wheezing.

Allergic Reactions

Call your doctor immediately if you think you may be allergic to the medicine or if you develop a skin rash, hives, itching, swelling of the face or difficulty in breathing. If you cannot reach your doctor, phone a hospital emergency department.

Storage

Store the capsules in a cool, dry, dark place. Do not refrigerate the capsules. Do not freeze the solution.

Store FIVENT INHALER at room temperature. Do not place it in hot water or near radiators, stoves, or other sources of heat. Do not puncture, burn or incinerate the container (even when it is empty).

CROMOGLYCATE SODIUM (NASAL)

RYNACROM CARTRIDGES, RYNACROM NASAL SOLUTION

Purpose

This nasal medicine is used to help prevent and treat allergic rhinitis. The medicine helps relieve the symptoms of nasal congestion, runny nose, sneezing, difficulty in breathing and postnasal drip.

Allergies/Warnings

If you have ever had an allergic reaction to CROMOGLYCATE, tell your doctor and pharmacist before you take any of this medicine. Tell your doctor and pharmacist if you have nasal polyps. This medicine may not be able to reach the nasal membranes if you have nasal polyps, and may not be effective.

How to Use This Medicine

Time of Administration

It is very important that you take this medicine exactly as your doctor has prescribed. Do not miss any doses during the treatment period and take the medicine even if you feel well. Try to take this medicine at the same time(s) every day so that you will have a constant level of medicine in your nose.

How to Administer

For RYNACROM NASAL SOLUTION:

- Assemble the unit according to the special instructions that come with the medicine and use the special RYNACROM device to administer the spray into the nose.

- Do not wash the pump unit before transferring it to the refill bottle.
- Before using the nasal spray, blow the nose gently. This will remove mucus from the nose and make it possible for the medicine to have better contact with the nasal membranes. If your nose is severely congested, your doctor may recommend that you use a nasal decongestant first.
- Insert the tip of the RYNACROM device into the nostril and press the bottle firmly upwards with the thumb in order to release one dose. One spray releases one dose. Sniff gently at the same time.
- If the unit does not spray properly, the outside case may be cleaned with warm water and thoroughly dried in order to remove any material that could clog the spray opening.
- When the bottle is empty, remove it from the plastic case, unscrew the pump and insert a refill.

Be sure to replace the cap on the RYNACROM pump after every use so that dirt cannot get into the solution.

For RYNACROM CARTRIDGES:

- Use the cartridge with the special RYNACROM Nasal Insufflator tube.
- Follow the instructions that come with the medicine.
- The manufacturer does NOT recommend that the device be cleaned. It is recommended that the special spray device be replaced every six months.

Special Instructions

Length of Therapy

It may take 1 to 4 weeks before the full benefit is noticed. Seasonal allergic rhinitis (often associated with high pollen counts during certain seasons) will usually respond after 1 week of treatment. Chronic or perennial allergic rhinitis (occurs year-round) may take up to 4 weeks before a response is seen.

Do not stop using this medicine suddenly. It is recommended that the dosage be reduced gradually over at least 7 days.

Pregnancy/Breastfeeding

Women who are pregnant, breastfeeding or planning to become pregnant should tell their doctor before taking this medicine.

Special Precautions

Some patients may experience nasal stinging or sneezing immediately after using the medicine. This is not unusual. Call your doctor if the stinging or sneezing becomes severe.

You may also experience occasional headache, cough and an unpleasant taste in the mouth. This is not unusual. Call your doctor if they become bothersome.

When to Call Your Doctor

Most people experience few or no side effects from this drug. However, any medicine can sometimes cause unwanted effects. Call your doctor if your symptoms do not improve or get worse, or if you develop nosebleeds, coughing, a rash, trouble swallowing, wheezing or difficulty breathing, increased sneezing or severe burning in the nose.

Allergic Reactions

Call your doctor immediately if you think you may be allergic to the medicine or if you develop a skin rash, hives, itching, swelling of the face or difficulty in breathing. If you cannot reach your doctor, phone a hospital emergency department.

Storage

Store at room temperature and in a dry, dark place.

CROMOGLYCATE SODIUM (OPHTHALMIC)

OPTICROM, VISTACROM

Purpose

This medicine is used to treat seasonal allergic disorders of the eye.

Allergies/Warnings

If you have ever had an allergic reaction to CROMOGLYCATE, tell your doctor and pharmacist before you take any of this medicine.

How to Use This Medicine

Time of Administration

It is very important that you use this medicine exactly as your doctor has prescribed. Do not miss any doses. Try to instill the drops at the same time(s) every day so that you will have a constant level of the medicine in your eye.

How to Administer

For eye drops and eye ointment: see How to Administer Medications (page 15).

Special Instructions

Length of Therapy

Decreased itching, tearing, redness and discharge is usually evident within a few days of treatment. Treatment may be required for up to 6 weeks.

Pregnancy/Breastfeeding

Women who are pregnant, breastfeeding, or planning to become pregnant should tell their doctor before taking this medicine.

Special Precautions

For eye drops:

- The manufacturer recommends that people who wear soft (hydrophilic) contact lenses should not wear them during treatment.

For eye ointment:

- OPTICROM OINTMENT should not be used when hard or soft contact lenses are in place.

This medicine may cause a mild stinging or burning sensation. This is not unusual.

Do not share this eye medicine with other people. Any germs or infections could be transferred.

Vision may be blurred for a few seconds after applying the ointment. Do not drive a car or operate dangerous machinery until your vision has cleared.

When to Call Your Doctor

Most people experience few or no side effects from this drug. However, any medicine can sometimes cause unwanted effects. Call your doctor if you develop severe swelling of the eye, unexplained burning or stinging, or if the condition does not improve.

Allergic Reactions

Call your doctor immediately if you think you may be allergic to the medicine or if you develop a skin rash, hives, itching, swelling of the face, or difficulty in breathing. If you cannot reach your doctor, phone a hospital emergency department.

Storage

Store in a cool, dark place.

Discard the medicine 4 weeks after opening the bottle or sooner if the label indicates an earlier expiration date.

CYCLOBENZAPRINE (ORAL)

FLEXERIL

Purpose

This medicine is used to relax muscles and to help relieve muscle pain and stiffness.

Allergies/Warnings

If you have ever had an allergic reaction to any medicine or if you have glaucoma, an enlarged prostate, difficulty urinating, hyperthyroidism, heart condition, or any other medical condition, tell your doctor and pharmacist before you take any of this medicine.

How to Use This Medicine

Time of Administration

This medicine may be taken with food or a glass of water.

Special Instructions

Length of Therapy

This medicine should only be used for short periods of time (generally up to 2 or 3 weeks).

Do not take any more of this medicine than your doctor has prescribed and do not stop taking this medicine suddenly without the approval of your doctor. It may be necessary for your doctor to reduce your dose slowly since your body may need time to adjust. If you suddenly stop taking the medicine, you may develop nausea, headache or tiredness.

Pregnancy/Breastfeeding

Women who are pregnant, breastfeeding or planning to become pregnant should tell their doctor before taking this medicine.

Drug Interactions

It is important that you obtain the advice of your doctor or pharmacist before taking any other prescription or nonprescription medicines including pain relievers, sleeping pills, tranquilizers, medicine for seizures, muscle relaxants, anesthetics, medicines for depression, medicines for allergies, colds or sinus products. Combining this medicine with some of these drugs could cause drowsiness or dizziness.

There are other drug interactions that can occur. If you are taking any other medicines, be sure to check first with your pharmacist or doctor.

Alcohol

Do not drink alcoholic beverages while taking this drug without the approval of your doctor because the combination could cause severe drowsiness.

Special Precautions

If your mouth becomes dry, drink water, suck ice chips or a hard, sour candy (sugarless) or chew gum (sugarless). Sugarless products are recommended in order to avoid dental problems. You may wish to ask your pharmacist about special solutions, called artificial saliva, that can also be used to help restore moisture in the mouth. It is especially important to brush and floss your teeth regularly if you develop a dry mouth to help prevent gum problems.

This drug commonly causes dizziness and drowsiness. Do not drive a car, pilot an airplane, operate dangerous machinery or do jobs that require you to be alert until you know how you are going to react to the drug. You should also be careful going up and down stairs. Sit or lie down at the first sign of dizziness. Tell your doctor if the drowsiness or dizziness continues.

This medicine may cause some people to become constipated. To help prevent constipation, try increasing the amount of bulk in your diet (for example, bran, fresh fruits and salads), exercising more often or drinking more fluids (unless otherwise directed). Call your doctor if the constipation continues.

When to Call Your Doctor

Most people experience few or no side effects from this drug. However, any medicine can sometimes cause unwanted effects. Call your doctor if you develop fast or irregular heartbeats, difficulty breathing, numbness of the hands or feet, stomach pain or constipation, trembling, difficulty in urinating (passing your water), eye pain, unusual sweating, seizures, unusual nervousness or if you become confused or depressed.

Allergic Reactions

Call your doctor immediately if you think you may be allergic to the medicine or if you develop a skin rash, hives, itching, swelling of the face or difficulty in breathing. If you cannot reach your doctor, phone a hospital emergency department.

CYPROHEPTADINE HCl (ORAL)

PERIACTIN

Purpose

This medicine is often used to help relieve symptoms (such as itching) of certain types of allergic conditions. This drug has several other uses (such as increasing the appetite and promoting weight gain) and the reason it was prescribed depends upon your condition. Check with your doctor if you do not understand why you are taking it.

Allergies/Warnings

If you have ever had an allergic reaction to any medicine or if you have asthma, glaucoma, an enlarged prostate, urinary retention (a type of bladder problem), high blood pressure or diabetes, tell your doctor and pharmacist before you take any of this medicine.

This medicine is not recommended for children under 2 years of age.

How to Use This Medicine

Time of Administration

It is best to take this medicine with food to help prevent stomach upset.

For syrup:

- *See* How to Administer Medications (page 15).

Special Instructions

Length of Therapy

Do not take this medicine more often or longer than recommended by your doctor. To do so may increase your chance of developing side effects.

Pregnancy/Breastfeeding

Women who are pregnant, breastfeeding or planning to become pregnant should tell their doctor before taking this medicine. Safe use during pregnancy has not been established.

Drug Interactions

It is important that you obtain the advice of your doctor or pharmacist before taking any other prescription or nonprescription medicines including pain relievers, sleeping pills, tranquilizers, medicine for seizures, muscle relaxants, anesthetics, medicines for depression or other medicines for allergies. Combining this medicine with some of these drugs could cause drowsiness or dizziness.

There are other drug interactions that can occur. If you are taking any other medicines, be sure to check first with your pharmacist or doctor.

Alcohol

Do not drink alcoholic beverages while taking this drug without the approval of your doctor because the combination could cause drowsiness. One drink may have the same effect that 2 or 3 drinks normally would have.

Special Precautions

In some people, this drug may initially cause dizziness or drowsiness. Do not drive a car, pilot an airplane, operate dangerous machinery or do jobs that require you to be alert until you know how you are going to react to the drug. If you become dizzy or drowsy, you should be careful going up and down stairs. Sit or lie down at the first sign of dizziness. Tell your doctor if the dizziness or drowsiness continues.

People over 65 years of age may be more sensitive to these side effects.

If your mouth becomes dry, drink water, suck ice chips or a hard, sour candy (sugarless) or chew gum (sugarless). Sugarless products are recommended in order to avoid dental problems. You may wish to ask your pharmacist about special solutions, called artificial saliva, that can also be used to help restore moisture in the mouth. It is especially important to brush and floss your teeth regularly if you develop a dry mouth to help prevent gum problems.

When to Call Your Doctor

Most people experience few or no side effects from this drug. However, any medicine can sometimes cause unwanted effects. Call your doctor if you develop a skin rash, fast or irregular heartbeats, blurred vision, stomach pain, unexplained weakness or tiredness, unexplained sore throat, fever, or mouth sores, unusual bruising or bleeding, unexplained nervousness, restlessness or irritability (especially in children), trouble sleeping, difficulty in urinating (passing your water) or if mucus (lung secretions) becomes thicker than usual.

Storage

If you were prescribed PERIACTIN SYRUP, do not freeze the medicine.

ORAL:

DICLOFENAC SODIUM
VOLTAREN, VOLTAREN S.R.

FENOPROFEN CALCIUM
NALFON

FLURBIPROFEN
ANSAID, FROBEN

IBUPROFEN
AMERSOL, APO-IBUPROFEN, MOTRIN, NOVOPROFEN

KETOPROFEN
ORUDIS, ORUDIS E-50, ORUDIS E-100

NAPROXEN
APO-NAPROXEN, NAPROSYN, NAXEN, NOVONAPROX

NAPROXEN SODIUM
ANAPROX

PIROXICAM
APO-PIROXICAM, FELDENE, NOVOPIROCAM

SULINDAC
CLINORIL

TIAPROFENIC ACID
SURGAM

TOLMETIN SODIUM
TOLECTIN

RECTAL:

DICLOFENAC
VOLTAREN SUPPOSITORIES

KETOPROFEN
ORUDIS SUPPOSITORIES

NAPROXEN
NAPROSYN SUPPOSITORIES

PIROXICAM
FELDENE SUPPOSITORIES

Purpose

This medicine is used to help relieve pain. Some of the medicines are to help relieve inflammation, stiffness, swelling and joint pain in certain kinds of arthritis or rheumatism. Some of the products are used to relieve menstrual cramps, dental pain, and the symptoms of gout, bursitis, tendinitis, muscle sprains or strains.

Allergies/Warnings

If you have ever had an allergic reaction to ASA (acetylsalicylic acid) or any other medicine or if you suffer from hay fever, asthma, nasal polyps, ulcers or stomach problems (such as heartburn), heart, kidney or liver problems or high blood pressure, tell your doctor and pharmacist before you take any of this medicine.

Tell your doctor if you take diuretics (water pills).

How to Use This Medicine

Time of Administration

For tablets and capsules containing FENOPROFEN, FLURBIPROFEN, IBUPROFEN, KETOPROFEN (ORUDIS CAPSULES), NAPROXEN, PIROXICAM, TIAPROFENIC ACID *and* TOLMETIN:

- This medicine will work whether or not you take it with food. To help lessen stomach upset, your doctor may recommend that you take this medicine with some food, after a meal, or with a glass of milk. Always take the medicine with a full glass of water, unless otherwise directed. It also may be helpful not to lie down for 15 minutes after taking the medicine so that the medicine can reach the stomach. Call your doctor if you develop stomach upset (indigestion, nausea, vomiting, stomach pain) that does not go away.

Special Note for ORUDIS E-50, ORUDIS E-100: It is best to take this medicine with a glass of water—not with milk or antacids. Milk or antacids can interfere with the special coating on this medicine.

For tablets containing DICLOFENAC *and* SULINDAC:

- Always take this medicine with food or immediately after meals to help prevent stomach upset. If you develop persistent stomach pain, nausea, vomiting or indigestion, contact your doctor.

If you were prescribed ORUDIS E-50, ORUDIS E-100, VOLTAREN *or*

VOTAREN S.R.:

- This medicine must be swallowed whole. Do not crush, chew or break tablets into pieces. Do not take these tablets within 1 hour of milk or antacids as this will dissolve the enteric coating designed to prevent stomach irritation.

For suppositories:

- *See* How to Administer Medications (page 15).

Special Instructions

Length of Therapy

This medicine will not cure arthritis but it can help control inflammation that can increase damage to your joints. It is very important that you take this medicine regularly and that you *do not miss any doses.* If you miss a dose, the level of the medicine in your body will fall and the drug will not be as effective. Only if the drug is at the right level will it be able to decrease the inflammation and swelling in your joints and help prevent further damage.

If you are taking this medicine for a joint or bone problem, you may have to take the drug for a few weeks before you feel its full benefits. Long-term therapy is often required in arthritis.

This medicine does not replace any exercise or rest programs or use of heat/cold treatments your doctor may have prescribed.

Pregnancy/Breastfeeding

Women who are pregnant, breastfeeding or planning to become pregnant should tell their doctor before taking this medicine. Use of this medicine during pregnancy, especially the last three months, and during breastfeeding is not recommended.

Drug Interactions

Do not take any other medicines containing ASA (acetylsalicylic acid), or salicylates or other prescription medicines used to treat arthritis while you are taking this medicine without contacting your doctor.

It is usually safe to take acetaminophen for fever or the occasional headache. Check with your pharmacist.

Do not take TOLMETIN with antacids containing sodium bicarbonate or baking soda because you might take too much sodium.

Alcohol

Do not drink alcoholic beverages while taking this drug without the approval of your doctor because the combination could cause stomach problems.

Special Precautions

In some people, this drug may cause dizziness or blurred vision. Do not drive a car, pilot an airplane, operate dangerous machinery or do jobs that require you to be alert until you know how you are going to react to this drug. If you become dizzy, you should be careful going up and down stairs. Sit or lie down at the first sign of dizziness. Tell your doctor if you have been dizzy. Call your doctor if you develop blurred vision.

This medicine may cause some people to become constipated. To help prevent constipation, try increasing the amount of bulk in your diet (for example, bran, fresh fruits and salads), exercising more often or drinking more fluids (unless otherwise directed). Call your doctor if the constipation continues.

When to Call Your Doctor

Most people experience few or no side effects from this drug. However, any medicine can sometimes cause unwanted effects. Call your doctor if you develop a skin rash, sore throat or fever, chills, flulike symptoms, ringing or buzzing in the ears, hearing problems, a feeling of fullness in the ears, fast heartbeats, shortness of breath, wheezing or tightness in the chest, swelling of the legs or ankles or sudden weight gain, blurred vision or changes in your eyesight, hearing loss or ear pain, bloody or black stools, severe stomach pain, vomiting of blood, yellow color to the skin or eyes, unusual bruising or bleeding, unusual tiredness or weakness, depression, confusion, difficulty in urinating (passing your water), decrease in the amount of urine, blood in the urine or a persistent headache.

Allergic Reactions

Call your doctor immediately if you think you may be allergic to the medicine or if you develop a skin rash, hives, itching, fast or irregular heartbeats, fainting, swelling of the face or difficulty in breathing. If you cannot reach your doctor, phone a hospital emergency department.

Storage

For tablets and capsules:

- Store the medicine in a cool, dry, dark place.

For suppositories:

- *See* How to Administer Medications (page 15).

Did You Know That?

Beekeepers should think twice before taking some anti-inflammatory drugs. The drugs may reverse their immunity to bee stings.

During the last few years, several new nonsteroidal anti-inflammatory drugs have been developed to relieve pain and reduce stiffness, swelling and joint pain associated with inflammation. Such drugs include IBUPROFEN, FENOPROFEN, NAPROXEN, KETOPROFEN, SULINDAC, PIROXICAM, and TOLMETIN.

It is well known that beekeepers develop an immunity to bee stings and it has even been reported that some people get temporary relief from the pain of arthritis if they sustain several bee stings. The *British Medical Journal* recently reported that two people with an immunity to bee stings taking a nonsteroidal anti-inflammatory drug had suffered serious allergic reactions to bee and wasp stings.

A 66-year-old beekeeper had developed an apparent immunity to bee stings over six years. She was prescribed a nonsteroidal anti-inflammatory drug for osteoarthrosis. A few months after taking the drug, she was stung on the wrists while working around the beehives and within 15 minutes developed heart palpitations, a rash and swelling of the mouth and tongue, making it difficult for her to breathe. She stopped taking the drug and 48 hours later when she was stung again, she developed no reaction.

Another report describes the 48-year-old wife of a beekeeper who had been taking a nonsteroidal anti-inflammatory drug for five months for osteoarthritis. She had previously had only skin reactions to wasp stings but one day she developed widespread swelling; red, itchy rash; heart palpitations and shortness of breath within two minutes of being stung by a wasp. Hospitalization was necessary.

Until more is learned about the reason for these reactions, beekeepers should be aware of the potential hazard associated with these drugs and bee stings.

Refills

Do not stop taking this medicine without your doctor's approval and do not go without medicine between prescription refills. Call your pharmacist for a refill 2 or 3 days before you will run out of the medicine.

Discuss with your pharmacist the implications of dispensing all your refills for this medicine with the same manufacturer's product. (*See* Generic Drugs, page 12.)

Miscellaneous

Carry an identification card in your wallet or wear a medical alert bracelet indicating that you are taking this medicine as well as the names and phone numbers of your doctors. If you do not already carry such a card, complete the Medicine Card in this book. Always tell your dentist, pharmacist and other doctors who are treating you that you are taking this medicine.

DICYCLOMINE HCl (ORAL)

BENTYLOL, BENTYLOL DOSPAN, FORMULEX, LOMINE, PROTYLOL, SPASMOBAN, VISCEROL

DICYCLOMINE HCl-PHENOBARBITAL

BENTYLOL WITH PHENOBARBITAL, DICLOPHEN, SPASMOBAN-PH

Purpose

This medicine is used to help relax muscles and to help relieve cramps and spasms of the stomach and bowels. It is also used in infants (over 6 months of age) to treat infant colic.

Allergies/Warnings

If you have ever had an allergic reaction to atropine, a barbiturate, or any other drug used to relax the stomach or bowels or if you have glaucoma, enlarged prostate, difficulty urinating (passing your water) or any other medical condition, tell your doctor and pharmacist before you take any of this medicine.

How to Use This Medicine

Time of Administration

Take this medicine approximately 30 minutes before a meal unless otherwise directed.

How to Administer

If you were prescribed BENTYLOL DOSPAN TABLETS:

- These tablets are long-acting and must be swallowed whole. Do not crush or chew the tablets.

For infants (over 6 months of age):

- If the syrup form of the drug has been prescribed for a baby, the syrup may be diluted with an equal amount of water.
- Measure the dose very carefully for the baby. If a spoon is used to measure the dose, it is recommended that you use a medicine spoon or an oral liquid syringe that you can obtain from your pharmacist. These are more accurate than the average household teaspoon. *See* How to Administer Medications (page 15).

Special Instructions

Length of Therapy

Do not take this medicine more often or longer than recommended by your doctor. To do so may increase your chance of developing side effects.

If you were prescribed BENTYLOL WITH PHENOBARBITAL, DICLOPHEN *or* SPASMOBAN-PH:

- Do not stop taking this medicine suddenly without the approval of your doctor. It may be necessary for your doctor to reduce your dose slowly since your body may need time to adjust.
- Check with your doctor if you develop any of the following while you are slowly stopping the medicine: nausea or vomiting, feeling faint, trembling, seizures, changes in vision or trouble sleeping.

Pregnancy/Breastfeeding

Women who are pregnant or planning to become pregnant should tell their doctor before taking this medicine.

Women who are breastfeeding should tell their doctor before taking this medicine. This drug may decrease the amount of breast milk produced and may appear in the breast milk.

Drug Interactions

It is important that you obtain the advice of your doctor or pharmacist before taking any other prescription or nonprescription medicines including pain relievers, sleeping pills, tranquilizers, medicine for seizures, muscle relaxants, anesthetics, medicines for depression or medicines for allergies, colds or sinus conditions. Combining this medicine with some of these drugs could cause drowsiness or dizziness.

Do not take this medicine at the same time as an antacid or an antidiarrhea medicine. Try to space them at least 1 hour apart.

There are other drug interactions that can occur. If you are taking any other medicines, be sure to check first with your pharmacist or doctor.

Alcohol

Do not drink alcoholic beverages while taking this drug without the approval of your doctor because the combination could cause severe drowsiness or dizziness. One drink may have the same effect that 2 or 3 drinks normally would have.

Special Precautions

If your mouth becomes dry, drink water, suck ice chips or a hard, sour candy (sugarless) or chew gum (sugarless). Sugarless products are recommended in order to avoid dental problems. You may wish to ask your pharmacist about special solutions, called artificial saliva, that can also be used to help restore moisture in the mouth. It is especially important to brush and floss your teeth regularly if you develop a dry mouth to help prevent gum problems.

In some people, this drug may cause dizziness, drowsiness or blurred vision. Do not drive a car, pilot an airplane, operate dangerous machinery or do jobs that require you to be alert if you are dizzy or drowsy. You should also be careful going up and down stairs. Sit or lie down at the first sign of dizziness. Tell your doctor if these problems continue.

An urge to urinate (pass your water) with an inability to do so sometimes occurs with this drug. Urinating before taking the drug each time may help relieve this problem. Tell your doctor if you are having this problem.

You may become more sensitive to heat because your body may perspire less while you are taking this drug. Be careful not to become overheated during exercise or in hot weather. Try to avoid strenuous exercise, standing for long periods of time (especially in hot weather), hot showers, hot baths, saunas or Jacuzzis while taking this medicine.

If your eyes become more sensitive to sunlight, it may help to wear sunglasses.

This medicine may cause some people to become constipated. To help prevent constipation, try increasing the amount of bulk in your diet (for example, bran, fresh fruits and salads), exercising more often or drinking more fluids (unless otherwise directed). Call your doctor if the constipation continues.

Did You Know That?

You should not give any medicine to a child less than one year of age unless the medicine has been prescribed by your doctor.

Do not give any nonprescription drugs to children between 1 and 12 years of age unless the doses for the different age groups are listed on the package container. If you have any questions, check with your pharmacist.

When to Call Your Doctor

Most people experience few or no side effects from this drug. However, any medicine can sometimes cause unwanted effects. Call your doctor if you develop a skin rash, diarrhea or constipation, difficulty urinating (passing your water), unusual restlessness or confusion, flushing, blurred vision, eye pain or fast heartbeats.

If you were prescribed BENTYLOL WITH PHENOBARBITAL, DICLOPHEN, SPASMOBAN-PH:

- Also call your doctor if you develop a sore throat, fever, mouth sores, a staggering walk, a yellow color to the skin or eyes, unusual bruising or bleeding, slow heartbeats or shortness of breath, bothersome sleepiness or tiredness during the day, unusual nervousness, confusion or depression, hallucinations, trouble sleeping, nightmares or slurred speech.

Did You Know That?

If a person has diarrhea, some medicines may be absorbed poorly.

If a medicine is normally absorbed in the intestines, diarrhea can cause the medicine to move too quickly through the intestines for complete absorption to occur.

The same problem can occur if a person develops diarrhea after taking strong irritating laxatives.

Allergic Reactions

Call your doctor immediately if you think you may be allergic to the medicine or if you develop a skin rash, hives, itching, swelling of the face or difficulty in breathing. If you cannot reach your doctor, phone a hospital emergency department.

DIETHYLPROPION (ORAL)

NOBESINE-75, TENUATE, TENUATE DOSPAN

PHENTERMINE HCl

FASTIN, IONAMIN

Purpose

This medicine is used to help decrease the appetite in weight reduction programs. It can help you develop new eating habits but is only useful for a short time.

Allergies/Warnings

If you have ever had an allergic reaction to any medicine or if you have epilepsy, diabetes, hyperthyroidism, glaucoma, high blood pressure, a heart condition or any other medical condition, tell your doctor and pharmacist before you take any of this medicine.

How to Use This Medicine

Time of Administration

Do not take this medicine late in the day since it may cause insomnia (difficulty in sleeping). It is recommended that IONAMIN be taken 10 to 14 hours before going to bed. NOBESINE-75 and TENUATE DOSPAN should be taken mid-morning.

How to Administer

Take this medicine with a glass of water.

If you were prescribed IONAMIN, NOBESINE-75 *or* TENUATE DOSPAN:

- This medicine is long-acting and must be swallowed whole. Do not crush or chew.

Special Instructions

Length of Therapy

Do not take any more of this medicine than your doctor has prescribed and do not stop taking it suddenly without the approval of your doctor. If you have been taking the medicine for a few weeks and stopped taking it suddenly, you could develop unwanted side effects such as nausea or vomiting, stomach cramps, trembling, depression, or unusual tiredness or weakness. Call your doctor if any of these symptoms appear.

Pregnancy/Breastfeeding

Women who are pregnant, breastfeeding or planning to become pregnant should tell their doctor before taking this medicine.

Drug Interactions

Avoid drinking large amounts of coffee, tea, cocoa or cola drinks because you could be more sensitive to the caffeine in these beverages. Also check the label of nonprescription products, especially decongestants and pain relievers, to see if they contain caffeine. Check with your pharmacist if you have any questions.

It is important that you obtain the advice of your doctor or pharmacist before taking any other medicines including decongestants, cough/cold or allergy medicines or other diet or weight reducing medicines.

Alcohol

Do not drink alcoholic beverages while taking this drug without the approval of your doctor.

Special Precautions

It is very important that you follow the diet prescribed by your doctor.

If your mouth becomes dry, drink water, suck ice chips or a hard, sour candy (sugarless) or chew gum (sugarless). Sugarless products are recommended in order to avoid dental problems. You may wish to ask your pharmacist about special solutions, called artificial saliva, that can also be used to help restore moisture in the mouth. It is especially important to brush and floss your teeth regularly if you develop a dry mouth to help prevent gum problems.

In some people, this drug may cause dizziness. Do not drive a car, pilot an airplane, operate dangerous machinery or do jobs that require you to be alert if you are dizzy or drowsy. You should also be careful going up and down stairs. Sit or lie down at the first sign of dizziness. Tell your doctor if the dizziness continues.

When to Call Your Doctor

If you think the medicine is not working as well as it first did, do not increase the dose. Call your doctor.

Most people experience few or no side effects from this drug. However, any medicine can sometimes cause unwanted effects. Call your doctor if you develop a skin rash, sore throat, fever, mouth sores, unusual nervousness, fast or irregular heartbeats, difficulty in urinating (passing your water), nausea or vomiting, stomach cramps, trembling, change in sexual ability, convulsions or depression.

Did You Know That?

An alarming number of teenagers may be inducing vomiting and taking laxatives and diuretics in order to lose weight.

The *Journal of the American Medical Association* reports that in a study of 1728 tenth-grade students, 13% of the teenagers reported some form of purging behavior: diet pills, laxatives, diuretics and self-induced vomiting. They had a condition called bulimia which is characterized by a pattern of binge eating followed by fasting and/or some type of purging. This condition occurs in both men and women.

The pressure of society to be slim typically begins with weight loss attempts and dieting that results in hunger. The hunger is satisfied with binge eating. After the large meal, fear of weight gain and guilt take over and the person induces vomiting or some other method of removing the food from the body. This can lead to serious medical complications such as acute gastric dilation and rupture, aspiration pneumonitis, metabolic alkalosis, low potassium levels, tooth loss, erosion of tooth enamel, rupture of the esophagus, inflammation of the esophagus and enlargement of the parotid gland.

Any person who has abrupt swings in their food intake between dieting/fasting and then gorging themselves should seek medical advice.

DIFLUNISAL (ORAL)

DOLOBID

Purpose

This medicine is used to help relieve pain. It is also used to help relieve

NONPRESCRIPTION MEDICINES
I Am Taking the Following
Nonprescription Medicines:

Check with your pharmacist before you take any medicines that you can buy without a prescription. They could interact with your prescription medicines.

Carry this card in your wallet. It could save your life!

MEDICINE CARD

Name
Address

Home Phone Number ( )

In an Emergency Call:
Doctor Phone
Pharmacy Phone
Relative/Friend Phone
Allergies to Drugs:
Medical Problems:

From *Understanding Canadian Prescription Drugs*
Published by Key Porter Books Limited

NONPRESCRIPTION MEDICINES
I Am Taking the Following
Nonprescription Medicines:

Check with your pharmacist before you take any medicines that you can buy without a prescription. They could interact with your prescription medicines.

Carry this card in your wallet. It could save your life!

MEDICINE CARD

Name
Address

Home Phone Number ( ) -

In an Emergency Call:
Doctor Phone
Pharmacy Phone
Relative/Friend Phone
Allergies to Drugs:
Medical Problems:

From *Understanding Canadian Prescription Drugs*
Published by Key Porter Books Limited

NONPRESCRIPTION MEDICINES
I Am Taking the Following
Nonprescription Medicines:

Check with your pharmacist before you take any medicines that you can buy without a prescription. They could interact with your prescription medicines.

Carry this card in your wallet. It could save your life!

MEDICINE CARD

Name
Address

Home Phone Number ( ) -

In an Emergency Call:
Doctor Phone
Pharmacy Phone
Relative/Friend Phone
Allergies to Drugs:
Medical Problems:

From *Understanding Canadian Prescription Drugs*
Published by Key Porter Books Limited

NONPRESCRIPTION MEDICINES
I Am Taking the Following
Nonprescription Medicines:

Check with your pharmacist before you take any medicines that you can buy without a prescription. They could interact with your prescription medicines.

Carry this card in your wallet. It could save your life!

MEDICINE CARD

Name
Address

Home Phone Number ( ) -

In an Emergency Call:
Doctor Phone
Pharmacy Phone
Relative/Friend Phone
Allergies to Drugs:
Medical Problems:

From *Understanding Canadian Prescription Drugs*
Published by Key Porter Books Limited

PRESCRIPTION MEDICINES

Prescription No.	Name of Medicine	Strength	Date Started	Directions

PRESCRIPTION MEDICINES

Prescription No.	Name of Medicine	Strength	Date Started	Directions

PRESCRIPTION MEDICINES

Prescription No.	Name of Medicine	Strength	Date Started	Directions

PRESCRIPTION MEDICINES

Prescription No.	Name of Medicine	Strength	Date Started	Directions

inflammation, stiffness, swelling and joint pain in certain kinds of arthritis.

Allergies/Warnings

If you have ever had an allergic reaction to ASA or any other medicine or if you suffer from hay fever, asthma, nasal polyps, ulcers or other medical problems, tell your doctor and pharmacist before you take any of this medicine.

How to Use This Medicine

Time of Administration

This medicine will work whether or not you take it with food. However, if you develop stomach upset after taking the drug, take it with some food or a glass of milk. If the stomach upset continues, check with your doctor.

How to Administer

Swallow the tablets whole with a full glass of water. Do not crush, chew or break them into pieces.

Special Instructions

Length of Therapy

This medicine will not cure arthritis but it can help control inflammation that may damage your joints. It is very important that you take this medicine regularly and that you *do not miss any doses*. If you miss a dose, the level of the medicine in your body will fall and the drug will not be as effective. Only if the drug is at the right level will it be able to decrease the inflammation and swelling in your joints and help prevent further damage.

It may take up to 1 or 2 weeks before you feel the full benefit of the medicine.

Pregnancy/Breastfeeding

Women who are pregnant, breastfeeding or planning to become pregnant should tell their doctor before taking this medicine. Use of this medicine during pregnancy, especially the last three months, is not recommended.

Drug Interactions

Check with your doctor or pharmacist before taking any other medicines containing ASA, acetaminophen or salicylates or other medicines used to treat arthritis while you are taking this medicine.

Do not take antacids on a regular basis while you are taking this medicine because the antacids may decrease the effect of this medicine. Occasional doses of antacids may not interfere with your therapy. Check with your pharmacist or doctor.

Alcohol

Do not drink alcoholic beverages while taking this drug without the approval of your doctor because the combination could cause stomach problems.

Special Precautions

In some people, this medicine may cause dizziness. Do not drive a car, pilot an airplane, operate dangerous machinery or do jobs that require you to be alert until you know how you are going to react to this drug. If you become dizzy, you should be careful going up and down stairs. Sit or lie down at the first sign of dizziness. Tell your doctor if you have been dizzy.

When to Call Your Doctor

Most people experience few or no side effects from this drug. However, any medicine can sometimes cause unwanted effects. Call your doctor if you develop a skin rash, sore throat or fever, ringing or buzzing in the ears, a feeling of fullness in the ears, swelling of the legs or ankles or sudden weight gain, bloody or black stools, severe stomach pain, vomiting of blood, yellow color to the skin or eyes, unusual bruising or bleeding, sudden decrease in urination (passing of water), unusual tiredness or weakness or confusion.

Allergic Reactions

Call your doctor immediately if you think you may be allergic to the medicine or if you develop a skin rash, hives, itching, swelling of the face or difficulty in breathing. If you cannot reach your doctor, phone a hospital emergency department.

Refills

Do not stop taking this medicine without your doctor's approval and do not go without medicine between prescription refills. Call your pharmacist for a refill 2 or 3 days before you will run out of the medicine.

Miscellaneous

Carry an identification card in your wallet or wear a medical alert

bracelet indicating that you are taking this medicine as well as the names and phone numbers of your doctors. If you do not already carry such a card, complete the Medicine Card in this book. Always tell your dentist, pharmacist and other doctors who are treating you that you are taking this medicine.

DIGOXIN (ORAL)

LANOXIN, LANOXIN PEDIATRIC ELIXIR

Purpose

This medicine is used to help make the heartbeat strong and steady. This can also help improve blood circulation.

Allergies/Warnings

Be sure to tell your doctor and pharmacist if you are allergic to any medicine.

How to Use This Medicine

Time of Administration

Take the medicine at the time recommended by your physician.

How to Administer

Take the medicine with a full glass of water.

If you were prescribed LANOXIN PEDIATRIC ELIXIR:

- A dropper is used to measure the dose. If you do not fully understand how to use the dropper to measure an accurate dose, *see* How to Administer Medications (page 15).

Special Instructions

Length of Therapy

It is very important that you take this medicine exactly as your doctor has prescribed. Do not miss any doses and take the medicine even if you feel well. Try to take this medicine at the same time(s) every day so that you will have a constant level of medicine in your body. Do not take extra tablets without your doctor's approval. Note: Some people may only need to take the medicine every second or third day.

Pregnancy/Breastfeeding

Women who are pregnant, breastfeeding or planning to become

pregnant should tell their doctor before taking this medicine.

Drug Interactions

Some nonprescription drugs can interfere with this medicine or aggravate your heart condition. Do not take any of the following without the approval of your doctor or pharmacist: antacids; laxatives; cough, cold or sinus products; antidiarrhea products; asthma or allergy products.

There are other drug interactions that can occur. If you are taking any other medicines, be sure to check with your pharmacist or doctor.

Special Precautions

It is recommended that you learn how to check your pulse rate. Ask your doctor or nurse to teach you. Check your pulse regularly while you are taking this medicine. If your pulse becomes much slower than usual (or if it is less than 50 beats per minute) or if the rhythm and force of your pulse changes, check with your doctor. The dose of your medicine may have to be adjusted. A pulse rate that is too slow may cause circulation problems.

When to Call Your Doctor

Most people experience few or no side effects from this drug. However, any medicine can sometimes cause unwanted effects. Call your doctor immediately if you develop nausea, vomiting, diarrhea (loose bowel movements), loss of appetite, blurred vision, changes in color vision (such as yellow or green vision or halos around objects), depression, confusion, bothersome headaches, unusual tiredness or weakness, skin rash or hives or if your pulse rate becomes slower than normal or changes in rhythm or force.

Refills

Do not stop taking this medicine without your doctor's approval and do not go without medicine between prescription refills. Call your pharmacist for a refill 2 or 3 days before you will run out of the medicine.

Miscellaneous

Carry an identification card in your wallet or wear a medical alert bracelet indicating that you are taking this medicine as well as the names and phone numbers of your doctors. If you do not already carry such a card, complete the Medicine Card in this book. Always tell your dentist, pharmacist and other doctors who are treating you that you are taking this medicine.

TARTRAZINE-CONTAINING DRUGS

Tartrazine (FD&C Yellow No. 5) is a dye present in thousands of foods and drugs. A small number of people are hypersensitive to tartrazine and will experience asthma, itching of the skin, swelling and runny nose. Tartrazine hypersensitivity is frequently seen in patients who are also hypersensitive to ASA.

Many questions about tartrazine hypersensitivity remain unanswered. In the meantime, sensitive patients should avoid foods and drugs containing tartrazine. It is not sufficient to avoid yellow-colored foods or drugs since the dye is often included in many other color blends, such as turquoise, green or maroon.

If you think you are allergic to tartrazine, discuss this with your doctor and tell your pharmacist.

DILTIAZEM (ORAL)

CARDIZEM

NIFEDIPINE

ADALAT, ADALAT P.A. 20, APO-NIFED, NOVO-NIFEDIN

VERAPAMIL

ISOPTIN

Purpose

This medicine is a type of drug called a calcium channel blocker and is used to help relieve and control angina attacks (chest pains). It does this by improving the supply of blood and oxygen to the heart. It eases the work of the heart and relaxes and widens narrowed blood vessels in the heart. It will not relieve an angina attack that has already started because it starts to work too slowly.

These medicines are also used to treat high blood pressure and a number of other conditions. Check with your doctor if you do not know why it has been prescribed.

Allergies/Warnings

Be sure to tell your doctor and pharmacist if you are allergic to any medicine.

How to Use This Medicine

Time of Administration

This medicine can be taken with a little fluid during or after meals. It may also be taken with a glass of water on an empty stomach at least 1 hour before (or 2 hours after) eating food.

If dizziness, flushing, or swelling of the feet occurs (more common with NIFEDIPINE), it may help to take the medicine with some food.

How to Administer

If you were prescribed ADALAT P.A. 20:

- These tablets are long-acting and must be swallowed whole. Do not crush, chew or break them into pieces.
- ADALAT capsules and tablets are sensitive to light. Therefore, keep the medicine in the container in which they were dispensed.

Special Instructions

Length of Therapy

Do not take any more of this medicine than your doctor has prescribed and do not stop taking this medicine suddenly without the approval of your doctor. It may be necessary for your doctor to reduce your dose slowly since your body will need time to adjust. It could be harmful and could cause an angina attack if you suddenly stopped taking the medicine.

Aging and the Color of Medicines

As a person gets older, the lens of the eye tends to yellow. This makes vision less clear, glare becomes more of a problem and it is more difficult to distinguish between blue and green and white and yellow.

If a person has difficulty distinguishing between these colors and if he or she is taking medicines that are white and yellow (or blue and green), there is a chance that he or she will get the medicines mixed up and not take them correctly.

It is important to distinguish the white from the yellow tablets (or the blue from the green tablets) in some way. Possible solutions would be to have the pharmacist dispense the drugs in different size containers and to label the vials clearly with large lettering.

Pregnancy/Breastfeeding

Women who are pregnant, breastfeeding or planning to become pregnant should not take DILTIAZEM or NIFEDIPINE; and should tell their doctor before taking VERAPAMIL.

Drug Interactions

Some nonprescription drugs can aggravate your heart condition. Do not take any of the following without the approval of your doctor or pharmacist: cough, cold or sinus products; asthma or allergy products. Read the label of the product to see if there is a warning. If there is, check with your doctor or pharmacist before using the product.

Alcohol

Do not drink alcoholic beverages after taking this medicine because the combination may cause a serious drop in blood pressure, dizziness and/or fainting.

Special Precautions

During the first few days of taking NIFEDIPINE, you may experience a headache. It may be relieved by taking the capsules with some food or, if your doctor agrees, by taking ASA or acetaminophen. This is a normal side effect and it usually disappears within a few days. Call your doctor if it continues.

If this medicine causes dizziness, lightheadedness or fainting, you should be careful going up and down stairs and you should not change positions too rapidly. Sit or lie down at the first sign of dizziness. Do not drive a car, pilot an airplane or operate machinery if you experience dizziness.

Keep a record of the number of angina attacks you have as well as a list of the possible causes of the attack. This information will help your physician give you the best treatment. Be sure to tell your doctor if you have an increase in the number, length or severity of attacks.

Cigarette smoking can aggravate angina and is a special risk for people who have heart conditions.

Check with your doctor about the amount of exercise that is safe for you. This medicine can reduce chest pain resulting from too much exercise and make it difficult to tell when a person has exercised just the right amount.

This medicine may cause some people to become constipated. To help prevent constipation, try increasing the amount of bulk in your diet (for example, bran, fresh fruits and salads), exercising more often or drinking more fluids (unless otherwise directed). Call your doctor if the constipation continues.

For ADALAT, ADALAT P.A. 20, APO-NIFED *and* NOVO-NIFEDIN:

- If you have diabetes, your diabetes medication may have to be adjusted.
- If you think your blood sugar is not normal or harder to control, call your doctor.

For CARDIZEM *and* ISOPTIN:

- Ask your doctor how to check your pulse rate. Check your pulse regularly while you are taking this medicine. If your pulse becomes much slower than usual or if it is less than 50 beats per minute, check with your doctor about taking the drug that day. The dose of your medicine may have to be adjusted. A pulse rate that is too slow may cause circulation problems.

Travelling Overseas? Don't Forget Your Medicines

If you are planning a trip to a foreign country, here are some practical tips about your medicines:

- Be sure you take enough of your regular medicines with you on the trip. If you do not have enough medicine to last for the entire trip, ask your doctor to prescribe an additional quantity of the medicine.
- If your doctor gives you a new prescription, get it filled at a pharmacy *before* you leave the country. Foreign pharmacies will not accept prescriptions from Canadian physicians.
- Carry your medicines with you in your hand luggage. Do not put them in your suitcases since luggage can get lost and is often exposed to hot and cold temperatures at airports or in the baggage area of the plane.
- Carry a list of your medicines with you. This list should include the generic name of the medicine, the brand name of the medicine, the strength, the manufacturer, the prescription number and the phone number of your pharmacy at home.
- In foreign countries, the same brand name of a drug may

contain a different dose of the medicine or may even contain a different drug!

- If you are taking a narcotic or a habit-forming drug, it is a good idea to get a letter from your doctor stating that you must take this medicine. This will help avoid any problems when suspicious customs agents ask you about the narcotics. Always keep the medicines in the original prescription containers with the prescription label attached.
- If any of your medicines can make you more sensitive to the sun, take along sunglasses, a sunscreen agent and try to stay out of the sun for long periods of time.
- If you become ill in a foreign country and must take a foreign drug, be sure to get the foreign doctor to write down the name, dosage and manufacturer of the drug he or she is prescribing. Your doctor at home will need this information.

Reference: *American Druggist*

When to Call Your Doctor

Most people experience few or no side effects from this drug. However, any medicine can sometimes cause unwanted effects.

For ADALAT, ADALAT P.A. 20, APO-NIFED, NOVO-NIFEDIN: Call your doctor if you develop fainting spells, a skin rash, swelling of the ankles, legs or feet, difficulty in breathing, coughing, swelling or soreness of the gums, unusually fast heartbeats or if your chest pain is not relieved.

For CARDIZEM: Call your doctor if you develop fainting spells, a skin rash, unusually slow heartbeats, swelling of the ankles, legs or feet or if your chest pain is not relieved.

For ISOPTIN: Call your doctor if you develop fainting spells, a skin rash, difficulty in breathing, coughing, unusually fast or slow heartbeats, swelling of the ankles, legs or feet or if your chest pain is not relieved.

Allergic Reactions

Call your doctor immediately if you think you may be allergic to the medicine or if you develop a skin rash, hives, itching, swelling of the face or difficulty in breathing. If you cannot reach your doctor, phone a hospital emergency department.

Refills

Do not stop taking this medicine without your doctor's approval and do not go without medicine between prescription refills. Call your pharmacist for a refill 2 or 3 days before you will run out of the medicine.

Discuss with your pharmacist the implications of dispensing all your refills for this medicine with the same manufacturer's product. (*See* Generic Drugs, page 12.)

Miscellaneous

Carry an identification card in your wallet or wear a medical alert bracelet indicating that you are taking this medicine as well as the names and phone numbers of your doctors. If you do not already carry such a card, complete the Medicine Card in this book. Always tell your dentist, pharmacist and other doctors who are treating you that you are taking this medicine.

DIPHENHYDRAMINE HCl (ORAL)

ALLERDRYL, BENADRYL, INSOMNAL

DIPHENHYDRAMINE COMPOUNDS

BENYLIN COUGH SYRUP, BENYLIN DECONGESTANT, BENYLIN DM, BENYLIN DM-D, BENYLIN DM-D-E, CHILDREN'S BENYLIN-DM-D, BENYLIN DIETETIC (SUGARLESS)

Purpose

This medicine is an antihistamine that is used to help relieve symptoms of certain types of allergic conditions (such as itching). This drug has several other uses, such as promoting sleep, and the reason it was prescribed depends upon your condition. Check with your doctor if you do not understand why you are taking it. The BENYLIN products are used to treat coughs and congestion due to colds or allergies.

Allergies/Warnings

If you have ever had an allergic reaction to any medicine or if you have asthma, glaucoma, an enlarged prostate, urinary retention (a type of bladder problem), high blood pressure or diabetes, tell your doctor and pharmacist before you take any of this medicine.

How to Use This Medicine

Time of Administration

This medicine may be taken without regard to meals. Take it either with food or on an empty stomach. If stomach upset occurs, take it with some food or a glass of milk.

If you are taking this medicine for the prevention of motion sickness, take the first dose at least 30 minutes before you travel.

For liquid medicines:

- It is recommended that a medicine spoon be used to measure the dose. An average household teaspoon is not accurate.

Special Instructions

Length of Therapy

Do not take this medicine more often or longer than recommended by your doctor. To do so may increase your chance of developing side effects.

Pregnancy/Breastfeeding

Women who are pregnant, breastfeeding or planning to become pregnant should tell their doctor before taking this medicine. Some of the products should not be taken during pregnancy or while breastfeeding.

Drug Interactions

It is important that you obtain the advice of your doctor or pharmacist before taking any other prescription or nonprescription medicines including pain relievers, sleeping pills, tranquilizers, medicine for seizures, muscle relaxants, anesthetics, medicines for depression or other medicines for allergies. Combining this medicine with some of these drugs could cause drowsiness or dizziness.

There are other drug interactions that can occur. If you are taking any other medicines, be sure to check first with your pharmacist or doctor.

Alcohol

Do not drink alcoholic beverages while taking this drug without the approval of your doctor because the combination could cause drowsiness. One drink may have the same effect that 2 or 3 drinks normally would have.

Special Precautions

In some people, this drug may initially cause dizziness or drowsiness.

Do not drive a car, pilot an airplane, operate dangerous machinery or do jobs that require you to be alert until you know how you are going to react to the drug. If you become dizzy or drowsy, you should be careful going up and down stairs. Sit or lie down at the first sign of dizziness. Tell your doctor if the dizziness continues.

People over 65 years of age may be more sensitive to these side effects.

If your mouth becomes dry, drink water, suck ice chips or a hard, sour candy (sugarless) or chew gum (sugarless). Sugarless products are recommended in order to avoid dental problems. You may wish to ask your pharmacist about special solutions, called artificial saliva, that can also be used to help restore moisture in the mouth. It is especially important to brush and floss your teeth regularly if you develop a dry mouth to help prevent gum problems.

When to Call Your Doctor

Most people experience few or no side effects from this drug. However, any medicine can sometimes cause unwanted effects. Call your doctor if you develop a skin rash, fast or irregular heartbeats, blurred vision, stomach pain, unexplained weakness or tiredness, unexplained sore throat, fever, or mouth sores, unusual bruising or bleeding, unexplained nervousness, restlessness or irritability (especially in children), trouble sleeping, difficulty in urinating (passing your water) or if mucus (lung secretions) becomes thicker than usual.

DIPYRIDAMOLE (ORAL)

Apo-Dipyridamole, Persantine

DIPYRIDAMOLE-ASA

Asasantine

Purpose

This medicine is used to help prevent angina attacks (chest pains). It will not relieve an angina attack that has already started because it starts to work too slowly.

It is also used alone or combined with other drugs, such as ASA, after a heart attack to lessen the risk of another heart attack and after some types of blood vessel surgery to prevent clotting of the blood.

It may also be used to treat some other conditions. Check with your doctor if you do not know why the drug has been prescribed.

How to Use This Medicine

Time of Administration

Take this medicine with a glass of water on an empty stomach at least 1 hour before (or 2 hours after) eating food. The drug may be taken with a light snack or a glass of milk if it upsets your stomach.

Special Instructions

Length of Therapy

It may be necessary to take this medicine for 2 or 3 months before you feel its full benefit.

If you are taking this medicine for angina, do not stop taking it suddenly without the approval of your doctor. It will be necessary for your doctor to reduce your dose slowly since your body will need time to adjust. It could be harmful and make your condition worse if you suddenly stopped taking the medicine.

Pregnancy/Breastfeeding

Women who are pregnant, breastfeeding or planning to become pregnant should tell their doctor before taking this medicine.

Drug Interactions

Some nonprescription drugs can aggravate your condition. Do not take any of the following without the approval of your doctor or pharmacist: cough, cold or sinus products; asthma or allergy products. Read the label of the product to see if there is a warning. If there is, check with your doctor or pharmacist before using the product.

Alcohol

Do not drink alcoholic beverages without the approval of your doctor while you are taking this medicine as the combination may make you feel dizzy or faint.

Special Precautions

If you become dizzy or feel faint, sit or lie down until these effects pass. Always get up slowly after you have been sitting or lying down. Get out of bed slowly in the morning and dangle your feet over the edge of the bed for a few minutes before standing up. Do not drive a car, pilot an airplane or operate dangerous machinery or do jobs that require you to be alert if you are dizzy.

When you first start taking this drug, you may get a headache or flushing. These are common side effects and will usually disappear within a few days. Call your doctor if they continue.

Cigarette smoking can aggravate angina and is a special risk for people who have heart conditions.

When to Call Your Doctor

Most people experience few or no side effects from this drug. However, any medicine can sometimes cause unwanted effects. Call

> **Did You Know That?**
>
> If you are applying a topical anesthetic (pain killer) to the inside of the mouth or gums, you should spit out the medicine and not swallow it.
>
> The anesthetic could cause side effects if you swallowed it and it passed into your bloodstream.
>
> This is why topical anesthetics (for example, LIDOCAINE) should not be prescribed for the relief of teething discomfort in infants. Infants do not know how to expectorate (spit out) the medicines and will swallow the medicine. There is a report in *Clinical Pediatrics* of an 11-month-old infant who developed seizures after being treated with a topical LIDOCAINE 2% solution. The mother had applied the solution to the infant's gum with her finger 5 or 6 times a day for seven days. Approximately 80 ml of the solution had been used. It was not possible to determine whether the toxic LIDOCAINE blood level was due to absorption of the drug from the gums or from the infant swallowing the anesthetic.

your doctor if you develop a skin rash, chest pain, fainting spells, nausea or vomiting, severe headaches or persistent stomach cramps.

Refills

Do not stop taking this medicine without your doctor's approval and do not go without medicine between prescription refills. Call your pharmacist for a refill 2 or 3 days before you will run out of the medicine.

Discuss with your pharmacist the implications of dispensing all your refills for this medicine with the same manufacturer's product. (*See* Generic Drugs, page 12.)

Miscellaneous

Carry an identification card in your wallet or wear a medical alert bracelet indicating that you are taking this medicine as well as the names and phone numbers of your doctors. If you do not already carry such a card, complete the Medicine Card in this book. Always tell your dentist, pharmacist and other doctors who are treating you that you are taking this medicine.

DISOPYRAMIDE (ORAL)

NORPACE, NORPACE CR, RYTHMODAN, RYTHMODAN-LA

Purpose

This medicine is used to help make the heart beat at a regular, normal rate and rhythm.

Allergies/Warnings

Be sure to tell your doctor and pharmacist if you are allergic to any medicine or if you have glaucoma, diabetes, congestive heart failure, a prostate problem, difficulty urinating or any other medical condition.

How to Use This Medicine

Time of Administration

It is best to take this medicine with a glass of water on an empty stomach. However, if you develop stomach upset after taking the drug, take it with some food. Call your doctor if you continue to have an upset stomach.

How to Administer

Take the medicine with a full glass of water unless otherwise directed.

If you were prescribed NORPACE CR *or* RYTHMODAN-LA:

- These medicines are long acting and must be swallowed whole. Do not crush or chew them.

Special Instructions

Length of Therapy

It is very important that you take this medicine exactly as your doctor has prescribed. Do not miss any doses. Take the medicine even if you feel well. Try to take this medicine at the same time(s) every day so that you will have a constant level of medicine in your body. Do not take extra tablets without your doctor's approval.

Do not stop taking this medicine suddenly without the approval of your doctor. It will be necessary for your doctor to reduce your dose slowly since your body will need time to adjust. It could be harmful and make your condition worse if you suddenly stopped taking the medicine.

Pregnancy/Breastfeeding

Women who are pregnant, breastfeeding or planning to become pregnant should tell their doctor before taking this medicine.

Drug Interactions

Some nonprescription drugs can interfere with this medicine or aggravate your heart condition. Do not take any of the following without the approval of your doctor or pharmacist: antacids or baking soda; cough, cold or sinus products; asthma or allergy products.

Alcohol

Do not drink alcoholic beverages while taking this drug without the approval of your doctor because the combination could cause dizziness, fainting or, rarely, low blood sugar.

Special Precautions

If this medicine causes dizziness or lightheadedness, you should be careful going up and down stairs and you should not change positions too rapidly. Lightheadedness is more likely to occur if you stand up suddenly—this is due to blood collecting in the legs and lasts for a few seconds. Therefore, get up from a sitting or lying position more slowly and tighten and relax your leg muscles or wiggle your toes to help promote circulation. In the morning, get out of bed slowly and dangle your feet over the edge of the bed for a few minutes before standing up. Sit or lie down at the first sign of dizziness. Do not drive a car, pilot an airplane, operate dangerous machinery or do jobs that require you to be alert if you have been dizzy.

You may become more sensitive to heat because your body may perspire less while you are taking this drug. Be careful not to become overheated during exercise or in hot weather. Try to avoid strenuous exercise, standing for long periods of time (especially in hot weather), hot showers, hot baths, saunas or Jacuzzis while taking this medicine.

If your mouth becomes dry, drink water, suck ice chips or a hard, sour candy (sugarless) or chew gum (sugarless). Sugarless products are recommended in order to avoid dental problems. You may wish to ask your pharmacist about special solutions, called artificial saliva, that can also be used to help restore moisture in the mouth. It is especially important to brush and floss your teeth regularly if you develop a dry mouth to help prevent gum problems.

If your eyes become dry, ask your pharmacist or doctor to recommend a lubricating/wetting solution or artificial tears. This side effect is more common in elderly people.

This medicine may rarely cause the blood sugar to fall in some people. This side effect is more common in patients with congestive heart failure or diabetes. If you develop sweating, shaking, drowsiness, headache, excessive hunger, nausea, nervousness, chills, cold sweats, cool pale skin, confusion, unusual tiredness or weakness, eat or drink a food containing sugar and call your doctor right away.

This medicine may cause some people to become constipated. To help prevent constipation, try increasing the amount of bulk in your diet (for example, bran, fresh fruits and salads), exercising more often or drinking more fluids (unless otherwise directed). Call your doctor if the constipation continues.

When to Call Your Doctor

Most people experience few or no side effects from this drug. However, any medicine can sometimes cause unwanted effects. Call your doctor if you develop a sore throat, fever, mouth sores, fainting, difficulty urinating (passing your water), shortness of breath, chest pains, unusually slow or fast heartbeats, confusion or depression, unusual nervousness, a yellow color to the skin or eyes, eye pain, swelling of the legs or ankles, sudden weight gain of 5 pounds (2.5 kg) or more or muscle weakness.

Allergic Reactions

Call your doctor immediately if you think you may be allergic to the medicine or if you develop a skin rash, hives, itching, swelling of the face or difficulty in breathing. If you cannot reach your doctor, phone a hospital emergency department.

Refills

Do not stop taking this medicine without your doctor's approval and do not go without medicine between prescription refills. Call your pharmacist for a refill 2 or 3 days before you will run out of the medicine.

Discuss with your pharmacist the implications of dispensing all your refills for this medicine with the same manufacturer's product. (*See*

Generic Drugs, page 12.) The long-acting medicines (NORPACE CR and RYTHMODAN-LA) are not interchangeable.

Miscellaneous

Carry an identification card in your wallet or wear a medical alert bracelet indicating that you are taking this medicine as well as the names and phone numbers of your doctors. If you do not already carry such a card, complete the Medicine Card in this book. Always tell your dentist, pharmacist and other doctors who are treating you that you are taking this medicine.

DOXYCYCLINE (ORAL)

APO-DOXY, VIBRAMYCIN, VIBRA-TABS C-PAK

MINOCYCLINE

MINOCIN

Purpose

This medicine is an antibiotic used to treat certain types of infections and help control acne. Your doctor has prescribed this antibiotic for your present infection only. Do not use it for other infections or give it to other people.

Allergies/Warnings

If you have ever had an allergic reaction to TETRACYCLINE or any other medicine, tell your doctor and pharmacist before you take any of this medicine.

If you have ever had allergies, asthma, hay fever, or hives, tell your doctor or pharmacist before taking any of this medicine.

This medicine should not be given to children under 12 years of age unless directed by your doctor. The medicine may permanently discolor the child's teeth and slow down the growth of the teeth and bones.

How to Use This Medicine

Time of Administration

This medicine may be taken with food. This will help prevent stomach upset. Call your doctor if you develop stomach upset.

Space your doses of the medicine around the clock (throughout the entire day of 24 hours). For example, if you are to take 2 doses each day, space the doses 12 hours apart. This will keep a constant level of the medicine in your body.

How to Administer

For tablets and capsules:

- Take the tablets and capsules with a full glass (8 ounces) of water. This will help prevent irritation of the stomach and esophagus.

For APO-DOXY, VIBRAMYCIN *and* VIBRA-TABS:

- Sit up or stand up when you take each dose in order to help prevent "heartburn" or irritation of the esophagus. It is also best to take the evening dose at least 1 hour before going to bed.

Special Instructions

Length of Therapy

It is important to take all of this medicine plus any refills that your doctor told you to take. Do not stop taking this medicine earlier than your doctor has recommended even if you begin to feel better. If you stop taking the medicine too soon, the infection may return.

This is especially important if you are taking the medicine to cure a strep infection because if the infection is not completely cleared up, serious heart problems could develop later. After treatment for a strep infection, your doctor may want to do a test to make sure that the infection is gone.

Pregnancy/Breastfeeding

Women who are pregnant or planning to become pregnant should tell their doctor before taking this medicine.

This medicine is not recommended during pregnancy since it may cause permanent discoloration of the infant's teeth and may slow down the normal growth and development of the infant's teeth and bones.

Women who are breastfeeding should tell their doctor before taking this medicine. This medicine may pass into the breast milk and cause discoloration of the infant's teeth and may slow down the normal growth and development of the infant's teeth and bones.

Drug Interactions

Some antacids and laxatives can make this medicine less effective if they are taken at the same time. This includes products which contain aluminum, magnesium, bismuth, Epsom salt, sodium bicarbonate and baking soda. In addition, if you are taking minocycline, products containing calcium can make this drug less effective.

Check with your pharmacist before you purchase any antacids or laxatives. If you must take antacids or laxatives, they should be taken at least 2 hours before or after this medicine.

Iron pills or vitamins containing minerals can also make this medicine less effective. In addition, products containing zinc can make this drug less effective. If you must take these products, take them 3 hours before (or 2 hours after) this medicine.

There have been some reports that oral contraceptives (birth control pills) may not work as well while taking this medicine. Unplanned pregnancies may occur. Ask your doctor about using another form of birth control while you are taking these antibiotics. Also call your doctor if you develop spotting or breakthrough bleeding since these can be signs of decreased birth control effect.

Special Precautions

This medicine may make some people more sensitive to sunlight and various tanning lamps. When you begin taking this medicine, try to avoid too much sun until you see how you are going to react. If your skin does become more sensitive to sunlight, tell your doctor and try not to stay in direct sunlight for extended periods of time. While in the sun, wear protective clothing and sunglasses. You may wish to ask your pharmacist about suitable sunscreen products. Call your doctor if you become sunburned.

It has been reported that MINOCYCLINE may cause dizziness or lightheadedness. Do not drive a car, pilot an airplane, operate dangerous machinery or do jobs that require you to be alert until you know how you are going to react to the drug. If you become dizzy or drowsy, you should be careful going up and down stairs. Sit or lie down at the first sign of dizziness. Tell your doctor if the dizziness continues.

When to Call Your Doctor

Call your doctor if your symptoms do not improve within a few days (or a few weeks or months if you are taking the medicine for acne) or if they become worse.

Any medicine can sometimes cause unwanted effects. Call your doctor if you develop severe cramps or burning of the stomach, vomiting, severe watery diarrhea, skin rash, dark-colored tongue, sore mouth or tongue, itching of the rectal or genital areas or, in women, a vaginal discharge that was not present before starting the medicine.

Allergic Reactions

Call your doctor immediately if you think you may be allergic to the medicine or if you develop a skin rash, hives, itching, swelling of the face or difficulty in breathing. If you cannot reach your doctor, phone a hospital emergency department.

Storage

Store the medicine in a cool, dark place and keep the bottle tightly closed.

If for some reason you cannot take all of the medicine, discard the unused portion by flushing it down the toilet. Do not take or save old medicine. Outdated medicine can cause serious problems.

Refills

Do not go without medicine between prescription refills. Call your pharmacist for a refill 2 or 3 days before you will run out of the medicine.

Did You Know That?

Some drug interactions can be avoided by spacing the 2 drugs far enough apart so that they are not in the stomach at the same time.

For example, the antibiotic effect of TETRACYCLINE can be decreased if a person takes an iron supplement at the same time. The iron pill binds with the TETRACYCLINE and prevents some of the tetracycline from being absorbed from the stomach.

With this interaction, it is not necessary for the person to stop taking one of the drugs. This drug interaction can be avoided by simply taking the iron supplement at least 3 hours before or 2 hours after the TETRACYCLINE. A long-acting iron supplement must not be used, because the drug interaction can still occur.

This interaction also applies to other drugs related to TETRACYCLINE such as DEMECLOCYCLINE, DOXYCYCLINE and MINOCYCLINE.

ERYTHROMYCIN PRODUCTS (ORAL)

ERYTHROMYCIN BASE

Apo-Erythro Base, E-Mycin, Eryc 125, Eryc 250, Erythromid, Novo-Rythro Base

ERYTHROMYCIN ESTOLATE

Ilosone, Novo-Rythro Estolate

ERYTHROMYCIN ETHYL SUCCINATE

Apo-Erythro-ES, EES 200, EES 400, EES 600

ERYTHROMYCIN STEARATE

APO-ERYTHRO-S, ERYTHROCIN, NOVO-RYTHRO STEARATE

Purpose

This medicine is an antibiotic used to treat certain types of infections. Your doctor has prescribed this antibiotic for your present infection. Do not use it for other infections or give it to other people.

Allergies/Warnings

If you have ever had an allergic reaction to ERYTHROMYCIN or any other medicine or if you have liver problems, tell your doctor and pharmacist before you take any of this medicine.

How to Use This Medicine

Time of Administration

The time you take your medicine depends on the brand of medicine your doctor prescribed. Take your medicine according to the following instructions:

If you were prescribed APO-ERYTHRO BASE, ERYC 125, ERYC 250, ERYTHROCIN LIQUID, ERYTHROMID, NOVO-RYTHRO BASE, NOVO-RYTHRO STEARATE LIQUID:

- It is best to take this medicine with a glass of water on an empty stomach at least 1 hour before (or 2 hours after) eating food. Do not drink acidic fruit juices (such as orange or grapefruit juice) within 1 hour of taking this medicine. Take the medicine at the proper time even if you skip a meal. If you develop stomach upset after taking the drug, take it with some food. Call your doctor if you continue to have an upset stomach.

If you were prescribed APO-ERYTHRO-S, ERYTHROCIN TABLETS, *or* NOVO-RYTHRO STEARATE TABLETS:

- Take the medicine *immediately before* meals.

If you were prescribed APO-ERYTHRO-ES *or* EES:

- Take the medicine *immediately after* meals.

If you were prescribed ILOSONE *or* NOVO-RYTHRO ESTOLATE capsules *or* liquid:

- The medicine may be taken without regard to meals on either an empty stomach or with food.

How to Administer

Take the medicine with a full glass of water unless otherwise directed.

If you were prescribed EES CHEWABLE:

- Chew the tablets well before swallowing. Do not swallow the tablets whole. After you have chewed and swallowed the small pieces of the tablet, you may wish to drink some water.

If you were prescribed E-MYCIN:

- This medicine has a special coating and must be swallowed whole. Do not crush, chew or break it into pieces.
- Take it with a glass of water on an empty stomach 1 hour before or 2 hours after food.

If you or your child were prescribed ERYC 125:

- These capsules may be swallowed whole.
- Patients who have difficulty swallowing capsules may sprinkle the contents on food:
- Hold the capsule with the clear end down and the orange end up. Gently twist off the orange cap to open.
- Sprinkle ALL the medicine inside the capsule on a small amount (e.g. a spoonful) of applesauce, fruit jams or jellies, or ice cream.
- Swallow the spoonful of food containing the medicine. Do not crush or chew any of the pellets.
- Then drink a full glass of water to make sure all the pellets are swallowed.
- Note: If you accidentally spill the medicine, start over with a new capsule to make sure a full dose is taken.

For liquid medicines:

- If you were prescribed a suspension, shake the bottle well each time before pouring so that you can measure an accurate dose.
- If a spoon is used to measure the dose, it is recommended that you use a medicine spoon or an oral liquid syringe that you can obtain from your pharmacist. These are more accurate than the average household teaspoon. *See* How to Administer Medications (page 15).

Special Instructions

Length of Therapy

It is important to take all of this medicine plus any refills that your doctor told you to take. Do not stop taking this medicine earlier than your doctor has recommended even if you begin to feel better. If you stop taking the medicine too soon, the infection may return. This is especially important if you are taking the medicine to cure a strep infection because if the infection is not completely cleared up, serious heart problems could develop later. After treatment for a strep infection, your doctor may want to do a test to make sure that the infection is gone.

Pregnancy/Breastfeeding

Women who are pregnant, breastfeeding or planning to become pregnant should tell their doctor before taking this medicine.

Special Precautions

This medicine sometimes causes diarrhea. Call your doctor if the diarrhea becomes severe and watery or does not go away after a few days. Do not try to treat the diarrhea yourself without first discussing it with your doctor.

When to Call Your Doctor

Call your doctor if your symptoms do not improve within a few days or if they become worse.

Most people experience few or no side effects from this drug. However, any medicine can sometimes cause unwanted effects. Call your doctor if you develop an unexplained fever, chills, sore mouth or tongue, severe stomach cramps, dark-colored urine, unusual weakness or tiredness, severe nausea or vomiting, pale-colored stools or a yellow color of the skin or eyes, rectal or genital itching or, in women, a vaginal discharge that was not present before you started taking the medicine.

Allergic Reactions

Call your doctor immediately if you think you may be allergic to the medicine or if you develop a skin rash, hives, itching, swelling of the face or difficulty in breathing. If you cannot reach your doctor, phone a hospital emergency department.

Storage

For NOVO-RYTHRO ESTOLATE *and* NOVO-RYTHRO STEARATE SUSPENSIONS:

• Some liquid forms of ERYTHROMYCIN should be kept in the refrigerator.

Do not freeze. Follow the directions on the container.

Throw away any unused medicine after the discard (expiration) date on the bottle by flushing it down the toilet. Do not take outdated medicine since it may not work as well.

Refills

Do not go without medicine between prescription refills. Call your pharmacist for a refill 2 or 3 days before you will run out of the medicine.

What Can You Do If Your Child Refuses to Take a Medicine?

If a parent is having difficulty administering a medicine to a child, it may be easier to gain the cooperation of the child if a positive approach is used. For example, children love to imitate and may be more cooperative if the parent says, "Here is your medicine. Drink it and I will give you some special medicine for your teddy bear."

It may also help to let children choose which of their medicines they would like first and let them choose whether they want to take it on your lap or in their favorite chair.

It is also a good idea to let the child handle the oral liquid syringe or the medicine spoon before it is filled with the medicine. This gives the child an opportunity to become familiar with the device so that he or she is not frightened.

When you know that a medicine does not taste good, be honest with the child. Don't try to trick the child by telling him or her that the medicine tastes good. The child will soon find out that you have tricked him or her and will be less cooperative the next time.

After the child has taken the medicine, a flavored drink or a glass of water may help to remove any aftertaste of the medicine. Ask your pharmacist if there are any fruit juices that should not be given immediately after administering the medicine. Some medicines are destroyed by fruit juices.

If you are administering a liquid medicine by means of an oral liquid syringe, point the tip of the syringe to the inside of the cheek or the back side of the mouth. This will help prevent drooling or choking. *Slowly* squirt the medicine into the mouth and allow the child to swallow naturally.

ERYTHROMYCIN ETHYLSUCCINATE-SULFISOXAZOLE (ORAL)
PEDIAZOLE

Purpose
This medicine contains two antibiotics and is used to treat middle-ear infections (acute otitis media) in children.

Your doctor has prescribed this antibiotic for the present infection. Do not use it for other infections or give it to other people.

Allergies/Warnings
If the child has ever had an allergic reaction to erythromycin or sulfa drugs or any other medicine (including diabetes medicines) or if the child has any liver problems, tell your doctor and pharmacist before you take any of this medicine.

This medicine should not be used in infants less than 2 months of age.

How to Use This Medicine

Time of Administration

This medicine may be taken without regard to meals but it is best to take it *immediately* after meals.

Try to space the medicine throughout the day in equally spaced intervals. Try to space the doses "around the clock" (throughout the entire day of 24 hours). For example, if the child is to receive 4 doses each day, space the doses as close to 6 hours apart as possible. This will keep a constant level of the medicine in the body.

Do not forget to give the child any doses. Arrange a schedule so that the child will also be able to receive necessary doses at school.

How to Administer

This medicine should be taken with a full glass of water with or without food. The medicine has a strawberry-banana flavor.

Shake the bottle well each time before pouring so that an accurate dose can be measured.

If a spoon is used to measure the dose, it is recommended that you use a medicine spoon or an oral liquid syringe that you can obtain from your pharmacist. These are more accurate than the average household teaspoon. If you are using an oral liquid syringe, wash it thoroughly with warm water after each use.

Special Instructions

Length of Therapy

It is important to give the child all of this medicine plus any refills that your doctor told you to take. Do not stop this medicine earlier than your doctor has recommended even if the child starts to feel better. If you stop taking the medicine too soon, the infection may return.

Pregnancy/Breastfeeding

This medicine should not be used in the last stages of pregnancy and/or during breastfeeding.

Special Precautions

This medicine sometimes causes diarrhea. Call your doctor if the diarrhea becomes severe and watery or does not go away after a few days. Do not try to treat the diarrhea yourself without first discussing it with your doctor.

This medicine may make some people more sensitive to sunlight and various tanning lamps. When your child begins taking this medicine, try to have the child avoid too much sun until you see how he/she is going to react. If the skin does become more sensitive to sunlight, tell your doctor and try to keep the child out of direct sunlight for extended periods of time. While in the sun, wear protective clothing and sunglasses. You may wish to ask your pharmacist about suitable sunscreen products. Call your doctor if the child becomes sunburned.

Since this medicine contains a "sulfa" drug, it is important that the child drink an adequate amount of water/liquids in order to prevent kidney problems.

If the child becomes dizzy, warn him/her to be careful going up and down stairs. The child should sit or lie down at the first sign of dizziness. Tell your doctor if the dizziness continues.

When to Call Your Doctor

Call your doctor if the symptoms do not improve within a few days or if they become worse.

Most people experience few or no side effects from this drug. However, any medicine can sometimes cause unwanted effects. Call your doctor if your child develops an unexplained fever, chills, sore throat, mouth sores, severe stomach cramps, dark-colored urine, unusual weakness or tiredness, severe nausea or vomiting, unusual pale skin, unusual bruising or bleeding, swelling of the front part of the neck or eyes, difficulty in swallowing, hearing loss, unusual joint or lower back pain, blood in the urine, pain while urinating (passing your water), redness, blistering, peeling or loosening of the skin, pale-colored stools or a yellow color of the skin or eyes, or rectal or genital itching.

Allergic Reactions

Call your doctor immediately if you think your child may be allergic to the medicine or if he/she develops a skin rash, hives, itching, swelling of the face or difficulty in breathing. If you cannot reach your doctor, phone a hospital emergency department.

Storage

- Store the medicine in the refrigerator. Do not freeze.
- Throw away any unused medicine after the discard (expiration) date on the bottle by flushing it down the toilet. This is usually 14 days after the prescription was filled. Do not use outdated medicine since it may not work as well.

Refills

Do not go without medicine between prescription refills. Call your pharmacist for a refill 2 or 3 days before you will run out of the medicine.

ETHACRYNIC ACID (ORAL)

EDECRIN

FUROSEMIDE

APO-FUROSEMIDE, FUROSIDE, LASIX, NOVOSEMIDE, URITOL

Purpose

This medicine is used to help the body get rid of excess fluids and to decrease swelling in several types of medical conditions. The medicine does this by increasing the amount of urine and is commonly called a water pill or fluid pill. FUROSEMIDE is also used to treat high blood pressure.

Allergies/Warnings

Be sure to tell your doctor or pharmacist if you are allergic to sulfa drugs, thiazide diuretics or any medicine or if you have any medical conditions.

How to Use This Medicine

Time of Administration

Try to take this medicine at the same time(s) every day so that you have a constant level of the medicine in your body.

When you first start taking this medicine, you will probably urinate (pass your water) more often and in larger amounts than usual. Therefore, if you are to take 1 dose each day, take it in the morning after breakfast. Do not initially take a dose at bedtime or you may have to get up during the night to go to the bathroom.

If you are to take more than 1 dose each day, take the last dose approximately 6 hours before bedtime so that you will not have to get up during the night to go to the bathroom. This effect will usually lessen after you have taken the drug for a while.

How to Administer

Take this medicine with food, meals or milk if it upsets your stomach.

For LASIX SOLUTION:

- Measure the dose carefully using the dropper or the special spoon that comes with the medicine. For more information, *see* How to Administer Medications (page 15).

Special Instructions

Length of Therapy

For patients with high blood pressure:

- High blood pressure (hypertension) is a long-term condition and it will probably be necessary for you to take the drug for a long time even if you feel better. If high blood pressure is not treated, it can lead to serious problems such as heart failure, strokes, blood vessel problems or kidney problems.

It is very important that you take this medicine as your doctor has directed and that you do not miss any doses. Otherwise, you cannot expect the drug to keep your blood pressure down or remove excess fluid.

Pregnancy/Breastfeeding

Women who are pregnant or planning to become pregnant should tell their doctor before taking this medicine.

This medicine passes into the breast milk and breastfeeding should be stopped.

Drug Interactions

Some nonprescription drugs can aggravate high blood pressure. Do not take any of the following without the approval of your doctor or pharmacist: cough, cold or sinus products; asthma or allergy products since they may increase your blood pressure. Read the label of the nonprescription drug product to see if there is a warning. If there is, check with your doctor or pharmacist before using the product.

Do not take large doses of ASA or products containing ASA without the approval of your pharmacist.

Alcohol

Be careful drinking alcoholic beverages while taking this medicine because it could make the possible side effect of dizziness worse.

Special Precautions

This medicine normally causes your body to lose potassium. The body has warning signs to let you know if too much potassium is being lost. Call your doctor if you become unusually thirsty or if you develop leg cramps, unusual weakness, fatigue, vomiting, confusion or an irregular pulse. Since these symptoms may not be present in all patients, your doctor may wish to check your blood occasionally to see if it is low in potassium. Depending upon your dose, your doctor may prescribe some medicine to replace the potassium or he or she may recommend that you regularly eat foods that contain a lot of potassium (see Appendix A). *Do not change your diet unless your doctor tells you to.*

If this medicine causes dizziness or lightheadedness, you should be careful going up and down stairs and you should not change positions too rapidly. Lightheadedness is more likely to occur if you stand up suddenly—this is due to blood collecting in the legs and lasts for a few seconds. Therefore, get up from a sitting or lying position more slowly and tighten and relax your leg muscles or wiggle your toes to help promote circulation. In the morning, get out of bed slowly and dangle your feet over the edge of the bed for a few minutes before standing up. Sit or lie down at the first sign of dizziness. Do not drive a car, pilot an airplane, operate dangerous machinery or do jobs that require you to be alert if you are dizzy. Tell your doctor if you have been dizzy.

In order to help prevent dizziness or fainting, your doctor may also recommend that you avoid strenuous exercise, standing for long periods of time (especially in hot weather), hot showers, hot baths or saunas.

People more than 65 years of age may be more sensitive to the side effects of dizziness and potassium loss.

For FUROSEMIDE *only:*

- This medicine may make some people more sensitive to sunlight and various tanning lamps. When you begin taking this medicine, try to avoid too much sun until you see how you are going to react. If your skin does become more sensitive to sunlight, tell your doctor and try not to stay in direct sunlight for extended periods of time. While in the sun, wear protective clothing and sunglasses. You may wish to ask your pharmacist about suitable sunscreen products. Call your doctor if you become sunburned.

For patients with diabetes:

- This medicine may cause your blood sugar to rise. Carefully test your blood or urine for sugar while you are taking this medicine. Call your doctor if you think your blood sugar is higher than normal or harder to control.

When to Call Your Doctor

Most people experience few or no side effects from this drug. However, any medicine can sometimes cause unwanted effects. Call your doctor if you develop an unexplained sore throat, chills or fever, ringing or buzzing or a feeling of fullness in the ears, any loss of hearing, sharp stomach pain, chest pain, sharp joint pain, severe muscle or leg cramps, unusual fatigue, unusual sweating, mental confusion, headache, fainting, unusual bruising or bleeding, a yellow color to the skin or eyes or a sudden weight gain of 5 pounds (2.5 kg) or more. Also call your doctor if you become sick or develop vomiting or diarrhea.

For ETHACRYNIC ACID:

- Stop taking the medicine and call your doctor immediately if you develop severe, watery diarrhea.
- Also call your doctor if you develop red or black stools.

Allergic Reactions

Call your doctor immediately if you think you may be allergic to the medicine or if you develop a skin rash, hives, itching, swelling of the face or difficulty in breathing. If you cannot reach your doctor, phone a hospital emergency department.

Refills

Do not stop taking this medicine without your doctor's approval and do not go without medicine between prescription refills. Call your pharmacist for a refill 2 or 3 days before you will run out of the medicine.

Discuss with your pharmacist the implications of dispensing all your refills for this medicine with the same manufacturer's product. (*See* Generic Drugs, page 12.)

Did You Know That?

Blood pressure is highest just after a person goes to bed at night.

This is why some doctors recommend elevating the head of the bed to approximately 5 to 20 degrees.

ETHOSUXIMIDE (ORAL)
ZARONTIN

METHSUXIMIDE
CELONTIN

PHENSUXIMIDE
MILONTIN

Purpose
This medicine is used to help control absence (petit mal) seizures. It is commonly used in the treatment of epilepsy.

Allergies/Warnings
If you have ever had an allergic reaction to an anticonvulsant or seizure medicine, tell your doctor and pharmacist before you take any of this medicine.

How to Use This Medicine

Time of Administration

It is very important that you take this medicine exactly as your doctor has prescribed. Do not miss any doses and take the medicine even if you feel well. Try to take this medicine at the same time(s) every day so that you will have a constant level of medicine in your body. This is the only way that you can receive the full benefit of the medicine. If you forget to take this medicine, the amount of medicine in your blood will decrease and you may have seizures.

How to Administer

Take this medicine with food if it upsets your stomach. Call your doctor if you continue to have stomach upset.

For ZARONTIN SYRUP:

- If a dropper, oral liquid syringe or special measuring spoon is used to measure the dose and you do not fully understand how to use it, *see* How to Administer Medications (page 15).

Did You Know That?

Millions of dollars are spent annually on quack cures.

Quack cures cost us more than just money. They can cost us our lives. Quackery is health fraud and is the promotion of medical remedies which are ineffective or have not been proven to be effective.

Most people think that the government screens all health product advertising BEFORE it is released. This is not true except for those drugs and medical devices that require premarket approval by the Health Protection Branch. The only way that law enforcement authorities can take action is after the advertisements have appeared. Often this is too late.

Many quacks sell their products through post office boxes and are "fly-by-night" operators. They have usually moved to another location by the time refund requests have come in. They do this in order to avoid law enforcement officials.

There are some things you can do to protect yourself:

- Be wary of any "special", "secret," or "ancient" formulas that are only available through the mail from one supplier.
- Be wary of testimonials from satisfied users or famous people. You want scientific proof about a product's efficacy.
- Be wary of claims that one product can cure several types of ailments.
- Be wary of claims that the product will "cure" a condition.
- Be wary of door-to-door salesmen or people who sell their products at public lectures and who use high pressure sales tactics.
- Do not give your credit card number or send an order through the mail until you have assurance that the product is not a quack product. Check with your doctor or pharmacist.

Special Instructions

Length of Therapy

Do not stop taking this medicine suddenly without the approval of your doctor. It usually will be necessary for your doctor to slowly reduce your dose since your body will need time to adjust. You could develop seizures if you suddenly stopped taking the medicine.

Pregnancy/Breastfeeding

Women who are pregnant or planning to become pregnant should tell their doctor before taking this medicine.

Women should not breastfeed without their doctor's approval. This medicine can pass into the breast milk and cause side effects in the infant.

Drug Interactions

It is important that you obtain the advice of your doctor or pharmacist before taking any other prescription and nonprescription medicines including pain relievers, sleeping pills, tranquilizers, medicine for seizures, muscle relaxants, anesthetics, medicines for depression or medicines for allergies. Combining this medicine with some of these drugs could cause drowsiness or dizziness.

There are other drug interactions that can occur. If you are taking any other medicines, be sure to check first with your pharmacist or doctor.

Alcohol

Do not drink alcoholic beverages while taking this drug without the approval of your doctor because the combination could cause drowsiness or an increase in the frequency of your seizures. One drink may have the same effect that 2 or 3 drinks normally would have.

Special Precautions

Be sure to keep your doctor's appointments so that your doctor can check your progress. This is especially important during the first few months of therapy when the doctor will decide the best dose of this medicine for your condition. To make sure that your dose is correct, your doctor may wish to take a blood sample periodically to measure the amount of medicine in it.

This medicine may cause dizziness, drowsiness or blurred vision in some people. If you become dizzy, you should be careful going up and down stairs. Sit or lie down at the first sign of dizziness. Do not drive a car, use a sewing machine, operate dangerous machinery or do jobs that require you to be alert until you know how you are going to react to the drug. Tell your doctor if you are dizzy, drowsy or have blurred vision. It may be necessary to lower your dose.

If this medicine is for a child, do not let him or her ride a bike, climb trees, etc. until you can determine how he or she is going to react to this medicine. Children could hurt themselves if they participated in these activities when they were dizzy.

Avoid swimming alone or taking part in high-risk sports in which a sudden seizure could cause injury.

When to Call Your Doctor

Most people experience few or no side effects from this drug. However, any medicine can sometimes cause unwanted effects. Call your doctor if you develop a sore throat, fever, or mouth sores, skin rash and itching, swollen glands, persistent hiccups, unusual bruising or bleeding or if you become confused or depressed.

Call your doctor if you have an increase in the frequency of seizures.

Allergic Reactions

Call your doctor immediately if you think you may be allergic to the medicine or if you develop a skin rash, hives, itching, swelling of the face or difficulty in breathing. If you cannot reach your doctor, phone a hospital emergency department.

Refills

Do not stop taking this medicine without your doctor's approval and do not go without medicine between prescription refills. Call your pharmacist for a refill 2 or 3 days before you will run out of the medicine.

Miscellaneous

Carry an identification card in your wallet or wear a medical alert bracelet indicating that you are taking this medicine as well as the names and phone numbers of your doctors. If you do not already carry such a card, complete the Medicine Card in this book. Always tell your dentist, pharmacist and other doctors who are treating you that you are taking this medicine.

FLECAINIDE (ORAL)

TAMBOCOR

Purpose

This medicine is used to help regulate the heartbeat so that it is strong and steady.

Allergies/Warnings

If you have ever had an allergic reaction to a local anesthetic or any medicine, tell your doctor and pharmacist before you take any of this medicine.

How to Use This Medicine

Time of Administration

It is very important that you take this medicine exactly as your doctor has prescribed. Do not miss any doses and take the medicine even if you feel well. Do not take extra tablets without your doctor's approval.

Take the medicine at the same times every day so that you have a constant level of the medicine in your body.

How to Administer

Take the medicine with a glass of water.

Special Instructions

Pregnancy/Breastfeeding

Women who are pregnant, breastfeeding or planning to become pregnant should tell their doctor before taking this medicine.

Drug Interactions

It is important that you obtain the advice of your doctor or pharmacist before taking any other prescription or nonprescription medicines that can excite the heart (including pain relievers, sleeping pills, tranquilizers, or medicines for depression, cough/cold or sinus products, asthma or allergy products).

There are other drug interactions which can occur. If you are taking any other medicines, be sure to check first with your pharmacist or doctor.

Length of Therapy

Do not take any more of this medicine than your doctor has prescribed and do not stop taking this medicine suddenly without the approval of your doctor. It may be necessary for your doctor to slowly reduce your dose since your body may need time to adjust. It might be harmful if you suddenly stopped taking the medicine.

Special Precautions

If your mouth becomes dry, drink water, suck ice chips or a hard, sour candy (sugarless) or chew gum (sugarless). Sugarless products are recommended in order to avoid dental problems. You may wish to ask your pharmacist about special solutions, called artificial saliva, that can also be used to help restore moisture in the mouth.

It is especially important to brush and floss your teeth regularly if you develop a dry mouth to help prevent gum problems.

If this medicine causes dizziness or lightheadedness, you should be careful going up and down stairs and you should not change positions too rapidly. Lightheadedness is more likely to occur if you stand up suddenly—this is due to blood collecting in the legs and lasts for a few seconds. Therefore, get up from a sitting or lying position more slowly and tighten and relax your leg muscles or wiggle your toes to help promote circulation. In the morning, get out of bed slowly and dangle your feet over the edge of the bed for a few minutes before standing up. Sit or lie down at the first sign of dizziness. Do not drive a car, operate dangerous machinery or do jobs that require you to be alert if you are dizzy. Tell your doctor if you have been dizzy.

In order to help prevent dizziness or fainting, your doctor may also recommend that you avoid strenuous exercise, standing for long periods of time (especially in hot weather), hot showers, hot baths or saunas.

When to Call Your Doctor

Call your doctor if you develop swelling of the legs or ankles, sudden weight gain of 5 pounds (2.5 kg) or more, fast or irregular heartbeats, fainting, blurred or "double" vision, spots before the eyes, chest pain, difficulty urinating, tremors, convulsions, flushing, increased sweating, depression, nightmares, confusion, fever, chills, sore throat, joint or muscle pains, numbness or tingling, unusual bruising or bleeding, shortness of breath, difficulty breathing, or a skin rash.

Allergic Reactions

Call your doctor immediately if you think you may be allergic to the medicine or if you develop a skin rash, hives, itching, swelling of the face or difficulty in breathing. If you cannot reach your doctor, phone a hospital emergency department.

Refills

Do not stop taking this medicine without your doctor's approval and do not go without medicine between prescription refills. Call your pharmacist for a refill 2 or 3 days before you will run out of the medicine.

Miscellaneous

Carry an identification card in your wallet or wear a medical alert bracelet indicating that you are taking this medicine as well as the names and phone numbers of your doctors. If you do not already carry such a card, complete the Medicine Card in this book.

Always tell your dentist, pharmacist and other doctors who are treating you that you are taking this medicine.

FLURAZEPAM (ORAL)

APO-FLURAZEPAM, DALMANE, NOVOFLUPAM, SOMNOL, SOM-PAM

TEMAZEPAM

RESTORIL

TRIAZOLAM

HALCION

Purpose

This medicine is used to treat some types of sleep disorders.

Allergies/Warnings

If you have ever had an allergic reaction to any medicine or if you have depression or any medical problem, tell your doctor and pharmacist before you take any of this medicine.

How to Use This Medicine

Time of Administration

Take this medicine at least 20 to 30 minutes before you want to fall asleep. Go to bed after you have taken the medicine. Do not smoke in bed after you have taken it because you could fall asleep and cause a fire.

How to Administer

This medicine may be taken either with food or on an empty stomach.

Special Instructions

Length of Therapy

Sleeping medicines are only useful for a short time. If used for too long, they lose their effectiveness. Do not take any more of this medicine than your doctor has prescribed.

Do not stop taking this medicine suddenly without the approval of your doctor. It may be necessary for your doctor to reduce your dose slowly since your body may need time to adjust.

Check with your doctor if you develop any of the following while you are slowly stopping the medicine: nausea or vomiting, trembling, seizures, muscle cramps, stomach cramps, unusual sweating, fast heartbeats, trouble sleeping or if you become confused, irritable or nervous.

Pregnancy/Breastfeeding

Women who are pregnant, breastfeeding or planning to become pregnant should tell their doctor before taking this medicine. This medicine should generally not be used during pregnancy and is not generally recommended during breastfeeding.

Drug Interactions

It is important that you obtain the advice of your doctor or pharmacist before taking any other prescription or nonprescription medicines, including pain relievers, sleeping pills, tranquilizers or medicines for depression, or cough, cold or allergy medicines. Excessive drowsiness or confusion may occur when some of these drugs are taken together.

There are other drug interactions that can occur. If you are taking any other medicines, be sure to check first with your pharmacist or doctor.

Alcohol

Do not drink alcoholic beverages while taking this drug or for a few days after you have stopped taking the drug without the approval of your doctor. The combination could cause drowsiness. One drink (even during the day) may have the same effect that 2 or 3 drinks normally would have.

Special Precautions

Be careful if you have to get up during the night while taking this medicine. You may not feel as alert as usual.

If you have problems sleeping, you should avoid caffeinated beverages, certain cold decongestants and strenuous exercise in the evenings as they make it more difficult to fall asleep. There are other drug interactions that can occur. If you are taking any other medicines, be sure to check with your pharmacist or doctor.

If this medicine causes dizziness or drowsiness the next day after you take it, do not drive a car, pilot an airplane, operate dangerous machinery or do jobs that require you to be alert if you are dizzy or drowsy. You should also be careful going up and down stairs. Sit or lie down at the first sign of dizziness.

If this hangover drowsiness becomes bothersome, call your doctor.

If you do not fall asleep after taking the prescribed amount, do *not* take an additional dose unless advised by your doctor.

You may experience a sleep problem (insomnia) on the first night or two after stopping the drug. This is not a reason for restarting the medicine and your sleep should gradually return to normal.

When to Call Your Doctor

Most people experience few or no side effects from this drug. However, any medicine can sometimes cause unwanted effects. Call your doctor if you develop a sore throat, fever, mouth sores, a staggering walk, a yellow color to the skin or eyes, slow heartbeats or shortness of breath, unusual tiredness or nervousness, stomach pain, confusion or depression, seizures, hallucinations, trouble sleeping, slurred speech, severe drowsiness, ringing or buzzing in the ears or numbness or tingling of the hands or feet.

Allergic Reactions

Call your doctor immediately if you think you may be allergic to the medicine or if you develop a skin rash, hives, itching, swelling of the face or difficulty in breathing. If you cannot reach your doctor, phone a hospital emergency department.

HALOPERIDOL (ORAL)

APO-HALOPERIDOL, HALDOL, NOVOPERIDOL, PERIDOL

Purpose

This medicine has many uses and the reason it was prescribed depends upon your condition. Check with your doctor if you do not fully understand why you are taking it.

Allergies/Warnings

If you have ever had an allergic reaction to any medicine or if you have high blood pressure, seizures, heart problems, enlarged prostate, difficulty urinating (passing your water), Parkinson's disease, glaucoma or any other medical problem, tell your doctor and pharmacist before you take any of this medicine.

Also tell your doctor if you are hypersensitive to tartrazine (a yellow dye). HALDOL 1mg, 5mg and 10mg contain tartrazine.

How to Use This Medicine

How to Administer

Take this medicine with food or immediately after meals to help prevent stomach upset unless otherwise directed.

For liquid medicine:

- The liquid medicine may be mixed with milk, food or water. Do *not* mix it with tea or coffee or some juices because this may decrease the effect of the medicine.
- A dropper is used to measure the dose. If you do not fully understand how to use it, *see* How to Administer Medications (page 15).
- Do not get the liquid on your skin or clothing.

Special Instructions

Length of Therapy

It is important that you take the medicine regularly and that you do not miss any doses. The full benefit of the medicine may not be noticed immediately, but may take from a few days to a few weeks.

Do not stop taking this medicine suddenly without the approval of your doctor. It will be necessary for your doctor to reduce your dose slowly since your body will need time to adjust. It could make your condition worse if you suddenly stopped taking the medicine. After you have stopped taking this medicine, you must observe the following precautions (see Alcohol below) for 1 to 2 weeks since some of the medicine will still be in your body.

Pregnancy/Breastfeeding

Women who are pregnant, breastfeeding or planning to become pregnant should tell their doctor before taking this medicine.

Drug Interactions

It is important that you obtain the advice of your doctor or pharmacist before taking any other prescription or nonprescription medicines, including pain relievers, sleeping pills, other tranquilizers or medicines for depression, cough, cold or allergy medicines.

There are other drug interactions that can occur. If you are taking any other medicines, be sure to check first with your pharmacist or doctor.

Alcohol

Do not drink alcoholic beverages while taking this drug without the approval of your doctor. The combination could irritate your stomach and could cause drowsiness or dizziness. One drink may have the same effect that 2 or 3 drinks normally would have.

If you have been taking this medicine regularly for several days or weeks, it is recommended not to drink alcohol for two weeks after you have stopped taking the medicine. Depending on your dose, it may take this long for the drug to be eliminated from your body.

Special Precautions

If this medicine causes dizziness or lightheadedness, you should be careful going up and down stairs and you should not change positions too rapidly. Lightheadedness is more likely to occur if you stand up suddenly—this is due to blood collecting in the legs and lasts for a few seconds. Therefore, get up from a sitting or lying position more slowly and tighten and relax your leg muscles or wiggle your toes to help promote circulation. In the morning, get out of bed slowly and dangle your feet over the edge of the bed for a few minutes before standing up. Sit or lie down at the first sign of dizziness. Tell your doctor if you have been dizzy.

In order to help prevent dizziness or fainting, your doctor may also recommend that you avoid strenuous exercise, standing for long periods of time (especially in hot weather), hot showers, hot baths or saunas.

In some people, this drug may cause drowsiness, especially after any increase in your dose. Do not drive a car, pilot an airplane, operate dangerous machinery or do jobs that require you to be alert until you know how you are going to react to this drug.

If your mouth becomes dry, drink water, suck ice chips or a hard, sour candy (sugarless) or chew gum (sugarless). Sugarless products are recommended in order to avoid dental problems. You may wish to ask your pharmacist about special solutions, called artificial saliva, that can also be used to help restore moisture in the mouth. It is especially important to brush and floss your teeth regularly if you develop a dry mouth to help prevent gum problems.

This medicine may cause some people to become constipated. To help prevent constipation, try increasing the amount of bulk in your diet (for example, bran, fresh fruits and salads), exercising more often or drinking more fluids (unless otherwise directed). Call your doctor if the constipation continues.

You may become more sensitive to heat because your body may perspire less while you are taking this drug. Be careful not to become overheated during exercise or in hot weather. Try to avoid strenuous exercise, standing for long periods of time (especially in hot weather), hot showers, hot baths, saunas or Jacuzzis while taking this medicine.

Some patients may also become more sensitive to cold and should dress warmly during cold weather and limit exposure to cold temperatures.

This medicine often makes some people more sensitive to sunlight and various tanning lamps. When you begin taking this medicine, try to avoid too much sun until you see how you are going to react. If your skin does become more sensitive to sunlight, tell your doctor and try not to stay in direct sunlight for extended periods of time. While in the sun, wear protective clothing and sunglasses. You may wish to ask your pharmacist about suitable sunscreen products. Call your doctor if you become sunburned.

When to Call Your Doctor

Any medicine can cause unwanted effects. Call your doctor if you develop a sore throat, fever, mouth sores, changes in vision, difficulty in urinating (passing your water), decreased sexual ability, a yellow color in the skin or eyes, fast heartbeats, a skin rash, nausea or vomiting, fainting spells or seizures.

Call your doctor if you become restless or unable to sit still or sleep or if you develop drooling, fever, confusion, menstrual irregularities, difficulty breathing, speaking or swallowing, disturbed gait or shuffling walk, tremors, shakiness or unusual movements of the face, tongue or hands or stiffness of the face or body.

If you develop painful muscle spasms, call your doctor or go to the hospital emergency room since treatment can be given to provide rapid relief of this problem.

Storage

Store the liquid medicine in a cool, dark place.

Refills

Do not stop taking this medicine without your doctor's approval and do not go without medicine between prescription refills. Call your pharmacist for a refill 2 or 3 days before you will run out of the medicine.

Discuss with your pharmacist the implications of dispensing all your refills for this medicine with the same manufacturer's product. (*See* Generic Drugs, page 12.)

Miscellaneous

Carry an identification card in your wallet or wear a medical alert bracelet indicating that you are taking this medicine as well as the names and phone numbers of your doctors. If you do not already carry such a card, complete the Medicine Card in this book. Always tell your dentist, pharmacist and other doctors who are treating you that you are taking this medicine.

Chronic Hallucinosis From Nose Drops

There are now 2 reports in the medical literature suggesting that heavy use of decongestant nose drops may cause psychoses (bizarre behavior) in some patients.

A 61-year-old man had been using a variety of nasal decongestant drops and sprays for a sinus condition since the early 1940s. After several years, he used the products every 30 minutes because of an impending feeling of suffocation. He reported heavy threatening voices and frightening visual imagery, usually at night, for the last 20 years.

When the nose drops and sprays were stopped and appropriate treatment started, the nasal obstruction gradually decreased and the symptoms of psychoses and anxiety disappeared. The symptoms reappeared when the patient had the flu and started taking decongestants at high doses. The hallucinations and delusions once again stopped when the doctor stopped the decongestants.

The *Journal of the American Medical Association* reported that four months later, the patient had no nasal congestion and had sustained relief from hallucinations for the first time in 20 years.

As a general rule, never use nasal decongestant drops or sprays for more than a few days. The symptoms of nasal congestion that you are treating can also become a side effect of the decongestants. Rebound congestion can occur if the nasal decongestant drops or sprays are used too long.

HYDRALAZINE (ORAL)

APRESOLINE, NOVO-HYALAZIN

Purpose

This medicine is used to treat high blood pressure.

Allergies/Warnings

If you have ever had an allergic reaction to any medicine, tell your doctor and pharmacist before you take any of this medicine.

How to Use This Medicine

Time of Administration

Try to take the medicine at the same time(s) every day so that you have a constant level of the medicine in your body.

How to Administer

It is best to take this medicine with food because food helps the body to absorb more of the drug.

Special Instructions

High blood pressure (hypertension) is a long-term condition and it will probably be necessary for you to take the drug for a long time in spite of the fact that you feel better. If high blood pressure is not treated, it can lead to serious problems such as heart failure, strokes, blood vessel problems or kidney problems. It is very important that you take this medicine as your doctor has directed and that you do not miss any doses. Otherwise, you cannot expect the drug to keep your blood pressure down.

Do not take any more of this medicine than your doctor has prescribed and *do not stop taking this medicine suddenly without the approval of your doctor*. It will be necessary for your doctor to reduce your dose slowly since your body will need time to adjust. It could be harmful and make your condition worse if you suddenly stopped taking the medicine.

Pregnancy/Breastfeeding

Women who are pregnant, breastfeeding or planning to become pregnant should tell their doctor before taking this medicine.

Drug Interactions

Some nonprescription drugs can aggravate your condition. Do not take any of the following without the approval of your doctor or pharmacist: cough, cold or sinus products; asthma, allergy or hay fever products since they could increase your blood pressure. Read the label of the product to see if there is a warning. If there is, check with your doctor or pharmacist before using the product.

This medicine may lower vitamin B_6 levels in the body. Signs of low vitamin B_6 (pyroxidine) include numbness or tingling of the fingers or toes, or shakiness. Call your doctor if this occurs—he may want to consider vitamin B_6 supplements.

Alcohol

Do not drink alcoholic beverages while taking this drug without the approval of your doctor because the combination could make the possible side effect of dizziness worse.

Special Precautions

If this medicine causes dizziness or lightheadedness, you should be careful going up and down stairs and you should not change positions too rapidly. Lightheadedness is more likely to occur if you stand up suddenly—this is due to blood collecting in the legs and lasts for a few seconds. Therefore, get up from a sitting or lying position more slowly and tighten and relax your leg muscles or wiggle your toes to help promote circulation. In the morning, get out of bed slowly and dangle your feet over the edge of the bed for a few minutes before standing up. Sit or lie down at the first sign of dizziness. Tell your doctor you have been dizzy. In order to help prevent dizziness or fainting, your doctor may also recommend that you avoid strenuous exercise, standing for long periods of time (especially in hot weather), hot showers, hot baths or saunas.

If you become dizzy, you should not drive a car, pilot an airplane, operate dangerous machinery or do jobs that require you to be alert.

Follow any special diet your doctor may have ordered. He or she may want you to limit the amount of salt in your diet.

Headaches may occur during the first few days of therapy, but they usually disappear within the first week. If they continue, call your doctor.

When to Call Your Doctor

Most people experience few or no side effects from this drug. However, any medicine can sometimes cause unwanted effects. Call your doctor if you develop a sore throat, fever, itching, chest pains, fast heartbeats, swelling of the legs or ankles, sudden weight gain of 5 pounds (2.5 kg) or more, swelling of the glands in the neck or armpits or numbness or tingling in the hands or feet.

Stop taking this medicine and call your doctor immediately if you develop joint or muscle pain, a skin rash, fever, chest pains, unusual tiredness or weakness or other unexplained symptoms.

Refills

Do not stop taking this medicine without your doctor's approval and do not go without medicine between prescription refills. Call your pharmacist for a refill 2 or 3 days before you will run out of the medicine.

Discuss with your pharmacist the implications of dispensing all your refills for this medicine with the same manufacturer's product. (*See* Generic Drugs, page 12.)

Miscellaneous

Carry an identification card in your wallet or wear a medical alert bracelet indicating that you are taking this medicine as well as the names and phone numbers of your doctors. If you do not already carry such a card, complete the Medicine Card in this book. Always tell your dentist, pharmacist and other doctors who are treating you that you are taking this medicine.

Did You Know That?

Blood pressure and stomach acid secretion are highest during the night.

Stomach acid secretion reaches a peak during the night between 10 P.M. and 2 A.M. The lowest point is during late morning just before lunch. Anti-ulcer drugs that block the secretion of stomach acids may have their greatest effect during the sleeping hours.

Blood pressure tends to be highest in the morning and lowest in the evening. The blood pressure rises during the night. Blood pressure medications given at bedtime may play a very significant role in the lowering of blood pressure during the night.

HYDROCHLOROTHIAZIDE (ORAL)

APO-HYDRO, DIUCHLOR H, HYDRODIURIL, NATRIMAX, NEO-CODEMA, NOVOHYDRAZIDE, UROZIDE

BENDROFLUMETHIAZIDE

NATURETIN

CHLORTHALIDONE

APO-CHLORTHALIDONE, HYGROTON, NOVOTHALIDONE, URIDON

INDAPAMIDE

LOZIDE

METHYCHLOTHIAZIDE

DURETIC

METOLAZONE

ZAROXOLYN

Purpose

This medicine is used to treat high blood pressure and heart and kidney problems. It helps rid the body of excess fluids and decreases swelling. The medicine works by increasing the amount of urine and is commonly called a water pill or fluid pill.

Allergies/Warnings

Be sure to tell your doctor and pharmacist if you are allergic to sulfa drugs, thiazide diuretics or any other medicine or if you have a history of gout.

How to Use This Medicine

Time of Administration

Try to take this medicine at the same time(s) every day so that you have a constant level of the medicine in your body.

When you first start taking this medicine, you will probably urinate (pass your water) more often and in larger amounts than usual. Therefore, if you are to take 1 dose each day, take it in the morning after breakfast. Do not initially take a dose at bedtime or you may have to get up during the night to go to the bathroom. If you are to take more than 1 dose each day, take the last dose approximately 6 hours before bedtime so that you will not have to get up during the night to go to the bathroom. This effect will usually lessen after you have taken the drug for a while.

How to Administer

Take this medicine with food, meals or milk if it upsets your stomach.

Special Instructions

Length of Therapy

For patients with high blood pressure:

- High blood pressure (hypertension) is a long-term condition and it will probably be necessary for you to take the drug for a long time even if you feel better. If high blood pressure is not treated, it can lead to serious problems such as heart failure, strokes, blood vessel problems or kidney problems.

It is very important that you take this medicine as your doctor has directed and that you do not miss any doses. Otherwise, you cannot expect the drug to keep your blood pressure down or remove excess fluid.

Pregnancy/Breastfeeding

Women who are pregnant, breastfeeding or planning to become pregnant should tell their doctor before taking this medicine.

Drug Interactions

Some nonprescription drugs can aggravate high blood pressure. Do not take any of the following without the approval of your doctor or pharmacist: cough, cold or sinus products; asthma or allergy products since they may increase your blood pressure. Read the label of the nonprescription drug product to see if there is a warning. If there is, check with your doctor or pharmacist before using the product.

Alcohol

Be careful drinking alcoholic beverages while taking this medicine because it could make the possible side effect of dizziness worse.

Special Precautions

This medicine normally causes your body to lose potassium. The body has warning signs to let you know if too much potssium is being lost. Call your doctor if you become unusually thirsty or if you develop leg cramps, unusual weakness, fatigue, vomiting, confusion or an irregular pulse. Since these symptoms may not be present in all patients, your doctor may wish to check your blood occasionally to see if it is low in potassium. Depending upon your dose, your doctor may prescribe some medicine to replace the potassium or he or she may recommend that you regularly eat foods that contain a lot of potassium (see Appendix A). *Do not change your diet unless your doctor tells you to.*

If this medicine causes dizziness or lightheadedness, you should be careful going up and down stairs and you should not change positions too rapidly. Lightheadedness is more likely to occur if you stand up suddenly—this is due to blood collecting in the legs and lasts for a few seconds. Therefore, get up from a sitting or lying position more slowly and tighten and relax your leg muscles or wiggle your toes to help promote circulation. In the morning, get out of bed slowly and dangle your feet over the edge of the bed for a few minutes before standing up. Sit or lie down at the first sign of dizziness. Do not drive a car, pilot an airplane, operate dangerous machinery or do jobs that require you to be alert if you are dizzy. Tell your doctor if you have been dizzy.

In order to help prevent dizziness or fainting, your doctor may also recommend that you avoid strenuous exercise, standing for long periods of time (especially in hot weather), hot showers, hot baths, Jacuzzis or saunas.

People more than 65 years of age may be more sensitive to the side effects of dizziness and potassium loss.

This medicine may make some people more sensitive to sunlight and various tanning lamps. When you begin taking this medicine, try to avoid too much sun until you see how you are going to react. If your skin does become more sensitive to sunlight, tell your doctor and try not to stay in direct sunlight for extended periods of time. While in the sun, wear protective clothing and sunglasses. You may wish to ask your pharmacist about suitable sunscreen products. Call your doctor if you become sunburned.

For patients with diabetes:

- This medicine may cause your blood sugar to rise. Carefully test your blood or urine for sugar while you are taking this medicine. Call your doctor if you think your blood sugar is higher than normal or harder to control.

Did You Know That?

At least one in ten people over the age of 65 years has a bladder problem, which can range from slight losses of urine to complete loss of bladder control.

Help for Incontinent People, a nonprofit organization to help people who are incontinent, lists the following ten warning signs of bladder control problems:

1. Leakage of urine that prevents the person from participating in daily activities
2. Leakage of urine that causes embarrassment
3. Leakage of urine that began or continued after an operation (hysterectomy, caesarean section, prostate surgery, lower intestinal or rectal surgery)
4. Inability to urinate (retention of urine) following an operation
5. Urinating more frequently than usual without a proven bladder infection
6. Needing to rush to the bathroom and/or losing urine if you do not "arrive in time"

7. Pain related to filling the bladder and/or pain related to urination (in the absence of a bladder infection)
8. Frequent bladder infections
9. Progressive weakness of the urinary flow with or without a feeling of incomplete bladder emptying
10. Abnormal urination or changes in urination related to a nervous system abnormality (stroke, spinal cord injury, multiple sclerosis, etc.)

What many people do not know is that, in some people, loss of bladder control can be successfully treated or cured. There are many different causes of bladder control problems. Transient or reversible incontinence is one type of incontinence that is temporary. Some people with transient incontinence appear to be more sensitive to the effects of certain medications on the bladder or the urethra. In these cases, simply changing the medications a person is taking can sometimes eliminate the problem and restore bladder control to normal. Always seek medical advice and never try to adjust your own drug therapy. Some medications, such as those for high blood pressure and heart conditions, could cause serious adverse effects if you tampered with the prescribed dosage.

If you, or anyone you know, has bladder control problems, ask your physician to refer you to a specialist in incontinence. Also ask your pharmacist about the newer incontinence products that are now available to help people continue to lead active lives.

When to Call Your Doctor

Most people experience few or no side effects from this drug. However, any medicine can sometimes cause unwanted effects. Call your doctor if you develop an unexplained sore throat or fever, sharp stomach pain, sharp joint pain, unusual bruising or bleeding, a yellow color to the skin or eyes, unusual weakness or tiredness or a sudden weight gain of 5 pounds (2.5 kg) or more. Also call your doctor if you become sick or develop persistent vomiting or diarrhea.

Allergic Reactions

Call your doctor immediately if you think you may be allergic to the medicine or if you develop a skin rash, hives, itching, swelling of the face

or difficulty in breathing. If you cannot reach your doctor, phone a hospital emergency department.

Refills

Do not stop taking this medicine without your doctor's approval and do not go without medicine between prescription refills. Call your pharmacist for a refill 2 or 3 days before you will run out of the medicine.

Discuss with your pharmacist the implications of dispensing all your refills for this medicine with the same manufacturer's product. (*See* Generic Drugs, page 12.)

HYDROCODONE AND PHENYLTOLOXAMINE-RESIN COMPLEXES (ORAL)

TUSSIONEX

Purpose

This is a strong cough medicine used to help relieve dry irritating coughs that have not responded to other cough medicines.

Allergies/Warnings

If you have ever had an allergic reaction to HYDROCODONE or CODEINE medicine or if you have asthma, glaucoma, an enlarged prostate or difficulty urinating (passing your water), tell your doctor before you take any of this medicine.

This medicine should not be used in children under the age of 1 year or weighing less than 9 kg.

How to Use This Medicine

Time of Administration

This medicine may be taken without regard to meals. Take it either with food or on an empty stomach. If stomach upset occurs, take it with some food or a glass of milk.

How to Administer

For tablets:

- Take with a glass of water or with food.

For liquid medicine:

- Shake the bottle well each time before pouring so that you can measure an accurate dose.

- Since a spoon is used to measure the dose, it is recommended that you use a medicine spoon or an oral liquid syringe that you can obtain from your pharmacist. These are more accurate than the average household teaspoon. *See* How to Administer Medications (page 15).
- Do *not* dilute the liquid medicine or mix with other liquid medicines. This could change the way the medicine acts and could result in an overdose. Try not to drink other liquids immediately after taking this medicine so that the medicine will work properly.

Helpful Hint: Trouble Swallowing Pills?

Do you have trouble swallowing tablets and capsules? Try this technique the next time you have to swallow a medication:

Place a small piece of bread (or another piece of soft food) on your tongue. Place the tablet or capsule next to the piece of bread. Take a drink of water and swallow the bread.

Guess what? The chances are very high that you swallowed the medicine too!

The Reason:
Every day we swallow pieces of food—many of which are much larger than any of the tablets or capsules you will ever have to take. Many of the problems surrounding the inability to swallow tablets and capsules are psychological and this simple technique has helped many people to overcome this problem.

Special Instructions

Length of Therapy

Do not use this medicine for more than 1 week without the advice of your doctor. When used for a long period of time, the drug can become less effective. Also, when used in large doses for a long period of time, the drug can become habit forming.

If you have had to take this medicine for more than a few weeks, do not stop taking this medicine suddenly without the approval of your doctor. It may be necessary for your doctor to reduce your dose slowly since your body will need time to adjust. It could be harmful and make your condition worse if you suddenly did not receive the medicine.

Pregnancy/Breastfeeding

Women who are pregnant, breastfeeding or planning to become pregnant should not take this medicine.

Drug Interactions

It is important that you obtain the advice of your doctor or pharmacist before taking any other prescription or nonprescription medicines including pain relievers, sleeping pills, tranquilizers, medicine for seizures, muscle relaxants, anesthetics, medicines for depression or medicines for allergies. Combining this medicine with some of these drugs could cause drowsiness or dizziness.

There are other drug interactions that can occur. If you are taking any other medicines, be sure to check first with your pharmacist or doctor.

Alcohol

Do not drink alcoholic beverages while taking this drug without the approval of your doctor because the combination could cause drowsiness or dizziness. One drink may have the same effect that 2 or 3 drinks normally would have.

Does Half a Tablet Contain Half the Dose?

Not always!

In one study reported in a leading medical journal, researchers evaluated whether tablets broke evenly into 2 halves of equivalent and accurate doses. The tablets were broken along the score lines (indentations) and each half of a tablet was weighed. A tablet was classified as excellent if 95% of the halves were within 5% of the expected weight.

Of the 13 brands of antihypertensive medications tested, only 2 brands were rated as excellent and contained equal doses in each half of the tablets. Eight brands were classed as moderate (within 5 to 10% of the expected weight) and 3 brands showed more than a 10% error in weight.

Special Precautions

If you feel nauseated or sick to your stomach when you first start taking this medicine, it may help to lie down for a few minutes. Lying down may also help any dizziness go away.

In some people, this drug may initially cause dizziness or drowsiness. Do not drive a car, pilot an airplane, operate dangerous machinery or do jobs that require you to be alert until you know how you are going to react to the drug. If you have been dizzy, tell your doctor at your next visit. Your dose may have to be adjusted.

If this medicine causes dizziness or lightheadedness, you should be careful going up and down stairs and you should not change positions too rapidly. Lightheadedness is more likely to occur if you stand up suddenly—this is due to blood collecting in the legs and lasts for a few seconds. Therefore, get up from a sitting or lying position more slowly and tighten and relax your leg muscles or wiggle your toes to help promote circulation. In the morning, get out of bed slowly and dangle your feet over the edge of the bed for a few minutes before standing up. Sit or lie down at the first sign of dizziness. Tell your doctor if you have been dizzy.

In order to help prevent dizziness or fainting, your doctor may also recommend that you avoid strenuous exercise, standing for long periods of time (especially in hot weather), hot showers, hot baths or saunas.

If your mouth becomes dry, drink water, suck ice chips or a hard, sour candy (sugarless) or chew gum (sugarless). Sugarless products are recommended in order to avoid dental problems. You may wish to ask your pharmacist about special solutions, called artificial saliva, that can also be used to help restore moisture in the mouth. It is especially important to brush and floss your teeth regularly if you develop a dry mouth to help prevent gum problems.

This medicine may cause some people to become constipated. To help prevent constipation, try increasing the amount of bulk in your diet (for example, bran, fresh fruits and salads), exercising more often or drinking more fluids (unless otherwise directed). Call your doctor if the constipation continues.

When to Call Your Doctor

Call your doctor if the cough lasts longer than 1 week or if you develop a fever, skin rash or constant headache.

Most people experience few or no side effects from these drugs. However, any medicine can sometimes cause unwanted effects. Call your doctor if you develop a skin rash, fast or slow heartbeats, unexplained nervousness, restlessness or irritability, trouble sleeping, shortness of breath, fainting, confusion, hallucinations or depression, seizures, ringing or buzzing in the ears, difficulty in urinating (passing your water) or if mucus (lung secretions) becomes thicker than normal.

People over 65 years of age may be more sensitive to these side effects.

Children may be more sensitive to the breathing problems. Therefore, this medicine should not be used in children under 1 year.

Allergic Reactions

Call your doctor immediately if you think you may be allergic to the medicine or if you develop a skin rash, hives, itching, swelling of the face or difficulty in breathing. If you cannot reach your doctor, phone a hospital emergency department.

Attention Breastfeeding Women!

Topical application of lanolin or vitamin E are popular treatments for sore nipples when a woman begins breastfeeding. As with the use of any drugs during breastfeeding, there are important considerations which should be made.

Women who are breastfeeding and allergic to wool should not apply lanolin to their nipples. Lanolin is made from the wool of sheep and the woman could experience an allergic reaction.

Vitamin E oil applied to the nipples of breastfeeding women has been reported to be absorbed by babies and cause high blood levels in the babies. It is not known whether the infants directly ingested and absorbed the vitamin E or whether the vitamin E was absorbed by the mother and transferred to the infant through the breast milk. The risk of the elevated vitamin E levels in the infants has not been established.

HYDROXYZINE HCl (ORAL)

APO-HYDROXYZINE, ATARAX, MULTIPAX, NOVOHYDROXYZIN

Purpose

This medicine is used to help relieve the symptoms of anxiety and tension and certain types of emotional problems, allergic conditions, and skin rashes. This drug has several other uses and the reason it was prescribed depends upon your condition. Check with your doctor if you do not fully understand why you are taking it.

Allergies

If you have ever had an allergic reaction to any medicine, tell your doctor and pharmacist before you take any of this medicine.

How to Use This Medicine

How to Administer

For capsules:

- Take the medicine with food or a full glass of water unless otherwise directed.

For ATARAX SYRUP:

- It is rccommended that you use a medicine spoon or an oral liquid syringe that you can obtain from your pharmacist. These are more accurate than the average household teaspoon. *See* How to Administer Medications (page 15).

Special Instructions

Pregnancy/Breastfeeding

Women who are pregnant, breastfeeding or planning to become pregnant should tell their doctor before taking this medicine.

Drug Interactions

It is important that you obtain the advice of your doctor or pharmacist before taking any other prescription or nonprescription medicines, including pain relievers, sleeping pills, tranquilizers or medicines for depression, or cough, cold or allergy medicines. Excessive drowsiness may occur in some people.

There are other drug interactions that can occur. If you are taking any other medicines, be sure to check first with your pharmacist or doctor.

Alcohol

Do not drink alcoholic beverages while taking this drug or for a few days after stopping the drug without the approval of your doctor because the combination could cause drowsiness. One drink may have the same effect that 2 or 3 drinks normally would have.

Special Precautions

In some people, this drug may cause dizziness or drowsiness. Do not drive a car, pilot an airplane, operate dangerous machinery or do jobs that require you to be alert if you are dizzy or drowsy. You should also be careful going up and down stairs. Tell your doctor if the dizziness continues.

If your mouth becomes dry, drink water, suck ice chips or a hard, sour candy (sugarless) or chew gum (sugarless). Sugarless products are recommended in order to avoid dental problems. You may wish to ask your pharmacist about special solutions, called artificial saliva, that can also be used to help restore moisture in the mouth. It is especially important to brush and floss your teeth regularly if you develop a dry mouth to help prevent gum problems.

Did You Know That?

You should *not* double your next dose if you forget to take a previous one without checking with your doctor or pharmacist.

All medications are slightly different. In some cases, doubling the next dose will be advisable and will not cause any problems. However, with other drugs, doubling the next dose could put too much drug into the bloodstream and cause serious toxic effects. Examples of some drugs that should *not* be doubled are:

WARFARIN (a blood thinner)
THYROID medicines
DIGOXIN (medicine for the heart) and
PHENYTOIN (medicine for epilepsy)

So that you do not face the question of whether to double the next dose, the best advice is to try to keep track of your doses and do your best not to miss any doses. There are several aids available in pharmacies and you can prepare your own reminder list on a calendar.

When to Call Your Doctor

Most people experience few or no side effects from this drug. However, any medicine can sometimes cause unwanted effects. Call your doctor if you develop a skin rash, sore throat, fever, mouth sores, fainting, trembling, difficulty urinating (passing your water), shakiness or seizures.

Allergic Reactions

Call your doctor immediately if you think you may be allergic to the medicine or if you develop a skin rash, hives, itching, swelling of the face or difficulty in breathing. If you cannot reach your doctor, phone a hospital emergency department.

INDOMETHACIN (ORAL)

APO-INDOMETHACIN, INDOCID, INDOCID SR, NOVOMETHACIN

INDOMETHACIN (RECTAL)

INDOCID SUPPOSITORIES

Purpose

This medicine is used to help relieve certain types of pain. It is also used to help relieve inflammation, stiffness, swelling and joint pain in certain kinds of arthritis and gout.

The sustained release (INDOCID SR) capsules are not meant to treat gout.

Allergies/Warnings

If you have ever had an allergic reaction to ASA (acetylsalicylic acid) or any other medicine or if you suffer from hay fever, asthma, nasal polyps, ulcers or any other medical problems, tell your doctor and pharmacist before you take any of this medicine.

How to Use This Medicine

Time of Administration

Always take this medicine with food or a glass of milk or immediately after meals to help prevent stomach upset (indigestion, nausea, vomiting, stomach pain). It is recommended that you do not lie down within 15 minutes after taking the medicine so that the capsule can reach the stomach. If you develop persistent stomach pain, contact your doctor.

How to Administer

If you were prescribed INDOCID SR, these capsules must be swallowed whole. Do not crush or break them open.

If you were prescribed INDOCID SUPPOSITORIES: *See* How to Administer Medications (page 15).

Special Instructions

Length of Therapy

This medicine will not cure arthritis but it can help control inflammation that can increase damage to your joints. It is very important that you take this medicine regularly and that you *do not miss any doses*. If you miss a dose, the level of the medicine in your body will fall and the drug will not be as effective. Only if the drug is at the right level will it be able to decrease the inflammation and swelling in your joints and help prevent further damage.

If you are taking this medicine for a joint or bone problem, you may have to take the drug from a few days to 4 weeks before you feel its full benefits. Long-term therapy is often required in arthritis.

This medicine does not replace any exercise or rest programs or use of heat/cold treatments your doctor may have prescribed.

Pregnancy/Breastfeeding

Women who are pregnant, breastfeeding or planning to become pregnant should tell their doctor before taking this medicine. Use of this medicine during pregnancy, especially the last three months, and during breastfeeding is not recommended.

Drug Interactions

Do not take any other medicines containing ASA (acetylsalicylic acid) or salicylates while you are taking this medicine without the approval of your doctor. The combination could cause stomach problems.

It is usually safe to take acetaminophen for fever or the occasional headache. Check first with your pharmacist.

Alcohol

Do not drink alcoholic beverages while taking this drug without the approval of your doctor because the combination could cause stomach problems.

Special Precautions

In some people, this drug may cause dizziness or drowsiness. Do not drive a car, pilot an airplane, operate dangerous machinery or do jobs that require you to be alert until you know how you are going to react to this drug. If you become dizzy, you should be careful going up and down stairs. Sit or lie down at the first sign of dizziness. Tell your doctor if you have been dizzy.

This medicine may cause some people to become constipated. To help prevent constipation, try increasing the amount of bulk in your diet (for example, bran, fresh fruits and salads), exercising more often or drinking more fluids (unless otherwise directed). Call your doctor if the constipation continues.

When to Call Your Doctor

Most people experience few or no side effects from this drug. However, any medicine can sometimes cause unwanted effects. Call your doctor if you develop a skin rash, sore throat or fever, chills, "ringing" or "buzzing" in the ears, any loss of hearing, fast heartbeats, swelling of the legs or ankles or sudden weight gain, blurred vision or changes in your eyesight, bloody or black stools, severe stomach pain, vomiting, diarrhea (loose bowel movements), a yellow color to the skin or eyes, unusual bruising or bleeding, unusual tiredness or weakness, confusion or depression, seizures, blood in the urine or a persistent headache.

Allergic Reactions

Call your doctor immediately if you think you may be allergic to the medicine or if you develop a skin rash, hives, itching, swelling of the face or difficulty in breathing. If you cannot reach your doctor, phone a hospital emergency department.

Storage

For tablets and capsules:

- Store in a cool, dry, dark place.

For suppositories:

- *See* How to Administer Medications (page 15).

Refills

Do not stop taking this medicine without your doctor's approval and do not go without medicine between prescription refills. Call your pharmacist for a refill 2 or 3 days before you will run out of the medicine.

Miscellaneous

Carry an identification card in your wallet or wear a medical alert bracelet indicating that you are taking this medicine as well as the names and phone numbers of your doctors. If you do not already carry such a card, complete the Medicine Card in this book. Always tell your dentist, pharmacist and other doctors who are treating you that you are taking this medicine.

Did You Know That?

Laxatives should not be used for longer than 1 week unless directed by your doctor.

Laxatives are not designed for long-term use. Chronic overuse of harsh stimulant laxatives can lead to a lazy colon—and constipation—and the person may be unable to have a bowel movement without taking a laxative. Excessive use of some laxatives can also result in serious diarrhea, liver disease and electrolyte imbalance.

If you self-medicate with a laxative longer than 1 week and there has been no improvement in your condition, consult your doctor. In addition, pay special attention to your diet and eat foods containing a high amount of fiber, drink adequate amounts of liquids and get the proper amount of exercise.

ISOCARBOXAZID (ORAL)
MARPLAN

PHENELZINE
NARDIL

TRANYLCYPROMINE
PARNATE

Purpose
This medicine is used to help relieve the symptoms of depression and other conditions. It belongs to a group of medicines called Monoamine Oxidase Inhibitors or "MAO Inhibitors."

Allergies/Warnings
If you have ever had an allergic reaction to any medicine or if you have high blood pressure, seizures, heart problems or glaucoma or any other medical condition, tell your doctor and pharmacist before you take any of this medicine.

Before you take this medicine, be sure to tell your doctor if you have taken *any other medicines* (either prescription or nonprescription drugs) within the last 2 weeks.

How to Use This Medicine

How to Administer

Take this medicine with a glass of water.

Special Instructions

Length of Therapy

It is important that you take the medicine regularly and that you do not miss any doses. The full effect of the medicine will not be noticed immediately, but may take from a few days to several weeks. Early signs of improvement are increased appetite, better sleep, increased energy and improved mood. *Do not stop taking the medicine* when you first feel better or you may feel worse in 3 or 4 days.

Do not stop taking this medicine suddenly without the approval of your doctor. It will be necessary for your doctor to reduce your dose slowly since your body will need time to adjust. It could be harmful and make your condition worse if you suddenly stopped taking the medicine. After you have stopped taking this medicine, you must continue to observe the following precautions (see Special Precautions below) for 2 weeks since some of the medicine will still be in your body.

Pregnancy/Breastfeding

Women who are pregnant, breastfeeding or planning to become pregnant should tell their doctor before taking this medicine.

Drug Interactions

It is very important that you obtain the advice of your doctor or pharmacist before taking any other prescription or nonprescription medicines, including pain relievers, sleeping pills, tranquilizers or medicines for depression, cough, cold, sinus, hay fever or allergy medicines because the combination could cause drowsiness, high blood pressure or other complications. Also check the label to see if there is any warning about taking the product with Monoamine Oxidase Inhibitors or MAO Inhibitors.

Do not drink excessive amounts of caffeine (coffee, tea, colas, etc.) or take nonprescription medicines containing caffeine. Check with your pharmacist if you do not know if a product contains caffeine.

There are other drug interactions that can occur. If you are taking any other medicines, be sure to check first with your pharmacist or doctor.

Alcohol

Do not drink alcoholic beverages while taking this drug because the combination could cause a serious reaction.

Special Precautions

When you are taking this medicine and for *at least 2 weeks after* your treatment ends, you must be very careful about your diet. Eating some of the following foods (usually aged, fermented or smoked foods) or beverages could cause a very unpleasant reaction (severe headache, nausea, vomiting or chest pains) in some people:

Cheese and Dairy Products

Foods to Avoid:

- Aged and natural cheeses (for example, cheddar, blue, Camembert, Stilton, Gruyere, Brie, Swiss and Emmenthaler).
- In general, avoid foods in which aging is used to increase the flavor.
- Lasagna, pizza, etc.

Foods Allowed:

- All milk products except those listed to avoid.
- Cream cheese, processed cheese, ricotta cheese and cottage cheese are safe to eat.
- Sour cream or yogurt when used before the "Best Before" date on the carton.

Meat/Fish

Foods to Avoid:

- Game meat (such as duck and goose).
- Chicken livers or beef livers.
- Dry fermented sausage (such as fermented bolognas and salamis, pepperoni and summer sausage).
- Smoked or pickled fish.
- Pickled or kippered herring.
- Meats prepared with tenderizers.
- Bouillon and commercial gravies in large amounts.
- Caviar (controversial).

Foods Allowed:

- All meats except those listed to avoid.
- Eat fresh meats promptly or freeze until ready to use.

Fruits/Vegetables

Foods to Avoid:
- Canned figs or raisins (controversial).
- The pods of broad beans (also called fava beans, Italian beans).
- Avocados (particularly if overripe).
- Bananas (particularly if overripe).
- Overripe or decaying food.

Foods Allowed:
- All fruits and vegetables except those listed to avoid.

Foods/Medicines Containing Yeast

Foods to Avoid:
- Yeast extracts (such as Marmite, Bovril, Brewer's yeast, some packaged soups) or meat extracts.
- Vitamins containing yeast.

Foods Allowed:
- Baker's yeast is allowed.

Alcoholic Beverages

Avoid:
- Wines, especially Chianti and other heavy red wines.
- Alcoholic beverages, including sherry and beer and ale. These beverages can also cause flushing of the face and sweating.
- Discuss the use of alcoholic beverages with your physician.

Miscellaneous

Foods to Avoid:
- Any foods which are overripe, fermenting, or slightly "off."
- Excessive amounts of chocolate or cocoa (controversial).
- Excessive amounts of caffeine (for example, coffee, tea, cola beverages) (controversial).
- Soy sauce (controversial).
- Meat tenderizers (controversial).

Foods Allowed:
- All breads and cereals.

Did You Know That?

Foods can interact with some drugs.

If you are taking a prescription medicine, the food you eat may interact with the drug and cause the drug to work faster or slower or may even prevent it from working.

- If TETRACYCLINE is taken with a glass of milk, yogurt or some cheese, the calcium in these foods can bind with the antibiotic and prevent it from being absorbed maximally.
- Acidic fruit juices, such as grapefruit juice or orange juice, can interact with PENICILLIN G and prevent the drug from working as well.

Some foods must be strictly avoided with some drugs because the combination could cause a dangerous reaction.

- A group of antidepressant drugs, called Monoamine Oxidase Inhibitors, react with foods that contain a high amount of tyramine (such as aged cheeses, Chianti wine, pickled herring and chicken livers) to cause high blood pressure, severe headaches, nausea or vomiting, brain hemorrhage and, in extreme cases, death. These foods must also be avoided for at least 2 weeks after the drug has been stopped since it takes this long for the drug to be excreted from the body.

See Special Precautions above for a more complete listing of these foods.

Some foods help improve the absorption of drugs.

- GRISEOFULVIN, a drug that is used to treat certain types of fungal infections, works much better if the person eats fatty foods before taking the drug. The fat in the food stimulates the release of bile, which helps to dissolve the drug and improve absorption.

As a general rule, if you are prescribed a medicine, be sure you know if the drug should be taken with or without food.

Also be sure you know whether there are certain foods or beverages that should not be taken at the same time as the drug or avoided during the entire drug treatment.

If you took this medicine with any of these substances and nothing happened, do not assume that it will be safe for you to do it again. Foods, beverages and medicines vary greatly in their ability to cause the reaction.

If you feel that you will not be able to follow these dietary restrictions, you should talk with your doctor about alternative treatments.

Any medicine has a few unwanted side effects. Many of these side effects are annoying but you should try to keep taking this medicine unless your doctor tells you to stop it. Because this medicine takes a few weeks to work, the side effects show the doctor that the drug is starting to work. Most of these side effects will go away as your body adjusts to the medicine, but some may not.

If this medicine causes dizziness or lightheadedness, you should be careful going up and down stairs and you should not change positions too rapidly. Lightheadedness is more likely to occur if you stand up suddenly—this is due to blood collecting in the legs and lasts for a few seconds. Therefore, get up from a sitting or lying position more slowly and tighten and relax your leg muscles or wiggle your toes to help promote circulation. In the morning, get out of bed slowly and dangle your feet over the edge of the bed for a few minutes before standing up. Sit or lie down at the first sign of dizziness. Tell your doctor if you have been dizzy. In order to help prevent dizziness or fainting, your doctor may also recommend that you avoid strenuous exercise, standing for long periods of time (especially in hot weather), hot showers, hot baths, Jacuzzis or saunas.

Make sure you know how you are going to react to this medicine and whether it will make you dizzy or drowsy. Do not drive a car, pilot an airplane, operate dangerous machinery or do jobs that require you to be alert if you are dizzy or drowsy.

If your mouth becomes dry, drink water, suck ice chips or a hard, sour candy (sugarless) or chew gum (sugarless). Sugarless products are recommended in order to avoid dental problems. You may wish to ask your pharmacist about special solutions, called artificial saliva, that can also be used to help restore moisture in the mouth. It is especially important to brush and floss your teeth regularly if you develop a dry mouth to help prevent gum problems.

This medicine may cause some people to become constipated. To help prevent constipation, try increasing the amount of bulk in your diet (for example, bran, fresh fruits and salads), exercising more often or drinking more fluids (unless otherwise directed). Call your doctor if the constipation continues.

For patients with diabetes:

- This medicine may cause your blood sugar to fall and may also mask or hide some of the signs of low blood sugar (such as blood pressure changes and faster pulse rate). Be alert for the other signs of low blood sugar that are not masked (such as sweating, hunger, tiredness). If you think your blood sugar is lower than normal, call your doctor. It may be necessary to adjust the dose of your diabetes medications.

When to Call Your Doctor

Stop taking this medicine and call your doctor immediately if you develop severe, pounding headaches, chest pains, rapid heartbeats, nausea, vomiting, stiff neck, high fever, unexplained sweating or dilated (larger) pupils. If you cannot reach your doctor, call an Emergency Medical Service or a hospital emergency department.

Any medicine can cause unwanted effects. Call your doctor if you develop a skin rash, fever, fainting, difficulty in urinating (passing your water), swelling of the legs and ankles, eye pain, changes in ability to see red and green colors, dark-colored urine, diarrhea, insomnia, daytime sedation, decreased sexual response, hallucinations, unusual excitability or a yellow color to the skin or eyes.

Refills

Do not stop taking this medicine without your doctor's approval and do not go without medicine between prescription refills. Call your pharmacist for a refill 2 or 3 days before you will run out of the medicine.

Miscellaneous

Carry an identification card in your wallet or wear a medical alert bracelet indicating that you are taking this medicine as well as the names and phone numbers of your doctors. If you do not already carry such a card, complete the Medicine Card in this book. Always tell your dentist, pharmacist and other doctors who are treating you that you are taking this medicine.

ISOPROPAMIDE (ORAL)

DARBID

Purpose

This medicine is used to help relieve spasm and cramping by relaxing the muscles of the stomach and bowels as well as to decrease the amount of acid formed in the stomach. It is also used in the treatment of peptic ulcer.

Allergies/Warnings

If you have ever had an allergic reaction to iodine or any medicine or if you have high blood pressure, glaucoma, enlarged prostate, difficulty urinating (passing your water) or any other medical condition, tell your doctor and pharmacist before you take any of this medicine.

How to Use This Medicine

How to Administer

Take this medicine with a glass of water.

Special Instructions

Pregnancy/Breastfeeding

Women who are pregnant or planning to become pregnant should tell their doctor before taking this medicine.

Women who are breastfeeding should tell their doctor before taking this medicine. This medicine may decrease the amount of breast milk produced.

Drug Interactions

It is important that you obtain the advice of your doctor or pharmacist before taking any other prescription or nonprescription medicines, including pain relievers, sleeping pills, tranquilizers or medicines for depression, or cough, cold, sinus or allergy medicines.

Do not take antacids or medicine for diarrhea within 1 hour of taking the medicine as they could make this medicine less effective.

There are other drug interactions that can occur. If you are taking any other medicines, be sure to check first with your pharmacist or doctor.

Special Precautions

You may become more sensitive to heat because your body may perspire less while you are taking this drug. Be careful not to become overheated during exercise or in hot weather. Try to avoid strenuous exercise, standing for long periods of time (especially in hot weather), hot showers, hot baths, saunas or Jacuzzis while taking this medicine.

If your mouth becomes dry, drink water, suck ice chips or a hard, sour candy (sugarless) or chew gum (sugarless). Sugarless products are recommended in order to avoid dental problems. You may wish to ask your pharmacist about special solutions, called artificial saliva, that can also be used to help restore moisture in the mouth. It is especially important to brush and floss your teeth regularly if you develop a dry mouth to help prevent gum problems.

An urge to urinate (pass your water) with an inability to do so sometimes occurs with this drug. Urinating before taking the drug each time may help relieve this problem. Tell your doctor if you are having this problem.

This medicine may cause some people to become constipated. To help prevent constipation, try increasing the amount of bulk in your diet (for example, bran, fresh fruits and salads), exercising more often or drinking more fluids (unless otherwise directed). Call your doctor if the constipation continues.

If your eyes become more sensitive to sunlight, it may help to wear sunglasses.

When to Call Your Doctor

Check with your doctor if you develop constipation.

Any medicine can sometimes cause unwanted effects. Call your doctor if you develop a skin rash, diarrhea, unusual restlessness, flushing, hazy vision, eye pain, drooping of eyelids, weakness in hand muscles, fever or fast heartbeats.

Allergic Reactions

Call your doctor immediately if you think you may be allergic to the medicine or if you develop a skin rash, hives, itching, swelling of the face or difficulty in breathing. If you cannot reach your doctor, phone a hospital emergency department.

ISOPROTERENOL (INHALATION AND SUBLINGUAL)

Isuprel Sublingual Tablets, Isuprel Mistometer, Medihaler-Iso Inhaler

ORCIPRENALINE (ORAL AND INHALATION)

Alupent Metered Aerosol, Alupent Tablets, Alupent Syrup

SALBUTAMOL (ORAL AND INHALATION)

NOVOSALMOL, VENTOLIN INHALER, VENTOLIN ROTACAPS, VENTOLIN TABLETS, VENTOLIN NEBULES, VENTOLIN ORAL LIQUID, VENTOLIN RESPIRATOR SOLUTION

TERBUTALINE (ORAL AND INHALATION)

BRICANYL TABLETS, BRICANYL AEROSOL

Purpose

This medicine is used to help open the bronchioles (air passages in the lungs) to make breathing easier and to relieve wheezing and shortness of breath. It is used in the treatment of bronchial asthma and other lung conditions.

Salbutamol is also used to help prevent bronchospasm, shortness of breath and wheezing caused by exercise, and is taken shortly before exercise.

Allergies/Warnings

If you have ever had an allergic reaction to any medicine (including any cough/cold, allergy, heart, or weight-reducing medicines), tell your doctor and pharmacist before you take any of this medicine. Also tell your doctor and pharmacist if you have any heart problems, high blood pressure, diabetes, thyroid disease or epilepsy.

How to Use This Medicine

How to Administer

For VENTOLIN ROTACAPS:

- VENTOLIN ROTACAPS must NOT be swallowed. These capsules are to be perforated and used with the VENTOLIN ROTAHALER.

For tablets:

- The tablets may be taken with a glass of water or food. Food may help prevent stomach upset.

For sublingual tablets (ISUPREL SUBLINGAUL TABLETS):

- *See* How to Administer Medications (page 15).
- Rinse your mouth or brush your teeth after the tablet has dissolved completely in order to wash the medicine (which may turn pink) off the teeth.

For syrup:
- If a spoon is used to measure a dose, it is recommended that you use a medicine spoon or an oral liquid syringe that you can obtain from your pharmacist.
- *See* How to Administer Medications (page 15).

For aerosol inhaler:
- *See* How to Administer Medications (page 15).
- Follow the special instructions that come with the inhaler. Some inhalers must be turned upside down when used. Some inhalers come with an extender device.
- Shake the inhaler well each time before use.
- The mouthpiece of the inhaler should be kept clean and dry. The metal canister must be fully and firmly positioned in the outer "shell" and rotated occasionally.
- Do not inhale the medicine more often than directed by your doctor. If your doctor has prescribed a second puff, wait at least 1 to 2 minutes before shaking the container again and repeating the procedure.
- If difficulty in breathing persists or if relief is not obtained with your usual dosage, call your doctor immediately.

For nebulizer solutions:
- Be sure to use the type of nebulizer recommended by your doctor and learn how to use it correctly. Do not drink the solution.

Special Instructions

Length of Therapy

Do not use this medicine more often or longer than recommended by your doctor. To do so may increase your chance of developing side effects such as tremors or rapid heartbeats.

Pregnancy/Breastfeeding

Women who are pregnant, breastfeeding or planning to become pregnant should tell their doctor before taking this medicine.

Drug Interactions

Some nonprescription drugs can aggravate your condition. Do not take any of the following without the approval of your doctor or pharmacist: cough, cold, or sinus products; ASA-containing products; asthma or allergy products.

Read the label of the nonprescription drug product to see if there is a warning. If there is, check with your doctor or pharmacist before using the product.

If you have been prescribed the inhaler form of this medicine, do not take other inhaled medicines that have not been prescribed by your doctor while you are using this medicine.

Special Precautions

If you are using the inhaler form of this medicine and a steroid inhaler (e.g. BECLOMETHASONE or FLUNISOLIDE), use this medicine approximately 10 to 15 minutes before using the steroid inhaler as directed by your doctor. This medicine will help open up the air passages in the lungs and increase the action of the steroid medicine.

In some people, this drug may cause dizziness or drowsiness. Do not drive a car, pilot an airplane, operate dangerous machinery or do jobs that require you to be alert if you are dizzy or drowsy. You should also be careful going up and down stairs. Sit or lie down at the first sign of dizziness. Tell your doctor if the dizziness continues or becomes severe.

People over 60 years of age are more sensitive to the side effects of this medicine.

In some people this medicine may cause a bad taste in the mouth. This is only temporary and will go away after you have finished the medicine.

If dryness of the mouth or throat occurs after using the inhalation form of the medicine, rinsing or gargling with warm water after inhaling the medicine may help.

For ISOPROTERENOL:

- This medicine may cause the saliva to turn pink to red. This is not unusual.
- Do not use the solution if it has turned pink or brown or if it contains a sediment.

It is not unusual for mild flushing of the face or a slightly faster heartbeat to occur just after taking the medicine. This should not last long. If it does, call your doctor.

When to Call Your Doctor

Call your doctor if the medicine does not relieve your breathing problems, or if your sputum turns yellow or green.

Most people experience few or no side effects from this drug. However, any medicine can sometimes cause unwanted effects. Call your doctor if you develop chest pain, rapid or irregular heartbeats, continuing nausea/vomiting, muscle cramps, severe headaches, muscle tremors, coughing, flushing, unexplained nervousness, insomnia, severe dizziness/drowsiness.

Storage

For inhaler:

- *See* How to Administer Medications (page 15).
- Store these inhalers in a dry (not humid) place away from heat or heat source.

For nebulizer solutions:

- Protect nebulizer solutions from heat and light. Do not use nebulizer solutions if they turn brown or contain a precipitate (sediment) at the bottom of the bottle. Do not use after the discard (expiration) date.

Allergic Reactions

Call your doctor immediately if you think you may be allergic to the medicine or if you develop a skin rash, hives, itching, swelling of the face or difficulty in breathing. If you cannot reach your doctor, phone a hospital emergency department.

Refills

Discuss with your pharmacist the implications of dispensing all your refills for this medicine with the same manufacturer's product. (*See* Generic Drugs, page 12.)

To determine the amount of medicine left in the inhaler and when a refill will be needed, *see* How to Administer Medications (page 15).

ISOSORBIDE DINITRATE (SUBLINGUAL)

APO-ISDN, CORONEX, ISORDIL

ISOSORBIDE DINITRATE (ORAL)

APO-ISDN, CEDOCARD-SR, CORONEX, ISORDIL, NOVOSORBIDE

Purpose

This medicine is used to help prevent angina (chest pains). It does this by decreasing the demand by the heart for oxygen.

Allergies/Warnings

Be sure to tell your doctor and pharmacist if you are allergic to any medicine.

How to Use This Medicine

Time of Administration

For tablets to be placed under the tongue (Apo-Isdn, Coronex *and* Isordil sublingual tablets):

- Carry this medicine with you all the time.
- This medicine should be used at the *first* sign of an attack of angina (chest pains or tightness or squeezing in the chest). Do not wait until the pain becomes severe. *Sit down* as soon as you feel an attack of angina coming on.
- If your doctor recommends, you may help prevent angina by placing a tablet under the tongue 5 or 10 minutes before stressful activities such as strenuous exercise, sexual activity, emotional stress, a heavy meal, high altitudes or exposure to cold. Let your doctor know what things usually cause your angina so that he/she can advise about preventing attacks.

For medicine to be swallowed (Apo-Isdn, Cedocard-SR, Coronex, Isordil, Novosorbide oral tablets):

- It is best to take this medicine with a glass of water on an empty stomach at least 1 hour before (or 2 hours after) eating food.

How to Administer

The sublingual tablets work faster than the tablets that are swallowed.

For tablets to be placed under the tongue (Apo-Isdn, Coronex *and* Isordil sublingual tablets):

- Place a tablet *under your tongue* and let it dissolve completely. *Do not swallow or chew* the tablet since this drug works faster when it is absorbed through the lining of the mouth.
- Try not to swallow until the tablet is dissolved and do not rinse your mouth for a few minutes afterwards. Do not eat, drink or smoke while the tablet is dissolving.
- This tablet usually has an effect in 2 to 5 minutes. If your angina is not relieved within 5 to 10 minutes, you may dissolve a second tablet under your tongue. If the angina continues for another 5 to 10 minutes, you may dissolve a third tablet. If 3 doses do not relieve your chest pains, call your doctor or nearest Emergency Medical Service immediately or go to the nearest hospital emergency department.
- Try to relax for 15 to 20 minutes after taking the drug and remain calm since this will also help to relieve the attack sooner. If you become dizzy or feel faint, breathe deeply and bend forward with your head

between your knees. Always get up slowly after you have been sitting or lying down.

For long-acting medicine (CEDOCARD-SR):

- This medicine is long acting and must be swallowed whole. Do not crush or chew it.

Special Instructions

Length of Therapy

If you are taking this medicine daily, do not stop taking this medicine suddenly without the approval of your doctor. It will be necessary for your doctor to reduce your dose slowly since your body will need time to adjust. It could be harmful and cause an angina attack if you suddenly stopped taking the medicine.

Pregnancy/Breastfeeding

Women who are pregnant, breastfeeding or planning to become pregnant should tell their doctor before taking this medicine.

Drug Interactions

Some nonprescription drugs can aggravate your heart condition. Do not take any of the following without the approval of your doctor or pharmacist: cough, cold or sinus products; asthma or allergy products. Read the label of the product to see if there is a warning. If there is, check with your doctor or pharmacist before using the product.

Alcohol

Do not drink alcoholic beverages too soon after taking this medicine as the combination may cause a serious drop in blood pressure, dizziness and/or fainting.

Special Precautions

The first few doses of this medicine may cause dizziness, flushing or headache. This is normal and will usually disappear after you have taken the drug a few times. Sit or lie down until these effects pass. Breathe deeply and bend forward with your head between your knees if you feel faint. Get up slowly after you have been sitting or lying down. It may help to relieve the headache by taking the medicine with some food or, if your doctor agrees, by taking ASA or acetaminophen. However, if the dizziness or the headaches do not go away, tell your doctor. Your dose may have to be adjusted.

If you become dizzy, you should be careful going up and down stairs.

Do not drive a car, pilot an airplane, operate dangerous machinery or do jobs that require you to be alert.

Keep a record of the number of angina attacks and possible causes of the attack. This information will help your physician give you the best treatment. Be sure to tell your doctor if you have an increase in number, length or severity of attacks.

Cigarette smoking can aggravate angina and is a special risk for people who have heart conditions.

When to Call Your Doctor

Most people experience few or no side effects from this drug. However, any medicine can sometimes cause unwanted effects. Call your doctor if you develop a skin rash, fainting, nausea or vomiting, a fast pulse and persistent or severe headaches.

Storage

Store in a cool, dry place but not in the refrigerator.

Did You Know That?

Drug timing may be critical in the treatment of cancer.

Researchers at the University of Minnesota have found that the time of administration of certain cancer drugs has a profound effect on their toxicity and complications. Patients who were receiving doxorubicin in the morning and cisplatin in the evening had fewer dosage modifications, treatment delays and complications than patients who were receiving the two drugs at opposite times of the day.

Refills

Do not stop taking this medicine without your doctor's approval and do not go without medicine between prescription refills. Call your pharmacist for a refill 2 or 3 days before you will run out of the medicine.

Discuss with your pharmacist the implications of dispensing all your refills for this medicine with the same manufacturer's product. (*See* Generic Drugs, page 12.)

Miscellaneous

Carry an identification card in your wallet or wear a medical alert bracelet indicating that you are taking this medicine as well as the names and phone numbers of your doctors. If you do not already carry such a card, complete the Medicine Card in this book. Always tell your dentist, pharmacist and other doctors who are treating you that you are taking this medicine.

ISOTRETINOIN (ORAL)

ACCUTANE ROCHE

Purpose

This medicine is used in the treatment of cystic acne, conglobate acne and severe acne that has not responded to the usual acne treatments. It should not be used in mild cases of acne.

Allergies/Warnings

Be sure to tell your doctor and pharmacist if you are allergic to oral vitamin A or any medicine or have any other medical condition.

Also tell your doctor if you are hypersensitive to parabens. ACCUTANE contains parabens as a preservative.

Be sure to tell your doctor if you have diabetes, or if there is a history of diabetes in your family. It may be necessary to test your blood for sugar while you are taking this medicine.

Also tell your doctor if you have epilepsy, are taking any medicines for seizures, or if you have a history of high blood cholesterol or triglycerides.

How to Use This Medicine

Time of Administration

This medicine is usually given one or two times a day, usually for 15 to 20 weeks unless otherwise directed by your doctor.

How to Administer

Take the medicine with food or meals.

Be sure to read your prescription label carefully and be sure to take the right amount of medicine. Your dose may change when the prescription is refilled.

Special Instructions

Length of Therapy

It is important not to miss any doses. Try to take the medicine at the same times every day so that you have a constant level of medicine in your body. Do *not* take any more of this medicine than your doctor has prescribed because it will increase the chance of developing side effects.

It may take 1 to 2 months before you see a benefit from this medicine.

Pregnancy/Breastfeeding

Important: *Women must not become pregnant during therapy and at least one month after stopping the medicine because severe birth defects have occured in the babies of women who took* ACCUTANE *during pregnancy.*

Women *must not* take this medicine until they are sure they are not pregnant. It is strongly recommended that a pregnancy test be done two weeks *before* starting the drug. An effective form of birth control must be used at least one month *before* starting this medicine and throughout ACCUTANE therapy.

If you think you are pregnant after you have started taking the drug or one month after you have stopped the medicine, STOP taking the drug immediately and call your doctor. This medicine can cause serious birth defects.

Women of childbearing age should use an effective form of birth control for at least 1 month after stopping the drug or until a normal menstrual period has occurred. If you become pregnant during the first month after stopping the medicine, consult your doctor immediately.

Women taking this medicine should *not* breastfeed infants.

Drug Interactions

This medicine is related to vitamin A. Therefore, vitamin products and health food supplements containing vitamin A must be avoided while receiving this medicine. This is because the vitamin A in these products may add to the unwanted effects of ACCUTANE. If you have any questions about the contents of a vitamin preparation, check with your pharmacist.

While taking this medicine, avoid eating foods that contain very high amounts of vitamin A, such as liver. Foods containing moderate amounts of vitamin A should not cause any problem.

Alcohol

It is best not to drink any alcoholic beverages while taking this medicine.

Special Precautions

During the first few weeks of treatment, your acne may seem to get worse and you may have redness and itching. This usually disappears as you continue to take the medicine. Call your doctor if the redness or itching does not disappear. A late flare-up of acne during the last few weeks of therapy may be seen in some people. It is important to remember that your acne may continue to improve even after you stop the medicine.

Do not give ACCUTANE to anyone else. It has been prescribed for your condition only and may not be suitable for another person.

Because the lipid (fat) levels in the blood can increase while taking the medicine, large amounts of foods containing saturated fats (whole milk, cheese, eggs and red meats) should be avoided.

Your doctor will order blood tests when you first begin taking the medicine. These blood tests are usually repeated after 2 weeks and then monthly for the rest of the therapy or as ordered by your doctor. It is important that you keep your appointments for these blood tests and that you follow any special diet your doctor recommends before the tests. Do not drink any alcoholic beverages for at least 36 hours before the blood tests are done. You must not eat anything for 14 hours before the test. Usually it is requested that you eat supper and then have the blood test the next morning before eating breakfast.

Do not donate blood while you are taking this medicine or for one or two months after the treatment has been stopped. The medicine will be in the blood and could cause serious effects if a pregnant woman received the blood.

Do not use any skin drying agents or other acne treatments without the approval of your doctor.

Sometimes, skin that was normal (such as hands and feet) may peel. Check with your doctor if this becomes a problem.

If your mouth becomes dry, drink water, suck ice chips or a hard, sour candy (sugarless) or chew gum (sugarless). Sugarless products are recommended in order to avoid dental problems. You may wish to ask your pharmacist about special solutions, called artificial saliva, that can also be used to help restore moisture in the mouth. It is especially important to brush and floss your teeth regularly if you develop a dry mouth to help prevent gum problems.

Dry lips are a common problem especially during the first two weeks of therapy. Petroleum jelly may be helpful. Fruits and vegetables should be cut up and eaten with a fork. Juices should be drunk with a straw. If these simple measures do not relieve the lip tenderness or peeling, call your doctor.

Nosebleeds are also common while taking ACCUTANE. Petroleum jelly can be gently inserted with a Q-Tip. If nosebleeds persist or become difficult to stop, call your doctor.

Patients wearing contact lenses may notice that they are more sensitive to the lenses during and after treatment. Dry eyes and poor night vision have also been reported. Ask your pharmacist about eye drops, called "artificial tears," to lubricate your eyes. Do not drive a car at night if your night vision becomes poor.

This medicine may make you more sensitive to sunlight and various tanning lamps. When you begin taking the medicine, avoid too much sun until you see how you react. If your skin does become more sensitive, inform your physician and try to stay out of direct sunlight for extended periods of time. While in the sun, wear protective clothing and sunscreens in creamy bases with an SPF of 15 or higher and proper U-V filtered sunglasses.

This medicine may cause a change in your body's ability to metabolize substances called triglycerides (fats). Your doctor will measure the amount of the substances in your blood in order to determine how your body is responding.

When to Call Your Doctor

This medicine causes side effects that may be noticeable before healing begins. The most common side effects are dry skin and lips, sore, scaly, red, cracked, burning lips, redness, dryness, burning or itching of the eyes, blurred vision or eye pain, hair thinning, rash, peeling of the skin of the palms and soles, muscle, joint or bone aches and pains, dryness of nose, mild nosebleeds and itching. These effects are usually temporary and will usually disappear after you have finished the therapy. Call your doctor if they become bothersome. Your doctor may recommend a dosage change as a precautionary measure or may recommend that you stop taking the medicine.

Call your doctor if your acne becomes extremely tender or if you develop open sores that bleed.

This medicine can also cause some serious side effects. Stop taking the medicine and call your doctor immediately if you develop any unusual symptoms, a skin rash, infection, severe or persistent headache, blurred vision or changes in eyesight, nausea or vomiting, severe stomach pain, diarrhea, rectal bleeding or if you think you are pregnant.

Storage

ACCUTANE does not have to be refrigerated. However, do not expose the capsules to sunlight or excessive heat.

Keep away from the reach of children.

Miscellaneous

Carry an identification card in your wallet or wear a medical alert bracelet indicating that you are taking this medicine as well as the names and phone numbers of your doctors. If you do not already carry such a card, complete the Medicine Card in this book. Always tell your dentist, pharmacist and other doctors who are treating you that you are taking this medicine.

Did You Know That?

Pressing gently on the bridge of the nose and next to the inner corner of the eyes will help prevent eye drops from being drained away from the eye as quickly.

Tears are constantly drained from the eye through the puncta into the nasolacrimal ducts and then swallowed. Eye drops are drained from the eye in the same manner and this is the reason that eye drops can sometimes be tasted after they are administered.

To slow down the drainage of eye drops, apply gentle pressure on the bridge of the nose for a minute to help block the nasolacrimal duct and keep the medicine in contact with the eye a little bit longer. It also will help to try not to blink more often than usual since blinking will also remove the eye drops from the eye.

LEVOTHYROXINE SODIUM (ORAL)

ELTROXIN, SYNTHROID

LIOTHYRONINE

CYTOMEL

LIOTRIX

THYROLAR

THYROGLOBULIN

PROLOID

DESICCATED THYROID

THYROID

Purpose

This medicine is a hormone used to treat conditions in which the body is not producing enough thyroid hormone or if the thyroid gland has been removed.

Allergies/Warnings

If you have ever had an allergic reaction to any medicine or had any other medical condition, tell your doctor and pharmacist before you take any of this medicine.

Also tell your doctor if you are allergic to pork or beef. Some thyroid products are made from pork or beef.

How to Use This Medicine

Time of Administration

It is very important that you take this medicine exactly as your doctor has prescribed. Do not miss any doses and take the medicine even if you feel well. Try to take this medicine at the same time(s) every day so that you will have a constant level of the thyroid hormone in your body. Do not take extra tablets without your doctor's approval.

How to Administer

It is best to take this medicine with some water.

Special Instructions

Length of Therapy

It may take a few days or weeks before you begin to notice any effect from this medicine. Check with your doctor if you continue to have any clumsiness, tiredness, muscle aches, constipation, coldness or weight gain.

It will be several weeks before you will obtain the maximum effect of any dose of this medicine. It may be necessary for your doctor to make several dosage changes and check your blood thyroid level before the best dose is obtained.

Depending upon your condition, it may be necessary to take this medicine the rest of your life since the body needs thyroid hormone.

Do not stop taking this medicine suddenly without the approval of your doctor.

Pregnancy/Breastfeeding

Women who are breastfeeding should tell their doctor.

Drug Interactions

Some nonprescription drugs can aggravate your condition and cause unnecessary problems. Do not take any of the following without the approval of your doctor or pharmacist: cough, cold, or sinus products; asthma or allergy products. Read the label of the product to see if there is a warning. If there is, check with your doctor or pharmacist before using any of these products.

Special Precautions

It is important to stay in touch with your doctor, especially in the weeks after any dosage change. Blood tests may be needed and the doses of all your medicines may have to be adjusted.

For patients with diabetes:

- This medicine may affect your blood sugar. Carefully test your blood or urine for sugar while you are taking this medicine. Call your doctor if you think your blood sugar is not normal or more difficult to control.

When to Call Your Doctor

Most people experience few or no side effects from this drug. However, any medicine can sometimes cause unwanted effects. Call your doctor if you develop chest pain, shortness of breath, fever, headaches, leg cramps, difficulty sleeping, changes in menstrual periods, fast heartbeats, shakiness, persistent diarrhea, vomiting, unusual nervousness, excessive sweating or sensitivity to heat.

Allergic Reactions

Call your doctor immediately if you think you may be allergic to the medicine or if you develop a skin rash, hives, itching, swelling of the face or difficulty in breathing. If you cannot reach your doctor, phone a hospital emergency department.

Refills

Do not stop taking this medicine without your doctor's approval and do not go without medicine between prescription refills. Call your pharmacist for a refill 2 or 3 days before you will run out of the medicine.

Do not change brands of this medicine without consulting your doctor and pharmacist. Your dosage requirements may vary from one product to another.

Miscellaneous

Carry an identification card in your wallet or wear a medical alert bracelet indicating that you are taking this medicine as well as the names and phone numbers of your doctors. If you do not already carry such a card, complete the Medicine Card in this book. Always tell your dentist, pharmacist and other doctors who are treating you that you are taking this medicine.

Tip for Ostomy Odors

A very simple, yet effective, method of deodorizing the wastes inside an ostomy pouch is to place a few drops of vanilla extract, peppermint oil or a commercial deodorant on several squares of toilet or facial tissue. The scented tissue can be slipped inside the ostomy pouch where it will deodorize the wastes and can later be flushed down the toilet.

LINDANE (TOPICAL)

GBH, KWELLADA

Purpose

This medicine is used to treat scabies and lice infestations of the skin or scalp.

Allergies/Warnings

Be sure to tell your doctor and pharmacist if you are allergic to LINDANE or any medicine.

This medicine is pesticidal and potentially toxic. Do not use it without your doctor's or pharmacist's permission.

Carefully read all the package instructions that come with the product you purchased.

How to Use This Medicine

How to Administer

Use plastic disposable gloves or rubber gloves when applying this product to another person.

Instructions for use of lotion or cream in scabies (on the skin):

- If crusts are present, take a warm bath or shower. (Hot water is not recommended because it can cause the blood vessels to dilate and increase the absorption of the product into the bloodstream.) Use a lot of soap to cleanse the skin well and to help remove loose scabs. Clean the tub or shower well after use. Allow the skin to cool before applying the drug.

- Dry the skin well. Shake the lotion well before applying. Then apply a thin layer of the cream or lotion over the entire skin surface. Start at the neck and work down. Rub in well. Do not miss any areas, especially between the fingers and toes, groin and genitals, anal area, as well as the bottom of your feet.
- Leave on for 8 to 12 hours (KWELLADA) or 12 to 24 hours (GBH), and then wash thoroughly.
- Put on freshly laundered or dry-cleaned clothing in order to prevent reinfestation.

Instructions for use of lotion or cream in pubic (crab) lice:

- Take a bath or shower that is cool or at room temperature. (Hot water is not recommended because it can cause the blood vessels to dilate and increase the absorption of the product into the bloodstream.) Use a lot of soap to cleanse the skin well and to help remove loose nits. Clean the tub or shower well after use. Allow the skin to cool before applying the drug.
- Dry the skin *thoroughly* and apply a thin layer of the cream or lotion over the affected skin and hair in the pubic area.
- Leave on for 8 to 12 hours (KWELLADA) or 12 to 24 hours (GBH), and then wash thoroughly.
- Put on freshly laundered or dry-cleaned clothing in order to prevent reinfestation.
- Your sexual partner should also be treated to prevent spread of the infestation.

Instructions for use of shampoo in head lice:

- Shampoo over the sink. Do not shampoo in the bathtub or shower since this will expose the rest of your body to the product.
- Keep the shampoo out of the eyes. If some does get into the eyes, flush it out with water immediately.
- Apply to dry hair.
- Pour about 1 to 2 tablespoonsful (1/2-1 ounce) for short or medium length hair and about 4 tablespoonsful (2 ounces) for long hair onto the affected scalp and rub in well for 4 minutes. Be sure to cover all hair areas.
- Then add small quantities of water to form a good lather. Continue to

lather and work through the hair vigorously for 4 minutes.

- Rinse the hair thoroughly and rub with a clean, dry towel. Some doctors recommend rinsing the hair with a solution of warm water and vinegar in equal amounts to help remove nits.
- When hair is dry, comb with a fine-tooth comb or use tweezers or scissors to remove any remaining nits (eggs) or nit shells. This is time consuming but *all nits must be removed.* This will prevent the nits that were not killed by the medicine from hatching into lice later. Combing the hair with a fine-tooth comb soaked in warm vinegar will help remove nits.
- This shampoo should also be used to clean the combs and brushes to prevent spread of the infestation.
- Do not let other members of the family use the comb used to remove the nits.
- The shampoo is *not* to be used as a regular shampoo.

Special Instructions

Length of Therapy

Usually only 1 treatment is necessary. Itching may continue for 1 week after you have applied the medicine. However, if it continues longer than 1 week, call your doctor. You may not have killed all the lice.

Do not use this product more frequently or leave on for a longer period than recommended by your doctor.

Pregnancy/Breastfeeding

Women who are pregnant, breastfeeding or planning to become pregnant should tell their doctor before taking this medicine.

Do not use this product on infants or in children younger than 6 years old without your doctor's permission.

Drug Interactions

If you normally use a hair dressing that has oil in it, shampoo, rinse and dry your hair thoroughly *before* applying the medicated shampoo. This is necessary because the oil on the hair can increase the absorption of the medicated shampoo.

Special Precautions

Disinfect or throw away combs and brushes immediately after using.

Put on freshly laundered clean clothing after each application of the medicine. Use fresh towels and fresh bed sheets after each application. Launder or dry-clean contaminated clothing since nits can live on clothes for up to 30 days. Clothing that can be washed should be washed in *hot* water and dried on a *hot* setting. Dry-clean the clothes if they cannot stand hot temperatures. This also applies to hats, caps, coats with fur collars or "fake fur" collars. Clothing or pillows that cannot be cleaned can be stored in a sealed bag for 2 weeks.

Carefully vacuum all rugs, upholstered furniture and mattresses to pick up any living lice or nits. Throw away the vacuum bag immediately.

Household pets should be examined for signs of lice and treated by a veterinarian if necessary. Do not use KWELLADA on a cat—you may kill it!

Keep this medicine away from the eyes, mouth, mucous membranes or open wounds such as cuts, scratches or open sores. If some does get into the eyes, flush it away with water immediately.

When to Call Your Doctor

Call your doctor if the condition for which you are using this medicine persists or becomes worse. Also call your doctor if you develop muscle cramps, clumsiness or unsteadiness, seizures, fast heartbeats, vomiting or unusual nervousness.

Storage

Throw away the empty bottle after you have used the medicine and be sure the discarded medicine is out of the reach of children. Do *not* reuse the bottle for anything.

Miscellaneous

This medicine is for external use only. It is poisonous if swallowed.

LITHIUM CARBONATE (ORAL)

CARBOLITH, DURALITH, LITHANE, LITHIZINE

Purpose

This medicine is used to help relieve the symptoms of certain types of mental and emotional conditions. It is also used to help prevent relapses of manic-depressive illness.

Allergies/Warnings

If you have ever had an allergic reaction to any medicine or if you have thyroid problems, diabetes, kidney disease or any other medical condition, tell your doctor and pharmacist before you take any of this medicine.

Be sure to tell your doctor if you are taking *any other medicines* (either prescription or nonprescription drugs).

How to Use This Medicine

How to Administer

Take this medicine with food or milk to help prevent stomach upset.

If you were prescribed DURALITH:

- This medicine must be swallowed whole. Do not crush or chew.

Special Instructions

Length of Therapy

It is important that you take the medicine regularly and that you do not miss any doses. The full effect of the medicine will not be noticed immediately, but may take from 1 week to several weeks. Early signs of improvement include restoration of normal appetite and sleep patterns and return of your mood and energy level to normal. *Do not stop taking* the medicine when you first feel better or you may feel worse in 3 or 4 days.

Since lithium is often used to help prevent relapses of manic episodes and depressive episodes, you may need to take lithium on a prolonged basis. You should discuss the length of your treatment with your doctor.

Pregnancy/Breastfeeding

Women who are pregnant, breastfeeding or planning to become pregnant should not take this medicine without their doctor's approval. Studies have indicated that lithium may cause birth defects, especially if taken during the first three months of pregnancy.

Drug Interactions

It is important that you obtain the advice of your doctor or pharmacist before taking any other prescription or nonprescription medicines, including pain relievers, asthma or allergy medicines, diuretics (water pills), laxatives, sodium bicarbonate (baking soda) or caffeine products.

There are other drug interactions that can occur. If you are taking any other medicines, be sure to check first with your pharmacist or doctor.

Do not drink large quantities of beverages containing caffeine (coffee, tea, colas) while taking this medicine. These beverages can decrease the effect of this medicine and make it less helpful.

Alcohol

Do not drink alcoholic beverages while taking this drug without the approval of your doctor.

Special Precautions

Use a normal amount of table salt in your diet unless otherwise directed. Do not alter your diet or use salt substitutes without first consulting your doctor.

Unless otherwise directed by your doctor, try to drink plenty of water or other liquids (but not beverages containing caffeine) every day while you are taking this medicine. This will help prevent kidney problems.

Keep your regular doctor appointments so that your doctor can check your progress and make sure you are getting the full benefit of this medicine. It is almost always necessary for dosages to be adjusted by the doctor.

It will also be necessary for your doctor to do regular laboratory tests. The *only* time *not* to take your lithium is the morning on the days you have a lithium blood test. Otherwise, your blood test will not give an accurate reading. Always make sure that you have your lithium blood test done as close as possible to 12 hours after your last lithium dose.

Any medicine has a few unwanted side effects. Side effects are annoying but you should try to keep taking the medicine unless your doctor tells you to stop it. Because this medicine takes a few weeks to work, the side effects show the doctor that the drug is starting to work. Some of these side effects will go away as your body adjusts to the medicine but some may not.

A mild hand tremor or shakiness is common when people start taking lithium and it is not harmful. Mild nausea and mild thirst may also occur during the first few days of treatment. These side effects are annoying but usually disappear within a few days. If they persist or become severe, check with your doctor.

If this medicine causes dizziness or lightheadedness, you should be careful going up and down stairs and you should not change positions too rapidly. Sit or lie down at the first sign of dizziness. Tell your doctor if you have been dizzy.

Your doctor may also recommend that you avoid strenuous exercise, standing for long periods of time (especially in hot weather), hot showers, hot baths or saunas. You could lose too much water and salt through increased sweating which can lead to serious side effects.

Do not drive a car, pilot an airplane, operate dangerous machinery or do jobs that require you to be alert if you are dizzy or drowsy.

When to Call Your Doctor

Call your doctor if you develop diarrhea, increased desire to urinate (pass your water) or pass large amounts of light colored urine, vomiting, slurred speech, increased trembling of the hands, jerking of the arms or legs, unusual weakness or drowsiness (sleepiness), blurred vision, stomach pains, ringing or buzzing in the ears, swelling of the hands or feet, slow or irregular heartbeats, lack of coordination, convulsions, stiffness of the muscles or confusion.

Check with your doctor if you develop the flu or other infection that is accompanied by vomiting and/or diarrhea, fever and/or sweating. The loss of too much body water may cause the amount of lithium in your system to increase and your doctor may have to adjust your lithium dose.

Refills

Do not stop taking this medicine without your doctor's approval and do not go without medicine between prescription refills. Call your pharmacist for a refill 2 or 3 days before you will run out of the medicine.

Do not change brands of this medicine without your doctor's approval. The dose you need could be different with different products. Also, do not change from tablets to capsules, or vice versa, unless prescribed by your doctor.

Miscellaneous

Carry an identification card in your wallet or wear a medical alert bracelet indicating that you are taking this medicine as well as the names and phone numbers of your doctors. If you do not already carry such a card, complete the Medicine Card in this book. Always tell your dentist, pharmacist and other doctors who are treating you that you are taking this medicine.

LOPERAMIDE (ORAL)

IMODIUM

Purpose

This medicine is used in the treatment of diarrhea, including Traveler's Diarrhea. It should not be used to treat diarrhea caused by intestinal toxins from bacteria (e.g. *E.coli, Salmonella* or *Shigella*) or diarrhea that develops sometimes while taking some types of antibiotics.

It is also used in the care of ileostomies, colostomies and other types of bowel surgeries.

Allergies/Warnings

If you have ever had an allergic reaction to any medicine, tell your doctor and pharmacist before you take any of this medicine.

This medicine should not be given to children under 2 years of age.

How to Use This Medicine

Time of Administration

The medicine should be taken after each unformed stool. Do not take more doses than recommended by your doctor.

How to Administer

For capsules: Take with food or a glass of water.

For liquid medicine: *See* How to Administer Medications (page 15).

Special Instructions

Length of Therapy

If the diarrhea does not stop or improve after 48 hours, check with your doctor. There are many causes of diarrhea.

Pregnancy/Breastfeeding

Women who are pregnant, breastfeeding or planning to become pregnant should tell their doctor before taking this medicine.

Special Precautions

In some people, this drug may cause dizziness or drowsiness. Do not drive a car, pilot an airplane, operate dangerous machinery or do jobs that require you to be alert if you are dizzy or drowsy. You should also be careful going up and down stairs. Sit or lie down at the first sign of dizziness. Tell your doctor if the dizziness or drowsiness continues.

If your mouth or skin becomes very dry, check with your doctor.

It is important to drink plenty of water or clear fluids when you have diarrhea and while you are taking this medicine.

Did You Know That?

Children who are taking a medicine in a syrup on a regular basis should brush their teeth or rinse their mouths with water after taking the medicine.

The syrup base of the medicine contains sugar. There is an increased risk of dental caries in children who are prescribed syrup-based medicines on a frequent dosage schedule for a long period of time.

When to Call Your Doctor

Call your doctor if you develop a fever, abdominal pain, bloating, constipation, nausea, vomiting, if the diarrhea continues, irregular heartbeats, severe muscle cramps, or if you have blood in the stools.

Allergic Reactions

Call your doctor immediately if you think you may be allergic to the medicine or if you develop a skin rash, hives, itching, swelling of the face or difficulty in breathing. If you cannot reach your doctor, phone a hospital emergency department.

MECLIZINE HCl (ORAL)

BONAMINE

Purpose

This medicine is used to help control nausea and vomiting and to help prevent motion sickness. MECLIZINE is also used to treat some types of dizziness.

Allergies/Warnings

If you have ever had an allergic reaction to any medicine or if you have glaucoma, enlarged prostate, difficulty urinating (passing your water), high blood pressure or diabetes, or any other medical condition, tell your doctor and pharmacist before you take any of this medicine.

How to Use This Medicine

Time of Administration

If you are taking this medicine to prevent motion sickness:

- Take this medicine 1 hour before you plan to travel.

If you are taking this medicine to help relieve nausea and vomiting of pregnancy:

- It is best to take the medicine at bedtime.

If you are taking this medicine to help prevent nausea and vomiting caused by radiation treatment:

- Take the medicine 2 to 12 hours before treatment, as directed by your doctor.

How to Administer

These tablets can be chewed, swallowed with water, or allowed to dissolve in the mouth.

Special Instructions

Pregnancy/Breastfeeding

Women who are pregnant, breastfeeding or planning to become pregnant should tell their doctor before taking this medicine.

Drug Interactions

It is important that you obtain the advice of your doctor or pharmacist before taking any other prescription or nonprescription medicines, including pain relievers, sleeping pills, tranquilizers or medicines for depression, cough, cold or allergy medicines, because the combination could cause drowsiness.

There are other drug interactions that can occur. If you are taking any other medicines, be sure to check first with your pharmacist or doctor.

Alcohol

Do not drink alcoholic beverages while taking this drug without the approval of your doctor because the combination could cause drowsiness. One drink may have the same effect that 2 or 3 drinks normally would have.

Special Precautions

If your mouth becomes dry, drink water, suck ice chips or a hard, sour candy (sugarless) or chew gum (sugarless). Sugarless products are recommended in order to avoid dental problems. You may wish to ask your pharmacist about special solutions, called artificial saliva, that can also be used to help restore moisture in the mouth. It is especially important to brush and floss your teeth regularly if you develop a dry mouth to help prevent gum problems.

In some people, this drug may cause drowsiness or blurred vision. Do not drive a car, pilot an airplane, operate dangerous machinery or do jobs that require you to be alert if you are dizzy or drowsy. You should also be careful going up and down stairs. Sit or lie down at the first sign of dizziness. Tell your doctor if these problems continue.

When to Call Your Doctor

Most people experience few or no side effects from this drug. However, any medicine can sometimes cause unwanted effects. Call your doctor if you develop a skin rash, sore throat, fever, mouth sores, difficulty in urinating (passing your water), blurred vision or fast heartbeats.

Allergic Reactions

Call your doctor immediately if you think you may be allergic to the medicine or if you develop a skin rash, hives, itching, swelling of the face or difficulty in breathing. If you cannot reach your doctor, phone a hospital emergency department.

METHYLDOPA (ORAL)

ALDOMET, APO-METHYLDOPA, DOPAMET, NOVOMEDOPA

METHYLDOPA-CHLOROTHIAZIDE

SUPRES

METHYLDOPA-HYDROCHLOROTHIAZIDE

ALDORIL, APO-METHAZIDE, NOVODOPARIL, PMS DOPAZIDE

Purpose

This medicine is used to treat high blood pressure.

Allergies/Warnings

Be sure to tell your doctor and pharmacist if you are allergic to any medicine.

How to Use This Medicine

Time of Administration

Try to take the medicine at the same time(s) every day so that you have a constant level of the medicine in your body.

How to Administer

Take the medicine with food or a glass of water.

Special Instructions

Length of Therapy

High blood pressure (hypertension) is a long-term condition and it will probably be necessary for you to take the drug for a long time in spite of the fact that you feel better. If high blood pressure is not treated, it can lead to serious problems such as heart failure, strokes, blood vessel problems or kidney problems.

It is very important that you take this medicine as your doctor has directed and that you do not miss any doses. Otherwise, you cannot expect the drug to keep your blood pressure down.

Pregnancy/Breastfeeding

Women who are pregnant, breastfeeding or planning to become pregnant should tell their doctor before taking this medicine.

Drug Interactions

Some nonprescription drugs can aggravate your condition. Do not take any of the following without the approval of your doctor or pharmacist: cough, cold, or sinus products; asthma, allergy or hay fever products since they could increase your blood pressure. Read the label of the product to see if there is a warning. If there is, check first with your doctor or pharmacist before using the product.

Alcohol

Do not drink alcoholic beverages while taking this drug without the approval of your doctor because the combination could make the possible side effect of dizziness worse.

Special Precautions

Drowsiness may occur during the first 2 or 3 days or after any increase in your dose and then usually disappears. If you become dizzy or drowsy, you should not drive a car, pilot an airplane, operate dangerous machinery or do jobs that require you to be alert.

If this medicine causes dizziness or lightheadedness, you should be careful going up and down stairs and you should not change positions too rapidly. Lightheadedness is more likely to occur if you stand up suddenly—this is due to blood collecting in the legs and lasts for a few seconds. Therefore, get up from a sitting or lying position more slowly and tighten and relax your leg muscles or wiggle your toes to help promote circulation. In the morning, get out of bed slowly and dangle your feet over the edge of the bed for a few minutes before standing up. Sit or lie down at the first sign of dizziness. Tell your doctor if you have been dizzy. In order to help prevent dizziness or fainting, your doctor may also recommend that you avoid alcohol, strenuous exercise, standing for long periods of time (especially in hot weather), hot showers, hot baths, Jacuzzis or saunas.

This medicine sometimes causes nasal congestion (stuffy nose). Do not try to treat it yourself but check with your doctor.

Follow any special diet your doctor may have ordered. He or she may want you to limit the amount of salt in your diet.

Your doctor will want to do laboratory tests to check your liver function, especially during the first 2 to 3 months of treatment.

If you were prescribed ALDORIL, APO-METHAZIDE, NOVODOPARIL, PMS DOPAZIDE *or* SUPRES, *the following special instructions also apply to these drugs:*

- This medicine normally causes your body to lose potassium. The body has warning signs to let you know if too much potassium is being lost. Call your doctor if you become unusually thirsty or if you develop leg cramps, unusual weakness, fatigue, vomiting, confusion or an irregular pulse. Since these symptoms may not be present in all patients, your doctor may wish to check your blood occasionally to see if it is low in potassium. Depending upon your dose, your doctor may prescribe some medicine to replace the potassium or he or she may recommend that you regularly eat foods that contain a lot of potassium (see Appendix A). *Do not change your diet unless your doctor tells you to.*
- This medicine may make some people more sensitive to sunlight and various tanning lamps. When you begin taking this medicine, try to avoid too much sun until you see how you are going to react. If your skin does become more sensitive to sunlight, tell your doctor and try not to stay in direct sunlight for extended periods of time. While in the sun, wear protective clothing and sunglasses. You may wish to ask your pharmacist about suitable sunscreen products. Call your doctor if you become sunburned.

For patients with diabetes who are taking ALDORIL, APO-METHAZIDE, NOVODOPARIL, PMS DOPAZIDE *or* SUPRES:

- This medicine may cause your blood sugar to rise. Carefully test your blood or urine for sugar while you are taking this medicine. Call your doctor if you think your blood sugar is higher than normal or harder to control.

When to Call Your Doctor

Most people experience few or no side effects from this drug. However any medicine can sometimes cause unwanted effects. Call your doctor if you develop a skin rash, sore throat, fever, chills, fast heartbeats, chest pains or difficulty in breathing, unusual tiredness or weakness, swelling of the legs or ankles, sudden weight gain of 5 pounds (2.5 kg) or more, severe diarrhea (loose bowel movements), stomach upset, unusual bruising or bleeding, a yellow color to the skin or eyes, dark-colored urine, impotence or decreased sexual ability, depression or confusion.

If you were prescribed ALDORIL, APO-METHAZIDE, NOVODOPARIL, PMS

DOPAZIDE *or* SUPRES:

- In addition to the previous symptoms, also call your doctor if you develop sharp stomach pain, sharp joint pain or yellow color to the skin or eyes. Call your doctor if you become sick or develop persistent nausea, vomiting or diarrhea.

Refills

Do not stop taking this medicine without your doctor's approval and do not go without medicine between prescription refills. Call your pharmacist for a refill 2 or 3 days before you will run out of the medicine.

Discuss with your pharmacist the implications of dispensing all your refills for this medicine with the same manufacturer's product. (*See* Generic Drugs, page 12.)

Miscellaneous

Carry an identification card in your wallet or wear a medical alert bracelet indicating that you are taking this medicine as well as the names and phone numbers of your doctors. If you do not already carry such a card, complete the Medicine Card in this book. Always tell your dentist, pharmacist and other doctors who are treating you that you are taking this medicine.

Did You Know That?

If you have difficulty opening child-proof caps and there are no children in your home, you may request a regular prescription vial cap from the pharmacist.

METOCLOPRAMIDE (ORAL)

EMEX, MAXERAN, REGLAN

Purpose

This medicine is used to treat certain types of stomach and intestinal disorders in which there is nausea, vomiting, and a persistent feeling of fullness after eating.

Allergies/Warnings

If you have ever had an allergic reaction to any medicine or if you have seizures or any other medical condition, tell your doctor and pharmacist before you take any of this medicine.

How to Use This Medicine

Time of Administration

Take this medicine 30 minutes *before* meals and at bedtime unless otherwise directed.

Relief of nausea should occur after the first few doses.

Did You Know That?

Taking a dose of baking soda with a large quantity of liquid can be dangerous or even fatal, according to a report in *Annals of Internal Medicine.*

A healthy 31-year-old man with no history of peptic ulcers, abdominal injury or surgery felt uncomfortably full after eating a large dinner. He had run out of Alka-Seltzer (his usual remedy) and decided to use ordinary baking soda. The package label of baking soda states that 1/2 teaspoon in a glass of water is effective as an antacid to help relieve heartburn, sour stomach and/or acid indigestion. The man recalled adding the recommended dose of 1/2 teaspoon to 1/2 glass of water and quickly drinking the solution. One minute later, he developed severe abdominal pain and was rushed to the hospital. An exploratory laparotomy was done and it was found that the stomach wall had ruptured and the peritoneal cavity surrounding the stomach was filled with food.

It was postulated that the baking soda when combined with water produced large quantities of gas that ruptured the stomach wall. This is very rare and it usually would take larger doses in larger quantities of water to release explosive amounts of carbon dioxide. There have been five reported cases of stomach rupture due to this home remedy in the medical literature.

Baking soda is another name for sodium bicarbonate. The powder is high in sodium and should not be taken by people who are on sodium-restricted diets, e.g. patients with high blood pressure or heart conditions.

How to Administer

For liquid medicines:

- If a spoon is used to measure the dose, it is recommended that you use a medicine spoon or an oral liquid syringe that you can obtain from your pharmacist. *See* How to Administer Medications (page 15).

Some Patients Should Fly with Caution

Some patients should be evaluated carefully by their doctors before traveling by airplane. Most of the medical problems associated with air travel are due to changes in the cabin pressure, concentration of oxygen in the blood and the volume of trapped gas in the body. As the airplane cabin pressure decreases with increasing altitude, gas that is normally in the person's body expands proportionately. Normally this does not create a problem. For some patients, however, the effects of air travel can be dangerous.

- If a patient has an obstructed bowel, trapped gas around the bowel obstruction can cause mild to severe pain, nausea, vomiting and potential rupturing of the bowel.
- Any patient who has recently had bowel surgery or a gallbladder operation should not fly for at least 2 weeks after surgery or until normal bowel function has been restored.
- People with a low vital capacity, heart conditions or severe anemia may not be able to tolerate the hypoxemia (low amounts of oxygen in the blood) caused by the changes in cabin pressure.
- Pneumothorax is a contraindication to flying. As the altitude of the plane increases, any gas trapped within the pleural cavity will expand and press against healthy lung tissue. Similarly, patients with lung cysts should avoid high altitude flying because expansion of trapped air in the cyst could result in rupture of the cyst.
- Patients with a sinus or ear infection, nasal tumor or nasal polyps, deviated septum or eustachian tube stenosis have an increased risk of developing sinus or ear problems due to the air pressure changes. If these patients must fly, they should ask their doctor or phar-

macist to recommend a nasal decongestant spray or drops that can be used before and during descent. Alternatively, an oral decongestant taken one hour before descent may help.

- A person with a dental abscess or a defective filling should have it repaired before flying. It is believed that expanding gas trapped in or near the defective tooth could press against a nerve.
- Patients who have had a myocardial infarction (heart attack) or stroke should not fly for at least 2 to 6 weeks.
- Patients who have severe angina at sea level may find that air travel may precipitate angina attacks.
- Scuba divers should be reminded not to fly for at least 12 hours after their last dive and 24 hours after deep or repeated dives.

In contrast, some people with asthma and chronic obstructive pulmonary disease breathe easier during airplane travel. The cabin air is less dense than air at sea level and as a result passes more easily through the obstructed bronchial tissues.

If you have a medical condition and wonder whether it is safe for you to travel by airplane, check with your doctor. It is better to know how safe it is to travel before you are aboard the plane!

Special Instructions

Length of Therapy

Do not take this medicine more often or longer than recommended by your doctor. To do so may increase your chance of developing side effects.

Pregnancy/Breastfeeding

Women who are pregnant, breastfeeding or planning to become pregnant should tell their doctor before taking this medicine.

Drug Interactions

Check with your pharmacist before purchasing any pain relievers, nonprescription drugs, sleeping pills, tranquilizers, medicine for seizures, muscle relaxants, anesthetics, medicines for diarrhea, medicines for glaucoma, medicines for depression or medicines for allergies without the permission of your doctor. Combining this medicine with some of these drugs could cause significant drowsiness or dizziness.

There are other drug interactions that can occur. If you are taking any other medicines, be sure to check first with your pharmacist or doctor.

Alcohol

Do not drink alcoholic beverages while taking this drug or for a few days after stopping the drug, as it may make the drowsiness worse.

Special Precautions

If you become dizzy, you should be careful going up and down stairs. Do not drive a car, pilot an airplane, operate dangerous machinery or do jobs that require you to be alert until you know how you are going to react to the drug. Sit or lie down at the first sign of dizziness. Tell your doctor if the dizziness continues.

When to Call Your Doctor

Most people experience few or no side effects from this drug. However, any medicine can sometimes cause unwanted effects. Call your doctor immediately if you develop unusual movements of the face, tongue, hands or eyes, trembling, shuffling walk, unusual muscle stiffness, stiff neck, depression or severe drowsiness.

Allergic Reactions

Call your doctor immediately if you think you may be allergic to the medicine or if you develop a skin rash, hives, itching, swelling of the face or difficulty in breathing. If you cannot reach your doctor, phone a hospital emergency department.

Storage

Store the medicine at room temperature away from heat and light.

METRONIDAZOLE (ORAL)

APO-METRONIDAZOLE, FLAGYL, NEO-METRIC, NOVONIDAZOL, PMS METRONIDAZOLE

Purpose

This medicine is used to treat certain types of infections.

Allergies/Warnings

Be sure to tell your doctor and pharmacist if you are allergic to any medicine.

How to Use This Medicine

Time of Administration

Take the tablets with food or a glass of milk to help prevent stomach upset. If stomach upset (nausea, vomiting, stomach pain or diarrhea) continues, call your doctor.

How to Administer

The tablets may be crushed if you cannot swallow them whole.

Special Instructions

Length of Therapy

It is very important that you take this medicine exactly as your doctor has prescribed. Do not miss any doses. Try to take this medicine at the same time(s) every day so that you will have a constant level of medicine in your body.

Take the medicine until it is finished even if you begin to feel better after a few days. If you stop taking the medicine too soon, the infection may return.

Pregnancy/Breastfeeding

This medicine should not be used during pregnancy, especially during the first 3 months of pregnancy.

Women who are pregnant, breastfeeding or planning to become pregnant should tell their doctor before taking this medicine.

Alcohol

Do not drink alcoholic beverages while taking this medicine because the combination could cause a very unpleasant reaction (headache, flushing, redness of the face or an upset stomach). Do not take cough syrups, cold preparations, elixirs or tonics that contain alcohol because they could cause the same problem.

Avoid alcohol for at least 1 day after you have finished the medicine.

Special Precautions

This medicine may cause your urine to turn red-brown or darker in color. This is not an unusual effect and will go away after you have finished taking the medicine.

If your mouth becomes dry, drink water, suck ice chips or a hard, sour candy (sugarless) or chew gum (sugarless). Sugarless products are recommended in order to avoid dental problems. You may wish to ask your pharmacist about special solutions, called artificial saliva, that can also be used to help restore moisture in the mouth. It is especially important to brush and floss your teeth regularly if you develop an unpleasant metallic taste in the mouth or if you develop a dry mouth to help prevent gum problems.

If you are taking this medicine for trichomoniasis (a genital infection):

- Your doctor may want to treat your sexual partner at the same time. In order to help prevent the infection from spreading, it is best to avoid having sexual intercourse (sex) until the infection is cured. If you do have sexual intercourse, the male partner should wear a condom.
- Women taking this medicine should not douche unless their doctor tells them to do so.
- It is recommended that women not wear panty hose or tight underwear while using this medicine. Wear cotton underwear until the infection is cured. Do not wear underwear made of silk, nylon, dacron or synthetic fabrics because these materials can cause increased sweating in the genital area that can make it more difficult to cure the infection.

When to Call Your Doctor

Call your doctor if your symptoms do not improve within a few days or if they become worse.

Most people experience few or no side effects from this drug. However, any medicine can sometimes cause unwanted effects. Call your doctor if you develop a skin rash, hives, redness, itching, severe diarrhea (lasting more than 24 hours), a sore throat and fever, sore mouth or tongue, a white coating on the tongue, confusion, insomnia, headache, numbness or tingling in the hands or feet, trembling, seizures, dizziness or drowsiness.

Allergic Reactions

Call your doctor immediately if you think you may be allergic to the medicine or if you develop a skin rash, hives, itching, swelling of the face or difficulty in breathing. If you cannot reach your doctor, phone a hospital emergency department.

MICONAZOLE NITRATE (TOPICAL)

MICATIN CREAM, MICATIN LOTION, MONISTAT DERM CREAM

MICONAZOLE NITRATE (VAGINAL)

MONISTAT, MONISTAT 5 TAMPONS, MONISTAT 7, MONISTAT 3 VAGINAL OVULES, MONISTAT 3 DUAL-PAK

Purpose

This medicine is used to treat fungal or yeast infections.

Allergies/Warnings

Be sure to tell your doctor and pharmacist if you are allergic to any medicine.

How to Use This Medicine

Time of Administration

For vaginal medicines:

- This medication is usually inserted into the vagina at bedtime to help prevent draining or leaking of the drug.

For topical creams and lotions:

- This medicine is usually applied to the skin twice daily, in the morning and evening.

How to Administer

For vaginal cream:

- *See* How to Administer Medications (page 15).

For vaginal suppositories or ovules:

- *See* How to Administer Medications (page 15) and read the instructions that come with the package.

For vaginal tampons:

- Insert the tampon into the applicator according to the package instructions.
- Insert the applicator containing the tampon into the vagina every day at bedtime. Leave in place over night and remove the next morning. Repeat for 5 days.

Special Instructions

Length of Therapy

It is important to use all of this medicine plus any refills that your doctor has recommended in spite of the fact that your symptoms seem to have improved. Do not stop using it earlier than your doctor has recommended or the infection may return.

Do not use this medicine more frequently or in larger quantities than prescribed by your doctor. To be effective, the vaginal medicine must be used *daily* for the length of time prescribed by your doctor.

Did You Know That?

Many health information brochures are written in language that many consumers cannot understand.

In a recent study reported in the *Journal of Family Practice,* several patient brochures prepared by various health organizations and pharmaceutical companies were evaluated. Many patients did not understand a wide variety of medical terms used in the brochures.

Word	Patients who did not understand meaning
"Symptom"	22%
"Orally"	38%
"Hereditary"	44%
"Hypertension"	56%
"Stroke"	76%
"Atherosclerosis"	96%

To be able to manage your drug therapy at home, you must first understand your doctor's and pharmacist's instructions. Medical terms are a "second language" to these health professionals and it is so easy for them to forget to translate these words for people who do not use them in their everyday language.

Whenever you do not understand a particular word, just ask your doctor or pharmacist to explain it. Do not be embarrassed to ask — just remember there are many, many other people who probably would not be able to understand the same word either. By not asking for clarification, there is the possibility that you could misinterpret an important instruction and suffer a serious consequence.

Pregnancy/Breastfeeding

Women who are pregnant, breastfeeding or planning to become pregnant should tell their doctor before using this medicine.

Caution: During pregnancy, the vaginal applicator should be used *only* on the advice of a doctor.

Special Precautions

For treatment of vaginal conditions:

- During treatment, your doctor may recommend that you do not have sexual intercourse (sex). If you do have sex, your partner should use a condom.
- It is recommended that you wear a sanitary napkin to prevent staining of your clothing by medicine that leaks from the vagina.
- Use this medicine continuously—even during your menstrual period. Do not use a menstrual tampon because it may absorb some of the drug. Wear a sanitary napkin during the menstrual period.
- Do not douche while using this medication unless your doctor tells you to.
- It is recommended that women not wear panty hose or tight underwear while using this medicine. Wear cotton underwear until the infection is cured. Do not wear underwear made of silk, nylon, dacron or synthetic fabrics because these materials can cause increased sweating in the genital area that can make it more difficult to cure the infection.
- Tell your doctor if you are using a diaphragm for birth control. The suppository form of this medicine has been reported to interact with certain latex products. The vaginal cream has not been reported to interact this way.

When to Call Your Doctor

Call your doctor if the condition for which this drug is being used continues or becomes worse or the medication causes a constant irritation such as itching or burning that was not present before you started using it.

Most people experience few or no side effects from this drug. However, any medicine can sometimes cause unwanted effects. If you are taking this medicine for a vaginal infection, call your doctor if you develop pelvic or abdominal cramps, hives, a skin rash or a severe headache.

Storage

For vaginal suppositories: *see* How to Administer Medications (page 15).

Miscellaneous

This drug is for external use only. Do not swallow it. Keep away from the eyes.

Did You Know That?

Some drugs can affect the way the body uses food.

Birth control pills are known to lower blood levels of certain vitamins, such as vitamin B_6 and folic acid. Usually the vitamin depletion is not serious enough to cause any symptoms, especially if the woman has a good diet. However, if a woman has a poor diet, eats primarily snack foods, or is always on a diet, there is a chance that she could develop a deficiency of folic acid and vitamin B_6.

It is important for any woman on "the pill" to eat a well-balanced diet including green leafy vegetables, which are a good source of folic acid.

NICOTINE RESIN COMPLEX (SMOKING CESSATION AID)

NICORETTE

Purpose

NICORETTE is a sugar-free chewing gum which contains nicotine and is a temporary aid to help you stop smoking. The nicotine in the gum is released only during chewing. This replaces the nicotine from smoking and makes it easier to break the habit of smoking.

The gum should be used as part of a total stop smoking program and is usually used for approximately 3 months or less.

Allergies/Warnings

NICORETTE is contraindicated in non-smokers and children.

Tell your doctor is you have a history of stomach ulcers, heart problems, circulation problems, or any other medical condition.

How to Use This Medicine

Time of Administration

Chew ONE piece of gum *slowly* whenever you have the urge to smoke.

Most people require about 10 pieces of gum each day during the first month of treatment. Never exceed 20 of the 2 mg or 10 of the 4 mg pieces of gum during one day.

As your desire to smoke disappears, gradually decrease the number of pieces of gum you chew each day. Unless your doctor tells you otherwise, do not attempt to stop chewing the gum until you are only using 1 or 2 pieces a day.

How to Administer

Chew the gum slowly and gently. As you chew the gum, nicotine is slowly released. If you chew too rapidly, the nicotine will be released too quickly and side effects similar to oversmoking can develop, e.g. nausea, vomiting, increased saliva, diarrhea, stomach upset (indigestion or heartburn), hiccoughs, lightheadedness, hearing and vision problems, throat irritation, or convulsions.

To receive the full effect of this drug, you must alternate between chewing the gum and not chewing the gum using the following steps:

- Chew one piece of gum slowly for up to 30 minutes. The first few pieces should be placed in the side of your mouth and chewed slowly at a rate of 2 or 3 bites per minute.
- If NICORETTE starts to taste "hot," you are releasing too much of the drug and should stop chewing.
- Start chewing again until it becomes uncomfortable, then stop again.
- Continue chewing this way for 30 minutes. After 30 minutes, most of the nicotine should be released from the gum and no warmth or tingling will occur during chewing.
- Then *throw away* this piece of gum and wait until you have an urge to smoke before using another piece of gum.
- Later in the treatment, you may be able to chew the gum a little more often. Follow your doctor's directions.
- Read carefully the patient instruction sheet that comes with this medicine. Ask your doctor or pharmacist for "How to Stop Smoking with NICORETTE" by Merrell Pharmaceuticals.

Special Instructions

Length of Therapy

Do not stop taking this medicine suddenly without the approval of your doctor. The medicine must be slowly stopped over a period of 1 to 2 weeks after the smoking habit has been broken. However, the nicotine gum should be carried for up to 3 months after it has been stopped in case you have a desire to smoke.

Pregnancy/Breastfeeding

NICORETTE contains nicotine which may cause fetal harm when

administered to a pregnant woman. Do not chew NICORETTE if you are pregnant or nursing. Take precautions to avoid pregnancy while using NICORETTE but if you suspect you are pregnant, stop the medication and tell your doctor at once.

Drug Interactions

Smoking can alter the response to some drugs (e.g. THEOPHYLLINE, IMIPRAMINE, PENTAZOCINE, FUROSEMIDE, PROPRANOLOL, PROPOXYPHENE). Therefore, when smoking is stopped, the response to these drugs can be changed. It is important to tell your pharmacist and doctor all the medications you are taking so that they can monitor your dose of these other medicines.

Special Precautions

You must have a sincere desire to quit smoking immediately before this medicine can be beneficial.

Carry the gum with you at all times.

Do not smoke while you are on this medicine. There could be a risk of a nicotine overdose.

Anyone needing the gum for longer than 3 months should be evaluated by his/her doctor because he/she may be using the gum as a substitute source of nicotine.

If the gum sticks to dentures, there is a possibility that it might damage the dentures. Check with your doctor or dentist.

If you swallow a piece of gum, you should not experience any adverse effects since the nicotine should not be released unless the gum is chewed. If you do develop side effects, however, call your doctor or a poison center immediately.

When to Call Your Doctor

Most people experience few or no side effects from this drug. However, any medicine can sometimes cause unwanted effects. Call your doctor if you develop mouth ulcers, heart palpitations, faintness, weakness, confusion, headaches, vision or hearing problems, convulsions, aching of teeth or jaw or problems with dentures.

Allergic Reactions

Call your doctor immediately if you think you may be allergic to the medicine or if you develop a skin rash, hives, itching, swelling of the face or difficulty in breathing. If you cannot reach your doctor, phone a hospital emergency department.

Storage

WARNING: Store this gum away from children. Nicotine is very toxic and children could be poisoned if they chewed only a few pieces of the gum.

NITROFURANTOIN (ORAL)

Apo-Nitrofurantoin, Macrodantin, Nephronex, Novofuran

Purpose

This medicine is used to treat certain types of infections of the bladder and kidneys.

Your doctor has prescribed this antibiotic for your present infection only. Do not use it for other infections or give it to other people.

Allergies/Warnings

If you have ever had an allergic reaction to any other medicine, tell your doctor and pharmacist.

Do not give this medicine to infants under 1 month of age.

How to Use This Medicine

Time of Administration

It is best to take all forms of this medicine with food or a full glass of milk. This will help your body absorb the drug better and will also help to prevent stomach upset.

How to Administer

For tablets and capsules:

- Swallow the tablets and capsules whole. Do not crush, chew or break them into pieces.

For liquid medicines:

- If you were prescribed a *suspension*, shake the bottle well each time before pouring so that you can measure an accurate dose.
- If a spoon is used to measure the dose, it is recommended that you use a medicine spoon or an oral liquid syringe that you can obtain from your pharmacist. *See* How to Administer Medications (page 15).

Special Instructions

Length of Therapy

It is important to take all of this medicine plus any refills that your doctor told you to take. Do not stop taking this medicine earlier than your doctor has recommended even if you begin to feel better. If you stop taking the medicine too soon, the infection may return.

Pregnancy/Breastfeeding

Women who are pregnant, breastfeeding or planning to become pregnant should tell their doctor before taking this medicine.

Drug Interactions

Some antacids and other nonprescription products containing magnesium can make this medicine less effective if they are taken at the same time. Check with your pharmacist before you purchase any nonprescription drugs.

Special Precautions

Try to drink at least six to eight 8-ounce glasses of water or other fluids a day, unless your doctor has otherwise directed. The extra intake of water will help to wash the bacteria causing the infection out into the urine.

In some people, this drug may cause dizziness or drowsiness. Do not drive a car, pilot an airplane, operate dangerous machinery or do jobs that require you to be alert if you are dizzy or drowsy. You should also be careful going up and down stairs. Sit or lie down at the first sign of dizziness. Tell your doctor if the dizziness or drowsiness continues.

In some people, this medicine may cause your urine to turn rust-yellow to brown in color. This is only temporary and will go away after you have finished the medicine.

When to Call Your Doctor

Call your doctor if your symptoms do not improve within a few days or if they become worse.

Most people experience few or no side effects from this drug. However, any medicine can sometimes cause unwanted effects. Call your doctor if you develop a skin rash, fever or chills, troublesome nausea or diarrhea, headache, unusual tiredness, cough, difficulty in breathing, chest pain, numbness or tingling in the mouth, face, fingers or toes, milky or foul-smelling urine, painful urination, unusually pale skin or a yellow color to the skin or eyes.

Allergic Reactions

Call your doctor immediately if you think you may be allergic to the medicine or if you develop a skin rash, hives, itching, swelling of the face

or difficulty in breathing. If you cannot reach your doctor, phone a hospital emergency department.

Storage

Store the medicine in a cool, dark place and keep the bottle tightly closed. Do not refrigerate or freeze the liquid medicine.

If for some reason you do not take all of the medicine, discard the unused portion by flushing it down the toilet. Do not take or save old medicine.

Refills

Do not go without medicine between prescription refills. Call your pharmacist for a refill 2 or 3 days before you will run out of the medicine.

Did You Know That?

Some drugs can change the color of the urine.

If you are taking a medicine and the color of your urine changes to orange, blue or green, it may be due to the medicine. Some drugs are capable of causing these color changes.

Call your doctor or pharmacist and ask if this abnormal urine color could be due to any of the medicines you are taking.

NITROGLYCERIN (ORAL)

NITRONG-SR

Purpose

This medicine is used to help prevent angina attacks (chest pains). It does this by easing the workload of the heart and decreasing the demand on the heart for oxygen. It will not relieve an angina attack that has already started because the medicine starts to work too slowly. Therefore, it will probably also be necessary for you to have a prescription for a quick-acting medicine to treat any angina attacks.

Allergies/Warnings

If you have ever had an allergic reaction to any medicine, tell your doctor and pharmacist before you take any of this medicine.

How to Use This Medicine

Time of Administration

Take this medicine on an empty stomach at least 1 hour before (or 2 hours after) eating food.

How to Administer

Take the medicine with a glass of water.

This medicine must be swallowed whole. Do not crush, chew or break it into pieces.

Special Instructions

Length of Therapy

Do not take any more of this medicine than your doctor has prescribed and do not stop taking this medicine suddenly without the approval of your doctor. It may be necessary for your doctor to reduce your dose slowly since your body will need time to adjust. It could be harmful and could cause an angina attack if you suddenly stopped taking the medicine.

Pregnancy/Breastfeeding

Women who are pregnant, breastfeeding or planning to become pregnant should tell their doctor before taking this medicine.

Drug Interactions

Some nonprescription drugs can aggravate your heart condition. Do not take any of the following without the approval of your doctor or pharmacist: cough, cold or sinus products; asthma or allergy products. Read the label of the product to see if there is a warning. If there is, check with your doctor or pharmacist before using the product.

Alcohol

Do not drink alcoholic beverages too soon after taking this medicine as the combination may cause a serious drop in blood pressure, dizziness and/or fainting.

Special Precautions

The first few doses of this medicine may cause dizziness, headache or flushing of the face. This is normal and will usually disappear after you have taken the drug a few times. Sit or lie down until these effects pass. Take slow, deep breaths and bend forward with your head between your knees if you feel faint. Get up slowly after you have been sitting or lying down. However, if the dizziness or the headaches do not go away, tell your doctor. Your dose may have to be adjusted.

If you become dizzy, you should be careful going up and down stairs. Do not drive a car, pilot an airplane, operate dangerous machinery or do jobs that require you to be alert.

Keep a record of the number of angina attacks and possible causes of the attack. This information will help your physician give you the best treatment. Be sure to tell your doctor if you have an increase in number, length or severity of attacks.

Cigarette smoking can aggravate angina and is a special risk for people who have heart conditions.

When to Call Your Doctor

Most people experience few or no side effects from this drug. However, any medicine can sometimes cause unwanted effects. Call your doctor if you develop a skin rash, fainting, blurred vision, dry mouth, nausea or vomiting, severe headaches or if you develop chest pains not relieved by quick-acting anti-anginal medicine.

Storage

Store in a cool, dry place but not in the refrigerator.

Refills

Do not stop taking this medicine without your doctor's approval and do not go without medicine between prescription refills. Call your pharmacist for a refill 2 or 3 days before you will run out of the medicine.

Miscellaneous

Carry an identification card in your wallet or wear a medical alert bracelet indicating that you are taking this medicine as well as the names and phone numbers of your doctors. If you do not already carry such a card, complete the Medicine Card in this book. Always tell your dentist, pharmacist and other doctors who are treating you that you are taking this medicine.

NITROGLYCERIN (SUBLINGUAL)

NITROGLYCERIN, NITROSTAT

NITROGLYCERIN (TRANSLINGUAL)

NITROLINGUAL SPRAY

Purpose

This medicine is used to relieve and prevent the chest pains of angina attacks. It does this by easing the workload of the heart and decreasing the demand on the heart for oxygen.

Allergies/Warnings

Be sure to tell your doctor and pharmacist if you are allergic to any medicine.

How to Use This Medicine

Time of Administration

Carry this medicine with you all the time but do not carry it in a pocket close to the body because body heat can destroy the drug.

This medicine should be used at the *first* sign of an attack of angina (chest pains or tightness or squeezing in the chest). The pain may travel to the arms, shoulders, neck and lower jaw. Do not wait until the pain becomes severe. *Sit down* as soon as you feel an attack of angina coming on.

NITROGLYCERIN and NITROSTAT SUBLINGUAL TABLETS may also be used 5 to 10 minutes before exercise or activities that might cause chest pain.

How to Administer

For sublingual tablets:

- Place a tablet *under your tongue* and let it dissolve completely. If your mouth is very dry and the tablet will not dissolve, add 1 ml (a few drops) of water under your tongue. Do not swallow or chew the tablet since this drug works faster when it is absorbed through the lining of the mouth.
- Always sit down while you are taking this medicine and waiting for it to dissolve.
- Try not to swallow until the tablet is dissolved and do not rinse your mouth for a few minutes. Do not eat, drink or smoke while the tablet is dissolving.
- The medicine may cause a tingling or burning sensation in the mouth while it is dissolving. This is not harmful.
- This medicine usually has an effect in 1 to 5 minutes. If your angina is not relieved within 5 minutes, you may dissolve a second tablet under your tongue. If the angina continues for another 5 minutes, you may dissolve a third tablet. If 3 doses do not relieve your chest pains, call your doctor or local Emergency Medical Service immediately or go to the nearest hospital emergency department.

For NITROLINGUAL SPRAY:

- Remove the plastic cap from the canister.
- DO NOT SHAKE canister before use because this will cause a smaller dose to be delivered.
- It is recommended that you sit down before using this medication.
- Hold the canister upright and place your forefinger on the top of the button.
- Open your mouth and bring the canister as close to the mouth as possible.
- Press the button firmly to release one spray—preferably onto or under the tongue.
- DO NOT INHALE THE SPRAY.
- Close your mouth. Try not to swallow and do not rinse your mouth for a few minutes. Do not eat, drink or smoke while the medicine is being absorbed.
- Replace the plastic cap on the canister.
- This medicine usually has an effect within 5 minutes. If your angina is not relieved within 5 minutes, you may use a second dose. If the chest pains continue, you may repeat the dose. Do not use more than 3 doses in 15 minutes. If 3 doses do not relieve your chest pains, call your doctor or local Emergency Medical Service immediately or go to the nearest hospital emergency department.

Try to relax for 15 to 20 minutes after taking the drug and remain calm since this will also help to relieve the attack sooner. If you become dizzy or feel faint, take slow, deep breaths and bend forward with your head between your knees. Always get up slowly after you have been sitting or lying down.

Special Instructions

Pregnancy/Breastfeeding

Women who are pregnant, breastfeeding or planning to become pregnant should tell their doctor before taking this medicine.

Drug Interactions

Some nonprescription drugs can aggravate your heart condition. Do not take any of the following without the approval of your doctor or pharmacist: cough, cold or sinus products; asthma or allergy products. Read the label of the product to see if there is a warning. If there is, check with your doctor or pharmacist before using the product.

Alcohol

Do not drink alcoholic beverages too soon after taking this medicine as the combination may cause a serious drop in blood pressure, dizziness and/or fainting.

Special Precautions

After using this medicine, you may get a headache or flushing of the face that will usually disappear within a few minutes. These are common side effects. If the headaches are severe or do not go away, tell your doctor.

Also keep a supply of the medicine at your bedside in case you need it during the night. Be sure you know how to operate the spray in the dark. Tell other family members where you are keeping this medicine so that they will be able to help you.

Keep a record of the number of angina attacks, number of tablets or sprays needed to relieve the chest pain and possible causes of the attack. This information will help your physician give you the best treatment.

You may help prevent angina attacks by taking a tablet 5 or 10 minutes before activities you know are likely to trigger attacks, such as strenuous exercise, sexual activity, emotional stress, a heavy meal, high altitudes or exposure to cold. Let your doctor know what things usually cause your angina so that he or she can advise you about preventing attacks.

Cigarette smoking can aggravate angina and is a special risk for people who have heart conditions.

When to Call Your Doctor

Most people experience few or no side effects from this drug. However, any medicine can sometimes cause unwanted effects. Call your doctor if you develop a skin rash, fainting, blurred vision, dry mouth, nausea or vomiting, severe headaches or if your chest pain is not relieved after you have taken the number of tablets that your doctor has prescribed.

Storage

For Sublingual Tablets:

This medicine must be fresh in order to work. It should be stored in the following way:

- Keep the tablets in the original *glass* container supplied by your pharmacist and keep the bottle tightly closed and away from moisture and light. This will help keep the tablets fresh. Do not put the tablets in containers made of metal, plastic or cardboard or mix the tablets with other medicines.

- Throw away the cotton that comes in the bottle and do not put labels, other drugs or any other material into the bottle.
- Carry the medicine with you *at all times* in the original glass container in a cool place, such as in a coat pocket or a purse. Do not carry the container close to your body because the body warmth may weaken the tablets.
- As soon as you remove a tablet, put the cap on the bottle tightly.
- Store unopened bottles of the medicine at room temperature away from direct heat or sunlight. Do *not* store it in the refrigerator or the bathroom medicine cabinet because the moisture in these areas could spoil the tablets. Do *not* store it in the glove compartment of your car.

For Spray:

- Store the inhaler at room temperature. Do not place it in hot water or near radiators, stoves, or other sources of heat. Do not puncture, burn, or incinerate the container (even when it is empty).
- The spray is stable for three years.

Refills

If you use the spray, it is a good idea to have an extra canister at home in case of an emergency. To test the amount of spray left in the canister, place the canister in a bowl of water. *See* How to Administer Medications (page 15).

Discuss with your pharmacist the implications of dispensing all your refills for this medicine with the same manufacturer's product. *See* Generic Drugs (page 12).

Miscellaneous

Carry an identification card in your wallet or wear a medical alert bracelet indicating that you are taking this medicine as well as the names and phone numbers of your doctors. If you do not already carry such a card, complete the Medicine Card in this book. Always tell your dentist, pharmacist and other doctors who are treating you that you are taking this medicine.

NITROGLYCERIN OINTMENT (TOPICAL)

NITRO-BID, NITROL, NITROL TSAR KIT, NITRONG

Purpose

This medicine is used to help prevent angina (chest pains). It does this by easing the workload of the heart and decreasing the demand on the heart for oxygen. Therefore, it will probably also be necessary for you to have a prescription for a quick-acting medicine to treat any angina attacks.

Allergies/Warnings

Be sure to tell your doctor and pharmacist if you are allergic to any medicine.

How to Use This Medicine

How to Administer

For ointment:

- Remove any old ointment before applying a new dose. Dry the skin completely before applying the ointment.
- This ointment must be carefully measured using the special dose-measuring papers that come with it. Use these papers to measure the length of ointment which you are to use.
- Place the printed side down and squeeze the prescribed amount of ointment onto the paper. Use this paper to spread the ointment on the skin—*do not use your fingers* to apply the ointment.
- Apply the ointment in a thin, even layer to any convenient part of the body *except* below the knee or below the elbow. Most people apply the ointment to the chest, abdomen, front of the thighs or upper arm. Do not use it on excessively hairy areas.
- Do not use the same spot all the time but rotate to different areas. This will help prevent skin irritation.
- Apply the ointment lightly—*do not rub or massage* the ointment into the skin because this would interfere with the constant slow release of the drug. Just spread it in a thin, even layer approximately the size of the special dose-measuring papers, unless otherwise directed by your doctor.
- Once the ointment is applied, use the application paper as a cover to prevent clothes from being soiled. Hold the paper in place with adhesive tape.
- If your doctor wants you to cover the ointment with transparent kitchen (plastic) wrap or other suitable material, be sure you understand the correct method. This can be held in place with adhesive or transparent tape.

For NITROL TSAR KIT:

- This medicine comes with a bandage backing so you do not have to cover it with plastic wrap.

- Tear off one TSAR patch from the roll.
- Measure the correct dose of ointment using the special dose-measuring ruler on the TSAR patch. Do not use more than 5 cm (2 inches) of ointment on each patch.
- Carefully fold the TSAR patch in half to spread the ointment. Do not get the ointment on the outer dotted border or you will not get the full dose.
- Peel off and discard the outer dotted border.
- Apply to any non-hairy area of the body *except* below the knee or below the elbow. Most people apply the patch to the upper chest, abdomen, back, or upper arm. Do not shave the area.
- Do not apply the patch over cuts, scrapes or areas with calluses or scars because this can change the absorption of the drug through the skin.
- Do not use the same spot all the time but rotate to different areas. This will help prevent skin irritation.
- Do not apply directly after showering, bathing or swimming. Wait until you are sure the skin is completely dry.
- Attach the patch to the skin and press firmly in place for 10 to 15 seconds. Run your finger along the outside edge and the center of the patch. Once the patch has been applied, do not test it by pulling on it.
- Remove and throw away the patch before applying the next dose. Discard patch in a garbage container.
- When you remove the patch from the skin, wash the area with soap and water.

Special Instructions

Length of Therapy

Do not use any more of this medicine than your doctor has prescribed and do not stop using this medicine suddenly without the approval of your doctor. It will be necessary for your doctor to reduce your dose slowly since your body will need time to adjust. It could be harmful and could cause an angina attack if you suddenly stopped using the medicine.

Pregnancy/Breastfeeding

Women who are pregnant, breastfeeding or planning to become pregnant should tell their doctor before taking this medicine.

Drug Interactions

Some nonprescription drugs can aggravate your heart condition. Do not take any of the following without the approval of your doctor or pharmacist: cough, cold or sinus products; asthma or allergy products.

Read the label of the product to see if there is a warning. If there is, check with your doctor or pharmacist before using the product.

Alcohol

Do not drink alcoholic beverages too soon after taking this medicine as the combination may cause a serious drop in blood pressure, dizziness and/or fainting.

Special Precautions

The first few doses of this medicine may cause dizziness, headache or flushing of the face. This is normal and will usually disappear after you have taken the drug a few times. Sit or lie down until these effects pass. Breathe deeply and bend forward with your head between your knees if you feel faint. Get up slowly after you have been sitting or lying down. However, if the dizziness or the headaches do not go away, tell your doctor. Your dose may have to adjusted.

If you become dizzy, you should be careful going up and down stairs. Do not drive a car, pilot an airplane, operate dangerous machinery or do jobs that require you to be alert.

Keep a record of the number of angina attacks and possible causes of the attack. This information will help your physician give you the best treatment. Be sure to tell your doctor if you have an increase in number, length or severity of attacks.

Cigarette smoking can aggravate angina and is a special risk for people who have heart conditions.

When to Call Your Doctor

Most people experience few or no side effects from this drug. However, any medicine can sometimes cause unwanted effects. Call your doctor if you develop a skin rash, fainting, blurred vision, dry mouth, nausea or vomiting, severe headaches or if you develop chest pains not relieved by sublingual nitroglycerin.

Storage

Keep tube tightly closed.

Store in a cool, dry place but not in the refrigerator.

Refills

Do not stop using this medicine without your doctor's approval and do not go without medicine between prescription refills. Call your pharmacist for a refill 2 or 3 days before you will run out of the medicine.

Discuss with your pharmacist the implications of dispensing all your refills for this medicine with the same manufacturer's product. (*See* Generic Drugs, page 12.)

Miscellaneous

Carry an identification card in your wallet or wear a medical alert bracelet indicating that you are taking this medicine as well as the names and phone numbers of your doctors. If you do not already carry such a card, complete the Medicine Card in this book. Always tell your dentist, pharmacist and other doctors who are treating you that you are taking this medicine.

PENICILLIN V (ORAL)

PEN-VEE, PVF

PENICILLIN V POTASSIUM

APO-PEN-VK, LEDERCILLIN-VK, NADOPEN-V, NOVOPEN-VK, PVF-K, VC-K 500, V-CILLIN K

PENICILLIN G POTASSIUM

MEGACILLIN, NOVOPEN-G-500

Purpose

This medicine is an antibiotic used to treat certain types of infections.

Your doctor has prescribed this antibiotic for your present infection. Do not use it for other infections or give it to other people.

Allergies/Warnings

If you have ever had an allergic reaction to penicillin, a cephalosporin, or any other medicine (including ASA) or if you have any allergies (for example, asthma or hay fever), tell your doctor and pharmacist before you take any of this medicine.

How to Use This Medicine

Time of Administration

It is best to take this medicine on an empty stomach 1 hour before (or 2 hours after) meals or food unless otherwise directed by your doctor. Take it at the proper time even if you skip a meal.

Space your doses of the medicine around the clock (throughout the entire day of 24 hours). For example, if you are to take 4 doses each day, space the doses 6 hours apart. This will keep a constant level of the medicine in your body.

How to Administer

For tablets:

- Take the tablets with a full glass of water (eight ounces) unless otherwise directed.
- If you were prescribed PENICILLIN G, do not drink acidic fruit juices, such as grapefruit juice, cranberry juice or orange juice, within 1 hour of the time you take the medicine. Acidic fruit juices may prevent the medicine from working as well as it should.

For liquid medicines:

- If you were prescribed a liquid medicine, shake the bottle well each time before pouring so that you can measure an accurate dose.
- If a spoon is used to measure the dose, it is recommended that you use a medicine spoon or an oral liquid syringe that you can obtain from your pharmacist. *See* How to Administer Medications (page 15).

Special Instructions

Length of Therapy

It is important to take all of this medicine plus any refills that your doctor told you to take. Do not stop taking this medicine earlier than your doctor has recommended even if you begin to feel better. If you stop taking the medicine too soon, the infection may return.

This is especially important if you are taking the medicine to cure a strep infection because if the infection is not completely cleared up, serious problems could develop later. After treatment for a strep infection, your doctor may want to do a test to make sure that the infection is gone.

Pregnancy/Breastfeeding

Women who are pregnant or planning to become pregnant should tell their doctor before taking this medicine.

Women who are breastfeeding should tell their doctor before taking this medicine. PENICILLIN can pass into the breast milk and may cause unwanted side effects in the baby.

Drug Interactions

There have been some reports that oral contraceptives (birth control pills) may not work as well while taking this medicine. Unplanned pregnancies may occur. Ask your doctor about another form of birth control while you are taking this antibiotic. Also call your doctor if you develop spotting or breakthrough bleeding since these can be signs of decreased birth control effect.

Special Precautions

In some people, this medicine may cause the tongue to become dark-colored. This is only temporary and will go away after you have finished the medicine.

If you develop diarrhea, do not treat it yourself without first checking with your doctor or pharmacist.

When to Call Your Doctor

Call your doctor if your symptoms do not improve within a few days or if they become worse.

Most people experience few or no side effects from this drug. However, any medicine can sometimes cause unwanted effects. Call your doctor if you develop fever, chills, severe watery diarrhea, yellow-green stools, nausea or vomiting, abdominal or stomach cramps, bloating, unusual thirst, unusual weakness or unusual weight loss. These effects are rare and may occur even after the medicine has been stopped. Also call your doctor if you develop rectal itching or, in women, vaginal itching or a vaginal discharge that was not present before you started taking the medicine.

Allergic Reactions

Call your doctor immediately if you think you may be allergic to the medicine or if you develop a skin rash, hives, itching, swelling of the face or difficulty in breathing. If you cannot reach your doctor, phone a hospital emergency department.

Storage

If for some reason you cannot take all of the medicine, discard the unused portion by flushing it down the toilet. Throw away any unused medicine after the discard (expiration) date on the bottle. Do not take or save old medicine.

For liquid medicines:

- Some liquid penicillin medicines must be stored in the refrigerator. Check with your pharmacist if you have any questions.

Refills

Do not go without medicine between prescription refills. Call your pharmacist for a refill 2 or 3 days before you will run out of the medicine.

Transdermal Patch Rubs Off on Baby

The parents of a nine-month-old infant took their baby into their bed one night after the child woke up with the symptoms of a cold and teething. The baby stayed in the bed for several hours until he was comforted.

When the father got up the following morning, he noticed that his transdermal patch containing a medicine was missing. The medicine in this patch was being used to control high blood pressure. A search of the bedding, shower and floor failed to locate the missing patch and it was decided that the patch must have been lost in the clothing.

According to a report in the *New England Journal of Medicine*, the baby was unusually irritable the next morning, less active than usual and slept frequently. He refused food and drank more than three times the normal amount of fluids. His urine output was also three times normal. While being prepared for his evening bath, the missing clonidine patch was noticed on his back. The patch was folded over and less than 1/10 of the surface of the patch containing the medicine was touching his skin. This means the baby received 1/10 the dose of the medicine being released from the patch.

The patch was immediately removed and the child began returning to normal within 6 hours. By the next day he was back to normal despite his cold and teething symptoms.

Even though this was a freak occurrence, it does alert us to the possibility that transdermal patches can be transferred between two people sleeping in the same bed. It also alerts us to the need to discard patches in a place where children cannot retrieve them. Children are attracted to "bandages" and it is quite possible that they would "play" with them if they found them in a wastepaper basket.

PENTOXIFYLLINE (ORAL)

TRENTAL

Purpose

This medicine is used in the treatment of intermittent claudication (a severe pain in calf muscles occurring during walking but which subsides with rest). The medicine improves blood flow to the legs and feet. It does this by making the red blood cells more flexible so that they can more easily carry oxygen to the tiny blood vessels called capillaries. This helps to reduce painful leg cramps that occur while walking and makes it possible to walk further with fewer rests.

Allergies/Warnings

If you have ever had an allergic reaction to this medicine or caffeine; any other xanthine drugs such as theophylline, theobromine or aminophylline or any drugs used to treat asthma, tell your doctor and pharmacist before you take any of this medicine.

How to Use This Medicine

Time of Administration

Take this medicine with food or immediately after meals to help prevent stomach upset (indigestion, heartburn), dizziness and headache unless otherwise directed by your doctor.

How to Administer

Take the medicine with a full glass of water unless otherwise directed.

This medicine has a special formulation so the drug is slowly released. It must be swallowed whole. Do not crush, chew, or break it into pieces.

Special Instructions

Length of Therapy

The full effect of the medicine may not be noticed immediately, but may take from 2 to 8 weeks. Be patient. Take the medicine regularly and try not to miss any doses.

Pregnancy/Breastfeeding

Women who are pregnant or planning to become pregnant should tell their doctor before taking this medicine.

Alcohol

Do not drink alcoholic beverages while taking this drug without the approval of your doctor. Thc combination could irritate your stomach and could cause drowsiness or dizziness. One drink may have the same effect that 2 or 3 drinks normally would have.

Special Precautions

The most common side effects are upset stomach (indigestion, heartburn), nausea, dizziness and headache. Taking the medicine with some food can usually help decrease these side effects.

If this medicine causes dizziness or lightheadedness, you should be careful going up and down stairs and you should not change positions too rapidly. Therefore, get up from a sitting or lying position more slowly and tighten and relax your leg muscles or wiggle your toes to help promote circulation. Sit or lie down at the first sign of dizziness. Do not drive a car, pilot a plane, operate dangerous machinery or do jobs that require you to be alert if you are dizzy. Tell your doctor if you have been dizzy.

It is recommended that you do not smoke while you are on this medicine because smoking can aggravate your condition.

You can monitor your own progress by keeping a daily record of how far you can walk without having to stop for a rest. This record will also be very useful to your doctor.

When to Call Your Doctor

Most people experience few or no side effects from this drug. However, any medicine can sometimes cause unwanted effects. Call your doctor if you develop vomiting/severe dizziness/severe headache, fainting, chest pains, flushing of the face, nosebleeds, flu-like symptoms, fever, fast or slow heartbeats, a yellow color to the skin or eyes or dark-colored urine, or a skin rash.

Allergic Reactions

Call your doctor immediately if you think you may be allergic to the medicine or if you develop a skin rash, hives, itching, swelling of the face or difficulty in breathing. If you cannot reach your doctor, phone a hospital emergency department.

Storage

Store this medicine in a cool, dry place.

Refills

Do not stop taking this medicine without your doctor's approval and do not go without medicine between prescription refills. Call your pharmacist for a refill 2 or 3 days before you will run out of the medicine.

PHENYLBUTAZONE (ORAL)

Apo-Phenylbutazone, Butazolidin, Intrabutazone, Novobutazone, Phenbuff

PHENYLBUTAZONE-ANTACIDS

Alka Butazolidin, Alkabutazone, Alka-Phenylbutazone, Phenylone Plus

Purpose

This medicine is used to help relieve the symptoms of ankylosing spondilitis and acute attacks of gout when other nonsteroidal anti-inflammatory drugs have not worked. This medicine is not recommended as an initial drug treatment.

The medicine is almost always used for a short time period and should be stopped as soon as possible.

Allergies/Warnings

If you have ever had an allergic reaction to ASA (acetylsalicylic acid) or any other medicine or if you suffer from hay fever, asthma, nasal polyps, ulcers, blood problems, heart or liver or kidney problems, high blood pressure, thyroid problems, or any other medical problems, tell your doctor and pharmacist before you take any of this medicine.

The medicine should not be used in children 14 years of age or less and in senile patients.

How to Use This Medicine

Time of Administration

Always take this medicine with food or a glass of milk or immediately after meals to help prevent stomach upset (indigestion, nausea, vomiting, stomach pain). If you develop persistent stomach pain, contact your doctor.

If you were prescribed Intrabutazone:

- These tablets have a special coating and must be swallowed whole. Do not crush or chew, or break into pieces. Do not take chipped tablets. Do not take the tablets with milk or antacids because they could dissolve the special coating.

Special Instructions

Length of Therapy

Do not use this medicine more often or longer than recommended by your doctor. If you do not feel better after 1 week, call your doctor. People with acute gout or over 60 years of age should not take this medicine for more than 1 week. (*See* When to Call Your Doctor, below.)

Pregnancy/Breastfeeding

Women who are pregnant, breastfeeding or planning to become pregnant should tell their doctor before taking this medicine. Use of this medicine during pregnancy, especially the last three months, or during breastfeeding is not recommended.

Drug Interactions

Do not take any other medicines containing ASA (acetylsalicylic acid) or salicylates while you are taking this medicine. The combination could cause stomach problems.

It is usually safe to take acetaminophen for fever or the occasional headache. Check with your pharmacist.

Alcohol

Do not drink alcoholic beverages while taking this drug without the approval of your doctor because the combination could cause stomach problems or make the drowsiness worse.

Special Precautions

In some people this medicine may cause drowsiness. Do not drive a car, pilot an airplane, operate dangerous machinery or do jobs that require you to be alert until you know how you are going to react to this drug.

Do not take antacids containing large amounts of sodium while you are taking this medicine. Check with your pharmacist.

This medicine does not replace any exercise or rest programs or use of heat/cold treatments your doctor may have prescribed.

When to Call Your Doctor

This medicine can sometimes cause serious side effects, especially if taken longer than one week and particularly in patients over 40 years of age. Patients over 60 years of age are even more sensitive to the side effects and should not take the medicine for more than 7 days. Some of these side effects may even occur many days or weeks *after* you have stopped taking the drug.

Call your doctor immediately if you develop a skin rash, sore throat, fever and joint pain, chills, swelling of the neck or throat, ringing or buzzing in the ears, any loss of hearing, fast heartbeats, swelling of the legs or ankles or sudden weight gain, blurred vision or changes in your eyesight, bloody or black stools, severe stomach pain, vomiting of blood or material that looks like coffee grounds, a yellow color to the skin or eyes, unusual bruising or bleeding, unusual tiredness or weakness, depression, seizures, difficulty or pain in urinating (passing your water) or sudden decrease in the amount of urine, bloody or cloudy urine or a persistent headache.

Allergic Reactions

Call your doctor immediately if you think you may be allergic to the medicine or if you develop a skin rash, hives, itching, swelling of the face or difficulty in breathing. If you cannot reach your doctor, phone a hospital emergency department.

Miscellaneous

Carry an identification card in your wallet or wear a medical alert bracelet indicating that you are taking this medicine as well as the names and phone numbers of your doctors. If you do not already carry such a card, complete the Medicine Card in this book. Always tell your dentist, pharmacist and other doctors who are treating you that you are taking this medicine.

PHENYTOIN (ORAL)

DILANTIN CAPSULES, DILANTIN INFATABS, DILANTIN-30 SUSPENSION, DILANTIN-125 SUSPENSION

MEPHENYTOIN

MESANTOIN

Purpose

This medicine is used to help control convulsions and seizures. It is commonly used in the treatment of epilepsy.

Allergies/Warnings

If you have ever had an allergic reaction to an anticonvulsant or seizure medicine, tell your doctor and pharmacist before you take any of this medicine.

How to Use This Medicine

Time of Administration

It is very important that you take this medicine exactly as your doctor has prescribed. Do not miss any doses and take the medicine even if you feel well. Try to take this medicine at the same time(s) every day so that you will have a constant level of medicine in your body. This is the only way that you can receive the full benefit of the medicine. If you forget to take this medicine, the amount of medicine in your blood will decrease and you may have seizures.

In adults, DILANTIN is taken in divided doses throughout the day or once daily. Be sure you know how your doctor wants you to take it.

In children, DILANTIN is given in divided doses throughout the day.

How to Administer

Take this medicine with a full glass of water.

Do not use DILANTIN Capsules if they have turned dark in color.

If you were prescribed DILANTIN INFATABS:

- This medicine can either be swallowed whole or chewed well before swallowing.

If you were prescribed DILANTIN SUSPENSION:

- Shake the bottle well each time before pouring so that you can measure an accurate dose.
- If a spoon is used to measure the dose, it is recommended that you use a medicine spoon or an oral liquid syringe that you can obtain from your pharmacist. *See* How to Administer Medications (page 15).

Special Instructions

Length of Therapy

Do not stop taking this medicine suddenly without the approval of your doctor. It usually will be necessary for your doctor to slowly reduce your dose since your body will need time to adjust. You could develop seizures if you suddenly stopped taking the medicine.

Pregnancy/Breastfeeding

Women who are pregnant or planning to become pregnant should tell their doctor before taking this medicine. There have been some reports of birth defects in infants born to women who were taking the medicine during pregnancy.

Women who are breastfeeding should tell their doctor before taking this medicine.

Drug Interactions

Do not take any other medicines without the approval of your doctor or pharmacist. This medicine can interact with several other medicines and cause serious reactions. This includes both prescription and non-prescription medicines, antacids, folic acid, vitamins, sleeping pills, tranquilizers, anticoagulants ("blood thinners"), medicine for seizures, muscle relaxants, anesthetics, medicines for depression or medicines for allergies.

Do not start taking medicines containing calcium (especially calcium supplements and antacids) or foods high in calcium without first checking with your doctor.

There have been some reports that oral contraceptives (birth control pills) may not work as well while taking this medicine. Unplanned pregnancies may occur. Ask your doctor about using another form of birth control or adjusting your dose of the birth control pills while you are taking this medicine. Also call your doctor if you develop spotting or breakthrough bleeding since these can be signs of decreased birth control effect.

Alcohol

Do not drink alcoholic beverages while taking this drug without the approval of your doctor because the combination could cause drowsiness or increase the frequency of your seizures. One drink may have the same effect that 2 or 3 drinks normally would have.

Special Precautions

Be sure to keep your doctor's appointments in order that your doctor can check your progress. This is especially important during the first few months of therapy, when the doctor will decide the best dose of this medicine for your condition. To make sure that your dose is correct, your doctor may wish to take a blood sample periodically to measure the amount of medicine in it.

If your doctor decides to switch you from capsules to suspension or tablets (or the other way), he/she will order a blood test to make sure you are getting the correct dose because all the different forms are not equal in strength.

This medicine may cause dizziness in some people. This side effect occurs more commonly with MEPHENYTOIN. If you become dizzy, you should be careful going up and down stairs. Sit or lie down at the first sign of dizziness. Do not drive a car, use a sewing machine, operate dangerous machinery or do jobs that require you to be alert until you know how you are going to react to the drug. Tell your doctor if you are dizzy. If this medicine is for a child, do not let him or her ride a bike, climb trees, etc. until you can determine how he or she is going to react to this medicine. Children can hurt themselves if they participate in these activities when they are dizzy.

While taking this medicine, brush your teeth and massage your gums regularly with a soft toothbrush. Also use dental floss daily. Visit your dentist regularly. The next time you visit your dentist, tell him or her that you are taking this medicine. Call your doctor if your gums become red, tender or swollen. This side effect occurs more commonly in younger patients receiving PHENYTOIN and after 2 to 3 months of therapy.

In some people, the medicine may rarely cause an increase in body and facial hair. If this becomes bothersome, tell your doctor. There are procedures that can be used to remove excessive hair.

For patients with diabetes:

- This medicine may cause your blood sugar to rise. Carefully test your blood or urine for sugar while you are taking this medicine. Call your doctor if you think your blood sugar is higher than normal or harder to control.

When to Call Your Doctor

Any medicine can sometimes cause unwanted effects. Call your doctor if you develop a sore throat, fever or mouth sores, persistent headache, severe nausea or vomiting, changes in vision, slurred speech, joint pain, swollen glands, swollen, tender or bleeding gums, increased facial hair, difficulty in walking, shakiness, easy bruising or bleeding, a yellow color to the skin or eyes, dark-colored urine, confusion or hallucinations, severe dizziness or drowsiness.

Call your doctor immediately if you develop a measles-like skin rash or any other type of rash, or if you develop continuous back-and-forth or rolling eye movements.

Call your doctor if you have an increase in the frequency of seizures.

Allergic Reactions

Call your doctor immediately if you think you may be allergic to the medicine or if you develop a skin rash, hives, itching, swelling of the face or difficulty in breathing. If you cannot reach your doctor, phone a hospital emergency department.

Refills

Do not stop taking this medicine without your doctor's approval and

do not go without medicine between prescription refills. Call your pharmacist for a refill 2 or 3 days before you will run out of the medicine.

First Aid for Epileptic Seizures

- Many patients with grand mal epilepsy may experience a warning (aura) before the onset of seizures. This aura may be in the form of unusual colors, smells or sounds, numbness, tingling or other disturbances. Some people will utter a short cry. If a patient experiences a seizure, place the patient where he or she cannot fall or be hurt. Sometimes the floor is the safest area. Clear the area of any furniture and hard, sharp or hot objects.
- Check the person's wrist or neck for an emergency medical information bracelet or necklace.
- Stay calm yourself! You cannot stop a seizure once it starts, so let the seizure run its course. Do not try to revive the person.
- Loosen tight clothing (especially around the neck) to make it easier for the person to breathe.
- Do not force anything between the patient's teeth since this could result in damage to the teeth or gums, aspiration of the material or bite injuries to the person administering the first aid. Remember it is physically impossible for a person to swallow his or her tongue during a seizure.
- Try to gently turn the patient on the side to allow mucus and often large amounts of saliva to drain from the mouth.
- Do not be alarmed if the person seems to stop breathing momentarily, but if the patient passes from one seizure to another without regaining consciousness, call an ambulance or seek medical assistance.
- After the seizure is over, the patient may be confused and/or incontinent (loss of bladder control). Allow him or her to sleep or rest. If the person remains groggy, weak or confused, he or she should not be allowed to go home alone. A relative should always be contacted if the patient is a child.
- The patient should inform his or her physician of the seizure.

Miscellaneous

Carry an identification card in your wallet or wear a medical alert bracelet indicating that you are taking this medicine as well as the names and phone numbers of your doctors. If you do not already carry such a card, complete the Medicine Card in this book. Always tell your dentist, pharmacist and other doctors who are treating you that you are taking this medicine.

POLYMYXIN (OPHTHALMIC)
AEROSPORIN OPHTHALMIC

POLYMYXIN B-NEOMYCIN-COMBINATIONS
NEOSPORIN EYE AND EAR SOLUTION, NEOSPORIN EYE OINTMENT

POLYMYXIN B-NEOMYCIN-STEROID COMBINATIONS
CORTISPORIN EYE DROPS, CORTISPORIN EYE OINTMENT, MAXITROL EYE DROPS, MAXITROL EYE OINTMENT

POLYMYXIN B-GRAMICIDIN
POLYSPORIN EYE/EAR DROPS

POLYMYXIN B-BACITRACIN
POLYSPORIN EYE/EAR OINTMENT

BACITRACIN
BACIGUENT

Purpose
This medicine is an antibiotic used to treat certain types of eye infections and used after eye surgery. It is to be used only for the eye infection you have now and should not be used for any eye infections that may develop later. CORTISPORIN and MAXITROL eye medicines contain a steroid that helps relieve redness and irritation of certain eye conditions.

Allergies/Warnings
Be sure to tell your doctor and pharmacist if you are allergic to neomycin or any medicine.

How to Use This Medicine

How to Administer
For eye drops and eye ointment see How to Administer Medications (page 15).

Special Instructions

Length of Therapy
It is important to use all of this medicine, plus any refills that your

doctor told you to use. Do not stop using it earlier than your doctor has recommended in spite of the fact that your symptoms seem to have improved. Otherwise, the infection may return.

Pregnancy/Breastfeeding

Women who are pregnant, breastfeeding or planning to become pregnant should tell their doctor before taking this medicine.

Drug Interactions

Do not use this medicine at the same time as any other eye medicine without the approval of your doctor. Some medicines cannot be mixed.

Special Precautions

If you are being treated for only one infected eye, do not touch the healthy eye to avoid spreading the infection.

Vision may be blurred for a few minutes after using the eye medicine, especially after using the eye ointments. Do not drive a car or operate dangerous machinery or do jobs that require you to be alert until your vision has cleared.

If you are prescribed CORTISPORIN and MAXITROL eye medicines for a long time, your doctor will want to do eye tests at regular intervals.

When to Call Your Doctor

Contact your doctor if the eye infection for which you are using this medicine does not begin to improve in 3 to 4 days, if increased eye redness or eye pain develops, if you develop any changes in vision or if the eye becomes irritated by the eye medicine for more than a few minutes. Many eye medicines sting for a short time immediately after use.

Miscellaneous

This medicine is for external use only. Do not swallow it.

Do not share this eye medication with family members or friends. The infection could be transferred.

POTASSIUM SUPPLEMENTS (ORAL)

APO-K, KALIUM DURULES, KAOCHLOR, KAOCHLOR-20 CONCENTRATE, KAON, KATO, KAY-CIEL, KCl 5%, K-LONG, K-LOR, K-LYTE, K-LYTE/Cl, K-10, K-MED, MICRO-K-10 EXTENCAPS, MICRO-K EXTENCAPS, NEO-K, NOVOLENTE-K, POTASSIUM-ROUGIER, POTASSIUM SANDOZ, ROYCHLOR 10%, ROYCHLOR 20%, ROYONATE, SLO-POT 600, SLOW-K

Purpose

This medicine is a potassium supplement that is used by people who have certain medical conditions or who are taking prescription medicines that can cause the body to be low in potassium.

Allergies/Warnings

Be sure to tell your doctor or pharmacist if you are allergic to any medicine.

How to Use This Medicine

Time of Administration

It is very important that you take this medicine exactly as your doctor has prescribed. Do not miss any doses and take the medicine even if you feel well. Try to take this medicine at the same time(s) every day so that you will have a constant level of medicine in your body.

Do not take extra doses without your doctor's approval. This is very important if you are also taking both diuretics (water pills) and digitalis medicines for your heart.

How to Administer

Always take this medicine immediately *after* food to help prevent stomach upset and diarrhea. Follow each dose with at least ½ glass (4 ounces) of water unless otherwise directed.

For liquid medicine:

- Mix each dose of the liquid with some water, root beer or orange juice. The amount of water, root beer, or orange juice used will depend on the brand of liquid medicine you were prescribed. Ask your pharmacist if you do not know how much water to use. Do not use tomato juice if you are on a low-salt diet.

For effervescent tablets (K-LYTE, POTASSIUM SANDOZ) *and for powders* (K-LOR, K-LYTE/C1, NEO-K EFFERVESCENT GRANULES):

- Dissolve each tablet or dose of the powder or granules in at least 1/2 glass of *cold* water or fruit juice. Let the bubbles disappear before drinking the solution. *Sip slowly* over a period of 5 to 10 minutes.

For KATO POWDER:

- Dissolve contents of 1 packet of powder in 1/2 glass of cold water.
- Allow mixture to stand 15 minutes before drinking.

For tablets to be swallowed (APO-K, KALIUM DURULES, K-LONG, K-MED, NOVOLENTE-K, SLO-POT-600, SLOW-K):

- This medicine must be swallowed whole. Do not crush, chew, or break it into pieces and do not take chipped tablets. Swallow with

plenty of water.
- Sit up or stand up when you take each dose in order to help prevent "heartburn" or irritation of the esophagus. It is also best to take any evening doses at least 1 hour before going to bed.

For MICRO-K EXTENCAPS, MICRO-K-10 EXTENCAPS:
- These capsules should be swallowed whole. Do not crush or chew.
- If you have difficulty swallowing the capsules, they may be opened and the contents sprinkled on a spoonful of soft food. The mouth should be rinsed well with water to remove any particles left in the mouth.

Special Instructions

Pregnancy/Breastfeeding

Women who are pregnant, breastfeeding or planning to become pregnant should tell their doctor before taking this medicine.

Special Precautions

Do not use salt substitutes, low-salt milk or low-salt soups without the approval of your doctor. They may contain large amounts of potassium.

Do not take laxatives without the permission of your doctor. Incorrect use of laxatives could interfere with the potassium level in your body. Some laxatives contain extra potassium and other laxatives could cause your body to lose too much potassium.

When to Call Your Doctor

Most people experience few or no side effects from this drug. However, any medicine can sometimes cause unwanted effects. Call your doctor if you develop sharp stomach pain, black or bloody stools, an unusual feeling of heaviness or weakness in the legs, numbness or tingling of the hands or feet, confusion, shortness of breath, unusual nervousness or irregular heartbeats.

Did You Know That?

If you must use more than 1 kind of eye drop, it is best to wait about 5 minutes between the drops.

This permits the buildup of the first drug in the cornea of the eye while allowing for minimal loss through drainage into the nasolacrimal ducts in the corner of the eye.

PRAZOSIN (ORAL)

MINIPRESS

Purpose

This medicine is used to treat high blood pressure.

Allergies/Warnings

Be sure to tell your doctor and pharmacist if you are allergic to any medicine.

How to Use This Medicine

Time of Administration

It is generally recommended that you lie down for approximately 1-2 hours after you take the first dose of this medicine or after the first dose of any dosage increases. The *first* dose of this medicine is generally taken at bedtime to help prevent dizziness or fainting, which may occur within 30 to 90 minutes after the first dose or any increase in the dosage. This is called the "first dose phenomenon" and is often decreased by starting with a low dose and gradually increasing it.

Check with your doctor if you do not know when to take the first dose. If you must get up during the night (especially after the first dose), get up very slowly (*see* Special Precautions below).

Try to take the medicine at the same time(s) every day so that you have a constant level of the medicine in your body.

How to Administer

It is best to take this medicine (especially the first dose) in a sitting position with some food or immediately after meals. This will help prevent dizziness or fainting.

Special Instructions

Length of Therapy

High blood pressure (hypertension) is a long-term condition and it will probably be necessary for you to take the drug for a long time in spite of the fact that you feel better. If high blood pressure is not treated, it can lead to serious problems such as heart failure, strokes, blood vessel problems or kidney problems.

It may take 4 to 6 weeks for you to feel the full effect of this medicine. It is very important that you take this medicine as your doctor had directed and that you do not miss any doses. Otherwise, you cannot expect the drug to keep your blood pressure down.

Pregnancy/Breastfeeding

Women who are pregnant, breastfeeding or planning to become pregnant should tell their doctor before taking this medicine.

Drug Interactions

Some nonprescription drugs can aggravate your condition. Do not take any of the following without the approval of your doctor or pharmacist: cough, cold, or sinus products; asthma, allergy or hay fever products since they could increase your blood pressure. Read the label of the product to see if there is a warning. If there is, check with your doctor or pharmacist before using the product.

Alcohol

Do not drink alcoholic beverages while taking this drug without the approval of your doctor because the combination could make the possible side effect of dizziness worse.

Special Precautions

In some people, this drug will cause dizziness, lightheadedness or drowsiness (especially during the first few days of therapy). Do not drive a car, pilot an airplane, operate dangerous machinery or do jobs that require you to be alert during the first 24 hours of starting this drug, when the dose is increased or until you have taken several doses and you know how you are going to react to the drug.

If you become dizzy, you should be careful going up and down stairs and you should not change positions too rapidly. Lightheadedness is more likely to occur if you stand up suddenly—this is due to blood collecting in the legs and lasts for a few seconds. Therefore, get up from a sitting or lying position more slowly and tighten and relax your leg muscles or wiggle your toes to help promote circulation. In the morning, get out of bed slowly and dangle your feet over the edge of the bed for a few minutes before standing up. Sit or lie down at the first sign of dizziness. Tell your doctor if you have been dizzy. You can help prevent dizziness or fainting by avoiding alcoholic beverages, strenuous exercise, standing for long periods of time (especially in hot weather), hot showers, hot baths or saunas.

Follow any special diet your doctor may have ordered. It may be necessary for you to limit the amount of salt in your diet.

If your mouth becomes dry, drink water, suck ice chips or a hard, sour candy (sugarless) or chew gum (sugarless). Sugarless products are recommended in order to avoid dental problems. You may wish to ask your pharmacist about special solutions, called artificial saliva, that can also be used to help restore moisture in the mouth. It is especially important to brush and floss your teeth regularly if you develop a dry mouth to help prevent gum problems.

Did You Know That?

People who are bedridden should sit up if at all possible to take their medicines.

British physicians have reported that esophageal ulceration occurred in a patient with no history of upper gastrointestinal disease who took a tetracycline tablet with no water and went to bed. He woke up during the night with severe pain that was later diagnosed as an ulceration of the wall of the esophagus (food pipe). This problem is also likely to occur if the person has a hiatal hernia, narrowed esophagus, or reflux of stomach contents back up the esophagus.

There is less of a chance that a medicine will lodge in the esophagus and fail to pass into the stomach if the person sits up for a few minutes and takes the medicine with a full glass of water (unless the patient has been told to restrict fluids). The water will quickly carry the drug into the stomach so that it does not get stuck in the esophagus or upper stomach (heartburn area). By sitting up, gravity can also assist in transporting medications past the esophagus and the heartburn area. For this reason, it is also a good idea to take bedtime doses of a medicine 20 to 30 minutes before lying down.

When to Call Your Doctor

Most people experience few or no side effects from this drug. However, any medicine can sometimes cause unwanted effects. Call your doctor if you develop a skin rash, fainting, fast heartbeats, swelling of the legs or ankles, sudden weight gain of 5 pounds (2.5 kg) or more, chest pains, or difficulty in breathing, difficulty in controlling urination (passing your water) or numbness or tingling in the hands or feet.

Refills

Do not stop taking this medicine without your doctor's approval and do not go without medicine between prescription refills. Call your pharmacist for a refill 2 or 3 days before you will run out of the medicine.

Miscellaneous

Carry an identification card in your wallet or wear a medical alert bracelet indicating that you are taking this medicine as well as the names and phone numbers of your doctors. If you do not already carry such a card, complete the Medicine Card in this book. Always tell your dentist, pharmacist and other doctors who are treating you that you are taking this medicine.

PROCAINAMIDE (ORAL)

APO-PROCAINAMIDE, PROCAN SR, PRONESTYL, PRONESTYL SR

Purpose

This medicine is used to help regulate the heartbeat so that it is strong and steady.

Allergies/Warnings

If you have ever had an allergic reaction to any local anesthetic or any medicine, tell your doctor and pharmacist before you take any of this medicine.

How to Use This Medicine

Time of Administration

It is very important that you take this medicine exactly as your doctor has prescribed. Do not miss any doses and take the medicine even if you feel well. Do not take extra tablets or capsules without your doctor's approval.

Take the medicine at the same times every day so that you have a constant level of the medicine in your body.

How to Administer

It is best to take this medicine with a glass of water on an empty stomach at least 1 hour before (or 2 hours after) eating food. Take it at the proper time even if you skip a dose. If you develop stomach upset after taking the drug, take it with some food. Call your doctor if you continue to have an upset stomach (indigestion or heartburn).

For PROCAN SR, PRONESTYL SR:

- This medicine has a special formulation so the drug is slowly released. It must be swallowed whole. Do not crush or chew it.

Special Instructions

Length of Therapy

Do not take any more of this medicine than your doctor has prescribed and do not stop taking this medicine suddenly without the approval of your doctor. It may be necessary for your doctor to slowly reduce your dose since your body may need time to adjust. It might be harmful if you suddenly stopped taking the medicine.

Pregnancy/Breastfeeding

Women who are pregnant, breastfeeding or planning to become pregnant should tell their doctor before taking this medicine.

Drug Interactions

It is important that you obtain the advice of your doctor or pharmacist before taking any other prescription or nonprescription medicines that can increase the heart rate (including pain relievers, sleeping pills, tranquilizers, or medicines for depression, cough/cold or sinus products, or asthma or allergy products).

There are other drug interactions which can occur. If you are taking any other medicines, be sure to check first with your pharmacist or doctor.

Special Precautions

If this medicine causes dizziness or lightheadedness, you should be careful going up and down stairs and you should not change positions too rapidly. Lightheadedness is more likely to occur if you stand up suddenly—this is due to blood collecting in the legs and lasts for a few seconds. Therefore, get up from a sitting or lying position more slowly and tighten and relax your leg muscles or wiggle your toes to help promote circulation. In the morning, get out of bed slowly and dangle your feet over the edge of the bed for a few minutes before standing up. Sit or lie down at the first sign of dizziness. Do not drive a car, pilot an airplane, operate dangerous machinery or do jobs that require you to be alert if you are dizzy. Tell your doctor if you have been dizzy.

In order to help prevent dizziness or fainting, your doctor may also recommend that you avoid strenuous exercise, standing for long periods of time (especially in hot weather), hot showers, hot baths or saunas.

If this medicine is taken for longer than one month, your doctor will want to do blood tests.

If you were prescribed PROCAN SR, do not become alarmed if you notice something that looks like a tablet in your stool. This medicine is contained in a wax core that has been designed to release the drug slowly in your body. The empty wax core is eliminated in the stool.

When to Call Your Doctor

Most people experience few or no side effects from this drug. However, any medicine can sometimes cause unwanted effects. Call your doctor if you develop a sore throat, fever, chills, nausea or vomiting, mouth sores, flu-like symptoms, muscle aches and joint pains, chest pains, coughing, skin lesions, fast heartbeats, depression, confusion, unusual bruising or bleeding, unexplained weakness, fainting or a skin rash.

Allergic Reactions

Call your doctor immediately if you think you may be allergic to the medicine or if you develop a skin rash, hives, itching, swelling of the face or difficulty in breathing. If you cannot reach your doctor, phone a hospital emergency department.

Refills

Do not stop taking this medicine without your doctor's approval and do not go without medicine between prescription refills. Call your pharmacist for a refill 2 or 3 days before you will run out of the medicine.

Discuss with your pharmacist the implications of dispensing all your refills for this medicine with the same manufacturer's product. (*See* Generic Drugs, page 12.)

Miscellaneous

Carry an identification card in your wallet or wear a medical alert bracelet indicating that you are taking this medicine as well as the names and phone numbers of your doctors. If you do not already carry such a card, complete the Medicine Card in this book.

Always tell your dentist, pharmacist and other doctors who are treating you that you are taking this medicine.

PROCHLORPERAZINE-ISOPROPAMIDE (ORAL)

COMBID

Purpose

This medicine is used to help relieve spasm and cramping by relaxing the muscles of the stomach and bowels. The medicine is also used to decrease the amount of acid formed in the stomach. It is also used to help decrease nausea or vomiting that is linked to gastrointestinal problems.

Allergies/Warnings

If you have ever had an allergic reaction to any medicine or iodine or if you have seizures, heart problems, liver disease, glaucoma, enlarged prostate, difficulty in urinating (passing your water) or any other medical condition, tell your doctor and pharmacist before you take any of this medicine.

How to Use This Medicine

How to Administer

These capsules must be swallowed whole. Do not open the capsules.

Special Instructions

Length of Therapy

Do not stop taking this medicine suddenly without the approval of your doctor. It may be necessary for your doctor to reduce your dose slowly since your body will need time to adjust.

Pregnancy/Breastfeeding

Women who are pregnant, breastfeeding or planning to become pregnant should tell their doctor before taking this medicine.

Drug Interactions

It is best not to take this medicine at the same time as an antacid or an antidiarrhea medicine containing aluminum. Try to space them 2 hours apart if you must take them while you are on this medicine.

It is important that you obtain the advice of your doctor or pharmacist before taking any other prescription or nonprescription medicines, including pain relievers, sleeping pills, tranquilizers or medicines for depression, or cough, cold or allergy medicines. There are other drug interactions which can occur. If you are taking any other medicines, be sure to check first with your pharmacist or doctor.

Alcohol

Do not drink alcoholic beverages while taking this drug without the approval of your doctor. The combination could irritate your stomach and could cause drowsiness. One drink may have the same effect that 2 or 3 drinks normally would have.

Special Precautions

If this medicine causes dizziness or lightheadedness, you should be careful going up and down stairs and you should not change positions too rapidly. Lightheadedness is more likely to occur if you stand up suddenly—this is due to blood collecting in the legs and lasts for a few seconds. Therefore, get up from a sitting or lying position more slowly and tighten and relax your leg muscles or wiggle your toes to help promote circulation. In the morning, get out of bed slowly and dangle your feet over the edge of the bed for a few minutes before standing up. Sit or lie down at the first sign of dizziness. Tell your doctor if you have been dizzy.

Do not drive a car, pilot an airplane, operate dangerous machinery or do jobs that require you to be alert if you are dizzy or drowsy.

You may become more sensitive to heat because your body may perspire less while you are taking this drug. Be careful not to become overheated during exercise or in hot weather. Try to avoid strenuous exercise, standing for long periods of time (especially in hot weather), hot showers, hot baths, saunas or Jacuzzis while taking this medicine.

Some patients may also become more sensitive to cold and should dress warmly during cold weather and limit exposure to cold temperatures.

If your mouth becomes dry, drink water, suck ice chips or a hard, sour candy (sugarless) or chew gum (sugarless). Sugarless products are recommended in order to avoid dental problems. You may wish to ask your pharmacist about special solutions, called artificial saliva, that can also be used to help restore moisture in the mouth. It is especially important to brush and floss your teeth regularly if you develop a dry mouth to help prevent gum problems.

This medicine may make some people more sensitive to sunlight and various tanning lamps. When you begin taking this medicine, try to avoid too much sun until you see how you are going to react. If your skin does become more sensitive to sunlight, tell your doctor and try not to stay in direct sunlight for extended periods of time. While in the sun, wear protective clothing and sunglasses. You may wish to ask your pharmacist about suitable sunscreen products. Call your doctor if you become sunburned.

This medicine may cause some people to become constipated. This side effect occurs more often in people over 65 years of age. To help prevent constipation, try increasing the amount of bulk in your diet (for example, bran, fresh fruits and salads), exercising more often or drinking more fluids (unless otherwise directed). Call your doctor if you develop constipation.

There have been some reports that this medicine may cause the urine to turn pink, red or red-brown. This is only temporary and will go away after you have finished the medicine.

This medicine may cause nasal congestion (stuffy nose). Do not try to treat this yourself with cold or allergy medicines. Check with your doctor or pharmacist.

When to Call Your Doctor

Stop taking the medicine and call your doctor if you become restless or unable to sit still or sleep.

Check with your doctor if you develop constipation.

Any medicine can sometimes cause unwanted effects. Call your doctor if you develop a sore throat, fever, mouth sores, eye pain or changes in vision, drooping of eyelids, difficulty in urinating (passing your water), a yellow color in the skin or eyes, dark yellow-colored urine, fast heartbeats, a skin rash, fainting spells, shuffling walk, confusion, weakness in hand muscles, shakiness or unusual movements of the face, tongue or hands, drooling, seizures or severe stiffness of muscles.

Allergic Reactions

Call your doctor immediately if you think you may be allergic to the medicine or if you develop a skin rash, hives, itching, scaling of the skin, increased sensitivity to sunlight, swelling of the face or difficulty in breathing. If you cannot reach your doctor, phone a hospital emergency department.

Refills

Do not stop taking this medicine without your doctor's approval and do not go without medicine between prescription refills. Call your pharmacist for a refill 2 or 3 days before you will run out of the medicine.

Miscellaneous

Carry an identification card in your wallet or wear a medical alert bracelet indicating that you are taking this medicine as well as the names and phone numbers of your doctors. If you do not already carry such a card, complete the Medicine Card in this book. Always tell your dentist, pharmacist and other doctors who are treating you that you are taking this medicine.

PROMETHAZINE (ORAL)

HISTANTIL, PHENERGAN, PMS PROMETHAZINE SYRUP

Purpose

This medicine is an antihistamine that is used to help relieve symptoms (such as itching) of certain types of allergic conditions. It is often used to treat nausea, vomiting and motion sickness. This drug has several other uses and the reason it was prescribed depends upon your condition. Check with your doctor if you do not understand why you are taking it.

Allergies/Warnings

If you have ever had an allergic reaction to any medicine or if you have asthma, glaucoma, an enlarged prostate or urinary retention (a type of bladder problem), high blood pressure or diabetes, tell your doctor and pharmacist before you take any of this medicine.

This medicine is not recommended for children less than 2 years of age.

How to Use This Medicine

Time of Administration

If you are taking this medicine to help prevent motion sickness, take it 30 minutes to 1 hour before travel and repeat if necessary according to your doctor's instructions.

How to Administer

This medicine may be taken without regard to meals. Take it either with food or on an empty stomach. If stomach upset occurs, take it with some food or a glass of milk.

If you were prescribed the syrup, see How to Administer Medications (page 15).

Special Instructions

Length of Therapy

Do not take this medicine more often or longer than recommended by your doctor. To do so may increase your chance of developing side effects.

Pregnancy/Breastfeeding

Women who are pregnant, breastfeeding or planning to become

pregnant should tell their doctor before taking this medicine.

Drug Interactions

It is important that you obtain the advice of your doctor or pharmacist before taking any other prescription or nonprescription medicines including pain relievers, sleeping pills, tranquilizers, medicine for seizures, muscle relaxants, anesthetics, medicines for depression or other medicines for allergies. Combining this medicine with some of these drugs could cause drowsiness or dizziness.

There are other drug interactions that can occur. If you are taking any other medicines, be sure to check first with your pharmacist or doctor.

Alcohol

Do not drink alcoholic beverages while taking this drug without the approval of your doctor because the combination could cause drowsiness. One drink may have the same effect that 2 or 3 drinks normally would have.

Special Precautions

In some people, this drug may initially cause dizziness or drowsiness. Do not drive a car, pilot an airplane, operate dangerous machinery or do jobs that require you to be alert until you know how you are going to react to the drug. If you become dizzy or drowsy, you should be careful going up and down stairs. Sit or lie down at the first sign of dizziness. Tell your doctor if the dizziness or drowsiness continues.

People over 65 years of age may be more sensitive to these side effects.

If your mouth becomes dry, drink water, suck ice chips or a hard, sour candy (sugarless) or chew gum (sugarless). Sugarless products are recommended in order to avoid dental problems. You may wish to ask your pharmacist about special solutions, called artificial saliva, that can also be used to help restore moisture in the mouth.

It is especially important to brush and floss your teeth regularly if you develop a dry mouth to help prevent gum problems.

This medicine may make some people more sensitive to sunlight and various tanning lamps. When you begin taking this medicine, try to avoid too much sun until you see how you are going to react. If your skin does become more sensitive to sunlight, tell your doctor and try not to stay in direct sunlight for extended periods of time. While in the sun, wear protective clothing and sunglasses. You may wish to ask your pharmacist about suitable sunscreen products. Call your doctor if you become sunburned.

When to Call Your Doctor

Most people experience few or no side effects from this drug. However, any medicine can sometimes cause unwanted effects. Call your doctor if you develop a skin rash, fast or irregular heartbeats, blurred vision, stomach pain, unexplained weakness or tiredness, unexplained sore throat, fever, mouth sores, unusual bruising or bleeding, unexplained nervousness, restlessness or irritability (especially in children), trouble sleeping, or difficulty in urinating (passing your water).

DID YOU KNOW THAT?

Too much vitamin A can cause weakness; muscle cramps; soreness, cracking and scaling around the mouth and anus; diffuse loss of scalp hair, eyebrows and eyelashes and unintentional weight loss.

These were the symptoms of a 41-year-old woman who had been taking high doses of vitamin A three months prior to admission to a hospital. According to the *American Journal of Medicine*, the medical staff calculated that she had ingested 22,190,000 International Units (IU) of vitamin A over the three month period. Seven months after stopping the vitamin A supplement, her scalp hair, eyebrows and eyelashes returned and her weakness and muscle cramps disappeared.

The Canadian Council on Nutrition recommends 2,600 IU to 3,000 IU per day of vitamin A in a mixed diet for adult men and adult women who are not pregnant or breastfeeding.

PROPOXYPHENE HCl (ORAL)

642's, Novopropoxyn

PROPOXYPHENE NAPSYLATE

Darvon-N

PROPOXYPHENE HCl-ASA-CAFFEINE

692's, Novopropoxyn Compound

PROPOXYPHENE NAPSYLATE-ASA

Darvon-N with ASA

PROPOXYPHENE NAPSYLATE-ASA-CAFFEINE

DARVON-N COMPOUND

Purpose

This medicine is used to help relieve pain or pain with fever.

Allergies/Warnings

If you have ever had an allergic reaction to caffeine, ASA (acetylsalicylic acid), propoxyphene or any other medicine, tell your doctor and pharmacist before you take any of this medicine.

Also tell your doctor if you have a stomach ulcer, asthma, hay fever or nasal polyps because some of these medicines contain ASA.

How to Use This Medicine

Time of Administration

This medicine works best if you take it when the pain first occurs. Do not wait until the pain becomes severe.

How to Administer

This medicine may be taken with food or a full glass of water.

For DARVON-N WITH ASA, DARVON-N COMPOUND, NOVOPROPOXYN COMPOUND *and* 692's:

- Do not take this medicine if it smells strongly like vinegar since this may mean the ASA in it is not fresh and may be losing strength.

Special Instructions

Length of Therapy

Do not take any more of this medicine than your doctor has prescribed. When used for a long period of time, the drug can become less effective. Also, when used in large doses for a long period of time, the drug can become habit forming. Call your doctor if you feel you need the medicine more often than it was prescribed. Do not take a larger dose without your doctor's approval.

If you have been taking this medicine for several weeks or more, do not stop taking it suddenly without the approval of your doctor. It may be necessary for your doctor to reduce your dose slowly. This will depend on the dose and the specific medicine you have been taking.

Pregnancy/Breastfeeding

Women who are pregnant, breastfeeding or planning to become pregnant should tell their doctor before taking this medicine.

Drug Interactions

It is important that you obtain the advice of your doctor or pharmacist before taking any other prescription and nonprescription medicines, including other pain relievers, sleeping pills, tranquilizers or medicines for depression, cough, cold or allergy medicines, or blood thinners.

Some drugs can interact with this medicine. If you are taking any other medicines, be sure to check with your pharmacist or doctor before starting this drug.

Alcohol

Do not drink alcoholic beverages while taking this drug without the approval of your doctor because the combination could cause drowsiness. One drink may have the same effect that 2 or 3 drinks normally would have.

Special Precautions

If you feel nauseated when you first start taking the medicine, it may help if you lie down for a few minutes.

In some people, this drug may cause dizziness or drowsiness. Do not drive a car, pilot an airplane, operate dangerous machinery or do jobs that require you to be alert if you are dizzy or drowsy. You should also be careful going up and down stairs. Get up slowly after you have been sitting or lying down. Sit or lie down at the first sign of dizziness. Tell your doctor if the dizziness or drowsiness continues.

This medicine may cause some people to become constipated. To help prevent constipation, try increasing the amount of bulk in your diet (for example, bran, fresh fruits and salads), exercising more often or drinking more fluids (unless otherwise directed). Call your doctor if the constipation continues.

For DARVON-N WITH ASA, DARVON-N COMPOUND, NOVOPROPOXYN COMPOUND *and* 692's:

• These products contain ASA which can thin the blood and prolong bleeding time; therefore, you may have to stop taking this medicine before surgery or dental work. Check with your doctor or dentist at least 1 week before you have any surgery or dental work.

When to Call Your Doctor

Most people experience few or no side effects from this drug. However, any medicine can sometimes cause unwanted effects. Call your doctor if you develop nausea, vomiting, stomach pain, unusual weakness or tiredness, confusion, seizures, depression, unusual nervousness, severe drowsiness, dizziness or trembling, blurred vision or changes in eyesight.

Also call your doctor if you are taking DARVON-N WITH ASA, DARVON-N COMPOUND, NOVOPROPOXYN COMPOUND or 692's and you develop unusual bruising or bleeding, a yellow color to the skin or eyes, red or black stools, ringing or buzzing in the ears or any difficulty in hearing, or vomiting of material that looks like coffee grounds.

Get emergency help at once if you think that anyone has taken an overdose of this medicine. Treatment may need to be started even before the symptoms of an overdose appear.

Allergic Reactions

Call your doctor immediately if you think you may be allergic to the medicine or if you develop a skin rash, hives, itching, swelling of the face or difficulty in breathing. If you cannot reach your doctor, phone a hospital emergency department.

Storage

Store the medicine in a cool, dark place.

Miscellaneous

Carry an identification card in your wallet or wear a medical alert bracelet indicating that you are taking this medicine as well as the names and phone numbers of your doctors. If you do not already carry such a card, complete the Medicine Card in this book. Always tell your dentist, pharmacist and other doctors who are treating you that you are taking this medicine.

PROPRANOLOL (ORAL)

APO-PROPRANOLOL, DETENSOL, INDERAL, INDERAL LA, NOVOPRANOL, PMS PROPRANOLOL

ACEBUTOLOL

MONITAN, SECTRAL

ATENOLOL

TENORMIN

LABETALOL

TRANDATE

METOPROLOL

APO-METOPROLOL, APO-METOPROLOL (TYPE L), BETALOC, BETALOC DURULES, LOPRESOR, LOPRESOR SR, NOVOMETOPROL

NADOLOL
CORGARD

OXPRENOLOL
TRASICOR, SLOW-TRASICOR

PINDOLOL
VISKEN

SOTALOL
SOTACOR

TIMOLOL
BLOCADREN

ATENOLOL-CHLORTHALIDONE
TENORETIC

METOPROLOL-HYDROCHLOROTHIAZIDE
CO-BETALOC

NADOLOL-BENDROFLUMETHIAZIDE
CORZIDE

PINDOLOL-HYDROCHLOROTHIAZIDE
VISKAZIDE

PROPRANOLOL-HYDROCHLOROTHIAZIDE
INDERIDE

TIMOLOL-HYDROCHLOROTHIAZIDE
TIMOLIDE

Purpose

All of these medicines are beta-blockers and may be used to lower the blood pressure.

PROPRANOLOL is also used in other medical conditions to keep the heartbeat regular and steady and to treat certain types of tremors.

The following medicines are also used to help prevent future heart attacks in people who have suffered a heart attack: METOPROLOL PROPRANOLOL and TIMOLOL.

The following medicines are also used to reduce chest pain (angina) by "calming" the heart so that it beats slower and less forcefully and requires less oxygen: ACEBUTOLOL, ATENOLOL, METOPROLOL,

NADOLOL, PINDOLOL, PROPRANOLOL, SOTALOL and TIMOLOL.

PROPRANOLOL is also used in some patients to help prevent migraine attacks.

Allergies/Warnings

Be sure to tell your doctor and pharmacist if you are allergic to any medicine or if you have a history of allergies (such as hay fever) or have any type of respiratory disease such as asthma, emphysema or bronchitis.

If you were prescribed Co-Betaloc, Corzide, Inderide, Tenoretic, Timolide, or Viskazide, be sure to tell your doctor and pharmacist if you are allergic to sulfa drugs, oral diabetes drugs, thiazide diuretics or any medicine.

Also tell your doctor if you burn easily when exposed to the sun.

How to Use This Medicine

Time of Administration

Try to take the medicine at the same time(s) every day.

If you were prescribed Co-Betaloc, Corzide, Inderide, Tenoretic, Timolide, *or* Viskazide:

- When you first start taking this medicine, you will probably urinate (pass your water) more often and in larger amounts than usual. Therefore, if you are to take 1 dose each day, take it in the morning after breakfast. Do not initially take a dose at bedtime or you may have to get up during the night to go to the bathroom.
- If you are to take more than 1 dose each day, ask your doctor if you can take the last dose approximately 6 hours before bedtime so that you will not have to get up during the night to go to the bathroom. This effect will usually decrease after you have taken the drug for awhile.

All of these medicines may be taken with food or on an empty stomach *except* Trandate, Viskazide and Visken which should be taken after food or meals.

How to Administer

Take this medicine with a full glass of water.

For Betaloc Durules, Inderal LA, Lopresor SR, *and* Slow-Trasicor:

- Swallow the medicine whole. Do not crush or chew it or cut it.

Special Instructions

Length of Therapy

It may be necessary for you to take this medicine for a long time in spite of the fact that you may feel better. It is very important that you take the medicine as your doctor has prescribed and that you do not miss any doses. Otherwise, you cannot expect the drug to work for you.

Do not take any more of this medicine than your doctor has prescribed and *do not stop taking this medicine suddenly without the approval of your doctor*. It will be necessary for your doctor to reduce your dose slowly since your body will need time to adjust. It could be harmful and make your condition worse if you suddenly stopped taking the medicine.

Pregnancy/Breastfeeding

Women who are pregnant, breastfeeding or planning to become pregnant should tell their doctor before taking this medicine.

Drug Interactions

Some nonprescription drugs can aggravate your condition. Do not take any of the following without the approval of your doctor or pharmacist: cough, cold, or sinus products; asthma, allergy or hay fever products since they could increase your blood pressure. Read the label of the product to see if there is a warning. If there is, check with your doctor or pharmacist before using the product.

Do not smoke while you are on PROPRANOLOL because smoking can make the drug less effective.

Be sure to tell your doctor and pharmacist if you are taking any nonprescription drugs containing ASA or salicylates. They may decrease the effect of this medicine.

PROPRANOLOL may interfere with the glaucoma screening test.

Special Precautions

Ask your doctor how to check your pulse rate. Check your pulse regularly while you are taking this medicine. If your pulse becomes much slower than usual or if it is less than 50 beats per minute, check with your doctor about taking the drug that day. The dose of your medicine may have to be adjusted. A pulse rate that is too slow may cause circulation problems.

Follow any special diet your doctor may have ordered. If you have high blood pressure, he or she may want to limit the amount of salt in your diet. Check with your pharmacist before using a salt substitute because it may contain potassium.

In some people, this drug may cause dizziness or drowsiness. Do not drive a car, pilot an airplane, operate dangerous machinery or do jobs that require you to be alert if you are dizzy or drowsy. You should also be careful going up and down stairs, getting out of bed or out of chairs. Sit or lie down at the first sign of dizziness. Tell your doctor if the dizziness or drowsiness continues.

If you were prescribed LABETALOL, it is recommended that you lie down for 2 to 4 hours after taking the first dose or any increase in dose. This will help prevent fainting.

If your mouth becomes dry, drink water, suck ice chips or a hard, sour candy (sugarless) or chew gum (sugarless). Sugarless products are recommended in order to avoid dental problems. It is especially important to brush and floss your teeth regularly if you develop a dry mouth to help prevent gum problems.

If your eyes become dry, ask your pharmacist or doctor to recommend a lubricating/wetting solution or artificial tears. This side effect is more common in elderly people.

If you were prescribed SLOW-TRASICOR, do not become alarmed if you notice something that looks like a tablet in your stool. This medicine is contained in a wax core that has been designed to release the drug slowly in your body. The empty wax core is eliminated in the stool.

If you become more sensitive to the cold, dress warmly during cold weather and do not stay outside for long periods of time in cold weather. Call your doctor if you develop cold hands or feet or numbness or tingling in the fingers or toes.

It is recommended that patients receiving this drug stop smoking.

For patients with angina:

- Check with your doctor about the amount of exercise that is safe for you. This medicine can reduce chest pain resulting from too much exercise and make it difficult to tell when a person has exercised just the right amount.

For patients with diabetes:

- This medicine may cause a change in your blood sugar level. It may also mask or hide some of the signs of low blood sugar (such as blood pressure changes and faster pulse rate). Be alert for the other signs of low blood sugar that are not masked (such as sweating, hunger or tiredness). If you think your blood sugar is lower than normal, call your doctor. It may be necessary to adjust the dose of your diabetes medications.

If you were prescribed Co Betaloc, Corzide, Inderide, Tenoretic, Timolide, *or* Viskazide, *the following special instructions also apply:*

- This medicine normally causes your body to lose potassium. The body has warning signs to let you know if too much potassium is being lost. Call your doctor if you become unusually thirsty or if you develop leg cramps, unusual weakness, fatigue, vomiting, confusion or an irregular pulse. Since these symptoms may not be present in all patients, your doctor may wish to check your blood occasionally to see if it is low in potassium. Depending upon your dose, your doctor may prescribe some medicine to replace the potassium or he or she may recommend that you regularly eat foods that contain a lot of potassium (see Appendix A). *Do not change your diet unless your doctor tells you to.*
- This medicine may make some people more sensitive to sunlight and various tanning lamps. When you begin taking this medicine, try to avoid too much sun until you see how you are going to react. If your skin does become more sensitive to sunlight, tell your doctor and try not to stay in direct sunlight for extended periods of time. While in the sun, wear protective clothing and sunglasses. You may wish to ask your pharmacist about suitable sunscreen products. Call your doctor if you become sunburned.
- Tingling of the scalp is common when you first start taking Trandate. This is temporary and will usually disappear after you have taken the drug for a while.

When to Call Your Doctor

For all drugs EXCEPT Trandate:

- Most people experience few or no side effects from this drug. However, any medicine can sometimes cause unwanted effects. Call your doctor if you develop a skin rash, shortness of breath, wheezing, fever or sore throat, unusual bruising or bleeding, swelling of the legs or ankles, sudden weight gain of 5 pounds (2.5 kg) or more, impotence or decreased sexual ability, changes in vision, if your pulse becomes slower than normal or is less than 50 beats per minute, cold hands or feet or numbness or tingling of the fingers or toes. Also call your doctor if you develop nightmares, depression, insomnia, unusual tiredness, headaches or if you become confused.

If you were prescribed Co-Betaloc, Corzide, Inderide, Tenoretic, Timolide, *or* Viskazide:

- In addition to the previous symptoms, also call your doctor if you develop sharp stomach pain, persistent nausea, vomiting or diarrhea, sharp joint pain, a yellow color to the skin or eyes or dark-colored urine.

If you were prescribed TRANDATE:

- Unlike the other medicines, this drug rarely affects the heart rate.
- Call your doctor if you develop shortness of breath, difficulty breathing, difficulty urinating (passing your water), impotence or decreased sexual ability, a yellow color to the skin or eyes, dark-colored urine, unusual weakness or tiredness, unusual bruising or bleeding, changes in vision, muscle or joint pain, nasal stuffiness, unusual dizziness or fainting, unpleasant taste in the mouth, swelling of the legs or ankles, or sudden weight gain of 5 pounds (2.5 kg) or more.

Did You Know That?

Tablets and capsules pass down the esophagus to the stomach at different rates.

The *Journal of Pharmacy and Pharmacology* reports that in a study of 112 women and 63 men, the time taken for tablets and capsules to reach the stomach was measured. The participants were told to swallow different shapes and sizes of tablets and capsules in both the upright and lying positions. The passage of the medication down the esophagus into the stomach was measured with a stop-watch during x-ray fluoroscopy. If a tablet or capsule remained in the espophagus for 5 minutes, its position was recorded and the subject was told to stand up and drink some more water in order to force the tablet or capsule into the stomach.

It is important that tablets and capsules do not become lodged in the esophagus because they could cause irritation leading to ulceration. Most people prefer to swallow capsules because of the smooth surface and the shape. However, it has been suggested that capsules are more prone to delayed passage through the esophagus because when the gelatin capsules become wet, they also become sticky and could adhere to the walls of the esophagus.

The results of the study were interesting:

- Large capsules passed more quickly down the esophagus than plain oval tablets in both the upright and lying positions.
- Heavy large capsules passed more quickly than light large capsules when the participants were upright.
- Film-coating of tablets significantly reduced the amount of time it took tablets to pass down the esophagus.
- In all cases, when the participants were lying down, it took both tablets and capsules longer to pass down the esophagus.

Tablets and capsules that became stuck in the esophagus were at the following locations: top third of the esophagus (5 times); level of the left main bronchus (35 times); level of the heart (73 times); above the lower esophageal sphincter (126 times); and more than one spot (6 times).

What does this study teach us? It is best to take tablets and capsules in the sitting or standing position so that gravity can help pull the medication down the esophagus into the stomach. It is important to take tablets and capsules with enough water to make it easier for the medication to pass down the esophagus. It also helps to swallow a little water in order to lubricate the esophagus before taking the medication.

Refills

Do not stop taking this medicine without your doctor's approval and do not go without medicine between prescription refills. Call your pharmacist 2 or 3 days before you will run out of the medicine for a refill.

Discuss with your pharmacist the implications of dispensing all your refills for this medicine with the same manufacturer's product. (*See* Generic Drugs, page 12.)

Miscellaneous

Carry an identification card in your wallet or wear a medical alert bracelet indicating that you are taking this medicine as well as the names and phone numbers of your doctors. If you do not already carry such a card, complete the Medicine Card in this book. Always tell your dentist, pharmacist and other doctors who are treating you that you are taking this medicine.

Did You Know That?

It is wise to keep the phone numbers of your doctors, pharmacy and nearest emergency center next to the telephone and on a card that you can carry in your wallet or purse. This simple step will help you be better prepared if an emergency occurs or if you have a problem with your medications.

QUINIDINE BISULFATE (ORAL)

BIQUIN DURULES

QUINIDINE GLUCONATE

QUINAGLUTE DURA-TABS, QUINATE

QUINIDINE POLYGALACTURONATE

CARDIOQUIN

QUINIDINE SULFATE

APO-QUINIDINE, NOVOQUINIDIN, QUINIDEX EXTENTABS

Purpose

This medicine is used to help make the heart beat at a regular and normal rate.

Allergies/Warnings

Be sure to tell your doctor and pharmacist if you are allergic to any medicine.

How to Use This Medicine

Time of Administration

It is best to take this medicine with a glass of water on an empty stomach at least 1 hour before (or 2 hours after) eating food. Take it at the proper time even if you skip a meal. However, if you develop stomach upset after taking the drug, take it with some food. Call your doctor if you continue to have an upset stomach.

How to Administer

Take the medicine with a full glass of water unless otherwise directed.

If you were prescribed BIQUIN DURULES, QUINAGLUTE DURA-TABS *or* QUINIDEX EXTENTABS:

- These tablets have a special coating and must be swallowed whole. Do not crush, chew or break them into pieces. Do not take chipped tablets.

Special Instructions

Length of Therapy

It is very important that you take this medicine exactly as your doctor has prescribed. Do not miss any doses and take the medicine even if you feel well. Try to take this medicine at the same time(s) every day so that you will have a constant level of medicine in your body. Do not take extra tablets without your doctor's approval.

Pregnancy/Breastfeeding

Women who are pregnant, breastfeeding or planning to become pregnant should tell their doctor before taking this medicine.

Drug Interactions

Some nonprescription drugs can interfere with this medicine or aggravate your heart condition. Do not take any of the following without the approval of your doctor or pharmacist: antacids or baking soda; cough, cold or sinus products; asthma or allergy products.

Do not use salt substitutes without the approval of your doctor. They may contain potassium, which could affect the way you respond to this medicine.

Special Precautions

The effect of a prescribed dose of QUINIDINE varies with each person and is not entirely predictable. Therefore, your doctor may wish to do a blood test to check the level of QUINIDINE in your serum or do a heart tracing or other tests to assess the effect of the drug in your body more thoroughly.

Tell your doctor if you become dizzy or feel faint. If you become dizzy or feel faint, you should be careful going up and down stairs, getting out of bed or out of chairs. Sit or lie down at the first sign of dizziness. Do not drive a car, pilot an airplane, operate dangerous machinery or do jobs that require you to be alert.

Some foods can affect the way your body handles this medicine. Avoid eating or drinking *excessive* amounts of citrus juices, milk and vegetables. Check with your doctor if you have any questions about your diet or before you make any drastic changes in your diet.

In some people, this medicine may cause a bitter taste. This problem is only temporary.

When to Call Your Doctor

Most people experience few or no side effects from this drug. However, any medicine can sometimes cause unwanted effects and some people may be more sensitive to QUINIDINE and develop side effects after taking the first few doses. Call your doctor if you develop ringing or buzzing in the ears or any loss of hearing, blurred vision, a skin rash, unexplained fever, irregular heartbeats, dizziness or feeling of faintness, severe headaches, nausea, vomiting, stomach cramps, troublesome diarrhea, shortness of breath, joint pain or unusual bruising or bleeding.

Allergic Reactions

Call your doctor immediately if you think you may be allergic to the medicine or if you develop a skin rash, hives, itching, swelling of the face or difficulty in breathing. If you cannot reach your doctor, phone a hospital emergency department.

Refills

Do not stop taking this medicine without your doctor's approval and do not go without medicine between prescription refills. Call your pharmacist for a refill 2 or 3 days before you will run out of the medicine.

Discuss with your pharmacist the implications of dispensing all your refills for this medicine with the same manufacturer's product. (*See* Generic Drugs, page 12.)

Did You Know That?

If you are suffering from a cold and have nasal congestion, ASA may make the nasal congestion worse.

ASA has been discovered to reduce air flow through the nasal passages by causing swelling and congestion of the nasal mucous membranes.

Miscellaneous

Carry an identification card in your wallet or wear a medical alert bracelet indicating that you are taking this medicine as well as the names and phone numbers of your doctors. If you do not already carry such a card, complete the Medicine Card in this book. Always tell your dentist, pharmacist and other doctors who are treating you that you are taking this medicine.

Did You Know That?

The cotton that is packed in many new bottles of nonprescription medicines and vitamins is meant to be discarded after the bottle is opened.

The cotton is used in many cases to prevent the tablets or capsules from rattling around and breaking during shipment. After the bottle has been opened, the cotton should generally be discarded. With some prescription medications, such as certain brands of sublingual nitroglycerin tablets, the cotton must be discarded to help ensure potency of the medicine. Ask your pharmacist if you have any questions.

SODIUM SULFACETAMIDE (OPHTHALMIC)

AK-SULF EYE DROPS, BLEPH-10 LIQUIFILM, CETAMIDE EYE OINTMENT, ISOPTO-CETAMIDE EYE DROPS, SODIUM SULAMYD EYE DROPS, SODIUM SULAMYD EYE OINTMENT, SULFEX 10% EYE DROPS

Purpose

This medicine is an antibiotic used to treat certain types of eye infections. It is to be used only for the eye infection you have now and should not be used for any other eye infections.

Allergies/Warnings

Be sure to tell your doctor and pharmacist if you are allergic to sulfa or sulfonamide medicines or any antibiotic medicine.

How To Use This Medicine

How to Administer

See How to Administer Medications (page 15).

Special Instructions

Length of Therapy

It is important to use all of this medicine, plus any refills that your doctor told you to use. Do not stop using it earlier than your doctor has recommended in spite of the fact that your symptoms seem to have improved. Otherwise, the infection may return.

Pregnancy/Breastfeeding

Women who are pregnant, breastfeeding or planning to become pregnant should tell their doctor before taking this medicine.

Drug Interactions

Do not use this medicine at the same time as any other eye medicine without the approval of your doctor. Some medicines cannot be mixed.

Special Precautions

Do not use eye drop solutions that have turned dark in color.

Vision may be blurred for a few minutes after using the eye medicine. Do not drive a car, pilot an airplane, operate dangerous machinery or do jobs that require you to be alert until your vision has cleared.

When to Call Your Doctor

Contact your doctor if the eye infection for which you are using this medicine does not begin to improve in 3 to 4 days, if increased eye redness or eye pain develops or if the eye becomes irritated by the medicine for more than a few minutes. Many eye medicines sting for a short time immediately after use.

Storage

Store this medicine in a cool place away from heat.

Miscellaneous

This medicine is for external use only. Do not swallow it.

Do not share this eye medication with family members or friends. The infection could be transferred.

SPIRONOLACTONE (ORAL)

ALDACTONE, NOVOSPIROTON, SINCOMEN

SPIRONOLACTONE-HYDROCHLOROTHIAZIDE

ALDACTAZIDE, NOVOSPIROZINE

Purpose

This medicine is used to help the body get rid of excess fluids and to decrease swelling. The medicine does this by increasing the amount of urine and is commonly called a water pill or fluid pill. It is commonly used to treat high blood pressure and other medical conditions.

Allergies/Warnings

Be sure to tell your doctor or pharmacist if you are allergic to any medicine.

How to Use This Medicine

Time of Administration

Try to take this medicine at the same time(s) every day so that you have a constant level of the medicine in your body.

When you first start taking this medicine, you will probably urinate (pass your water) more often and in larger amounts than usual. Therefore, if you are to take 1 dose each day, take it in the morning after breakfast. Do not initially take a dose at bedtime or you may have to get up during the night to go to the bathroom.

If you are to take more than 1 dose each day, take the last dose approximately 6 hours before bedtime so that you will not have to get up during the night to go to the bathroom. This effect will usually decrease after you have taken the drug for awhile.

How to Administer

Take this medicine with food, meals or milk to decrease stomach upset and increase the absorption of this medicine. If stomach upset occurs, call your doctor.

Special Instructions

Length of Therapy

For patients with high blood pressure:

- High blood pressure (hypertension) is a long-term condition and it will probably be necessary for you to take the drug for a long time even if you feel better. If high blood pressure is not treated, it can lead to serious problems such as heart failure, strokes, blood vessel problems or kidney problems.

It is very important that you take this medicine as your doctor has directed and that you do not miss any doses. Otherwise, you cannot expect the drug to keep your blood pressure down or remove excess fluid.

Pregnancy/Breastfeeding

Women who are pregnant, breastfeeding or planning to become pregnant should tell their doctor before taking this medicine.

Drug Interactions

Do not take large doses of ASA or other salicylates without the approval of your doctor or pharmacist.

Some nonprescription drugs can aggravate high blood pressure. Do not take any of the following without the approval of your doctor or pharmacist: cough, cold, or sinus products; asthma or allergy products since they may increase your blood pressure. Read the label of the nonprescription drug product to see if there is a warning. If there is, check with your doctor or pharmacist before using the product.

Alcohol

Be careful drinking alcoholic beverages while taking this medicine because it could make the possible side effect of dizziness worse.

Special Precautions

If this medicine causes dizziness or lightheadedness, you should be careful going up and down stairs and you should not change positions too rapidly. Lightheadedness is more likely to occur if you stand up suddenly—this is due to blood collecting in the legs and lasts for a few seconds. Therefore, get up from a sitting or lying position more slowly and tighten and relax your leg muscles or wiggle your toes to help promote circulation. In the morning, get out of bed slowly and dangle your feet over the edge of the bed for a few minutes before standing up. Sit or lie down at the first sign of dizziness. Do not drive a car, pilot an airplane, operate dangerous machinery or do jobs that require you to be alert if you are dizzy. Tell your doctor if you have been dizzy.

In order to help prevent dizziness or fainting, your doctor may also recommend that you avoid strenuous exercise, standing for long periods of time (especially in hot weather), hot showers, hot baths or saunas.

People more than 65 years of age may be more sensitive to the side effect of dizziness.

This medicine does not cause your body to lose potassium as some other types of water pills do. Therefore, it is not usually necessary for you to eat foods rich in potassium. In fact, too much potassium while you are taking this medicine could be harmful. Call your doctor if you develop any of the warning signs of too much potassium: irregular heartbeats, numbness or tingling in the hands, feet or lips, confusion, difficulty breathing, unusual tiredness or weakness, unexplained nervousness, weakness or a feeling of heaviness in the legs. Since not all patients develop these symptoms, your doctor may want to check your blood occasionally to see if the potassium level is normal.

Do not use salt substitutes, low-salt milk or low-salt soups without the approval of your doctor. They may contain large amounts of potassium, which could affect the way you respond to this medicine.

If you were prescribed ALDACTAZIDE *or* NOVOSPIROZINE:

- This medicine may make some people more sensitive to sunlight and various tanning lamps. When you begin taking this medicine, try to avoid too much sun until you see how you are going to react. If your skin does become more sensitive to sunlight, tell your doctor and try not to stay in direct sunlight for extended periods of time. While in the sun, wear protective clothing and sunglasses. You may wish to ask your pharmacist about suitable sunscreen products. Call your doctor if you become sunburned.
- If you are a diabetic, this medicine may cause your blood sugar to rise. Carefully test your blood or urine for sugar while you are taking this medicine. Call your doctor if you think your blood sugar is higher than normal or harder to control.

When to Call Your Doctor

Most people experience few or no side effects from this drug. However, any medicine can sometimes cause unwanted effects. Call your doctor if you develop a sore throat, fever, skin rash, a dry mouth (or if you become very thirsty), nausea, tiredness, drowsiness, weakness, swelling of the legs or ankles, stomach pain, a sudden weight gain of 5 pounds (2.5 kg) or more, swelling or tenderness of the breasts (men or women), increased facial hair (in women) or menstrual problems (in women).

Also call your doctor if you become sick or develop persistent vomiting or diarrhea.

If you were prescribed ALDACTAZIDE *or* NOVOSPIROZINE:

- Also call your doctor if you develop sharp joint pain, unusual bruising or bleeding, a yellow color to the skin or eyes or dark-colored urine.

Allergic Reactions

Call your doctor immediately if you think you may be allergic to the medicine or if you develop a skin rash, hives, itching, swelling of the face or difficulty in breathing. If you cannot reach your doctor, phone a hospital emergency department.

Refills

Do not stop taking this medicine without your doctor's approval and do not go without medicine between prescription refills. Call your pharmacist for a refill 2 or 3 days before you will run out of the medicine.

Discuss with your pharmacist the implications of dispensing all your refills for this medicine with the same manufacturer's product. (*See* Generic Drugs, page 12.)

DID YOU KNOW THAT?

It is important to tell your doctor if you did not have a prescription refilled.

When a person forgets or decides not to have a prescription refilled, the physician should be told so that he can take this into consideration when he is planning future treatment. If you stopped taking a medication but did not tell your doctor, he/she may decide that the medication is not producing the expected effect and may switch you to another medication.

The best policy is to tell your doctor when you have not taken the medication correctly. Patients usually have good reasons for being unable to continue with a therapy and it is important to tell your doctor your reasons. Once your doctor is aware of the problems the medication is causing, there are usually several things that can be done to help make the therapy more acceptable.
The most important thing to remember is that no medication — not even a "wonder drug" — can be effective if it is not taken correctly.

SUCRALFATE (ORAL)

SULCRATE

Purpose

This medicine is used in the treatment and prevention of duodenal and stomach ulcers.

Allergies/Warnings

If you have ever had an allergic reaction to SUCRALFATE or any other medicine, tell your doctor and pharmacist before you take any of this medicine.

How to Use This Medicine

Time of Administration

Take this medicine with a glass of water on an empty stomach at least

1 hour before meals and at bedtime unless otherwise directed.

Special Instructions

Length of Therapy

It is very important that you take this medicine for the full length of treatment as your doctor has prescribed. Try not to miss any doses because the medicine will not be as effective. It may take several days or a few weeks before you feel the full benefit of this medicine.

Pregnancy/Breastfeeding

Women who are pregnant, breastfeeding or planning to become pregnant should tell their doctor before taking this medicine.

Drug Interactions

If you develop stomach pain between doses of this medicine, ask your doctor if you may take an antacid between doses. If you do take an antacid, do not take the antacid within 1/2 hour before or after this medicine. Taking the two drugs too close together will keep the SUCRALFATE from producing as much benefit as it normally would.

If you are taking any other medicines, be sure to tell your doctor and pharmacist because this medicine can interact with certain prescription drugs. SULCRALFATE should not be taken within 2 hours of any other medicines.

Alcohol

Do not drink alcoholic beverages while taking this drug because it may make the ulcer pain worse and interfere with healing of the ulcer.

Special Precautions

People with ulcers should avoid ASA-containing medicines since they may interfere with healing of the ulcer. Also avoid those foods and beverages that cause your ulcer symptoms to reappear.

Rarely, this drug may cause dizziness or drowsiness. Do not drive a car, pilot an airplane, operate dangerous machinery or do jobs that require you to be alert until you know how you are going to react to the drug. If you become dizzy, you should be careful going up and down stairs. Sit or lie down at the first sign of dizziness. Tell your doctor if the dizziness or drowsiness continues.

This medicine may cause some people to become constipated. To help prevent constipation, try increasing the amount of bulk in your diet (for example, bran, fresh fruits and salads), exercising more often or drinking more fluids (unless otherwise directed). Call your doctor if the constipation continues.

If your mouth becomes dry, drink water, suck ice chips or a hard, sour candy (sugarless) or chew gum (sugarless). Sugarless products are recommended in order to avoid dental problems. You may wish to ask your pharmacist about special solutions, called artificial saliva, that can also be used to help restore moisture in the mouth. It is especially important to brush and floss your teeth regularly if you develop a dry mouth to help prevent gum problems.

When to Call Your Doctor

Most people do not develop side effects from this medicine. If side effects do occur, they are usually mild and usually disappear when you stop taking the medicine.

Call your doctor immediately if you are being treated for an ulcer and you develop fainting spells, unusual thirst, dizziness, sweating, vomiting of blood or bloody or black stools. This may mean your condition is getting worse.

Allergic Reactions

Most people experience few or no side effects from this drug. However, any medicine can sometimes cause unwanted effects. Call your doctor if you develop a skin rash, hives, itching, back pain, stomach pain or severe constipation.

DID YOU KNOW THAT?

Even though two drugs might look the same, this does not mean that they are the same. NEVER SHARE YOUR MEDICINES.

Even if a friend takes the same drugs as you, the drug could be a different strength and serious problems could result if your friend took one of your medicines.

SULFASALAZINE (ORAL)

PMS SULFASALAZINE, PMS SULFASALAZINE EC, SALAZOPYRIN, SALAZOPYRIN EN-TABS, S.A.S.-500, S.A.S. ENTERIC-500

Purpose

This medicine is used to treat certain conditions of the intestines involving diarrhea (loose bowel movements).

Allergies/Warnings

If you have ever had an allergic reaction to sulfa drugs, salicylates or

ASA, thiazide water pills, diabetes medicine that you take by mouth or glaucoma medicine that you take by mouth, tell your doctor and pharmacist before you take any of this medicine. Also tell your doctor if you have a condition known as porphyria or any other medical problems.

This medicine should *not* be given to children under 2 years of age.

How to Use This Medicine

Time of Administration

Space your doses of the medicine around the clock (throughout the entire day of 24 hours). For example, if you are to take 4 doses each day, space the doses 6 hours apart. This will keep a constant level of the medicine in your body.

The interval between the nighttime dose and the next morning dose should generally not be greater than 8 hours unless otherwise directed by your doctor.

How to Administer

It is best to take this medicine with food or immediately after meals to help prevent stomach upset. Call your doctor if you continue to have stomach upset.

Take each dose of medicine with a full glass (8 ounces) of water and try to drink 8 glasses of water or other fluids every day unless otherwise directed by your doctor. This will help prevent some unwanted side effects.

For PMS SULFASALAZINE EC, SALAZOPYRIN EN-TABS, S.A.S. ENTERIC-500, SULFASALAZINE (KENRAL):

- These tablets have a special coating and must be swallowed whole. Do not crush, chew or break them into pieces. Do not take chipped tablets.

Special Instructions

Length of Therapy

It is important to take all of this medicine plus any refills that your doctor told you to take. Do not stop taking this medicine earlier than your doctor has recommended even if you begin to feel better. Otherwise, you cannot expect the drug to work for you.

Pregnancy/Breastfeeding

Women who are pregnant or planning to become pregnant should tell their doctor before taking this medicine.

Women who are breastfeeding should tell their doctor before taking this medicine. This medicine can pass into the breast milk.

Special Precautions

Be sure to keep your doctor's appointments so that he or she can check your progress and make sure that you are getting the most benefit from this medicine.

This medicine may make some people more sensitive to sunlight and various tanning lamps. When you begin taking this medicine, try to avoid too much sun until you see how you are going to react. If your skin does become more sensitive to sunlight, tell your doctor and try not to stay in direct sunlight for extended periods of time. While in the sun, wear protective clothing and sunglasses. You may wish to ask your pharmacist about suitable sunscreen products. Call your doctor if you become sunburned.

In some people, this drug may cause dizziness or drowsiness. Do not drive a car, pilot an airplane, operate dangerous machinery or do jobs that require you to be alert until you know how you are going to react to this drug. You should also be careful going up and down stairs. Sit or lie down at the first sign of dizziness. Tell your doctor if the dizziness continues.

This medicine may cause the urine to turn orange-yellow. This is not an unusual effect and is not harmful. It will go away after you have finished the medicine.

When to Call Your Doctor

Call your doctor if your symptoms (including diarrhea) do not improve within 1 month or if they become worse.

Most people experience few or no side effects from this drug. However, any medicine can sometimes cause unwanted effects. Call your doctor if you develop a sore throat, fever, mouth sores, unusual bruising or bleeding, skin blisters or peeling or loosening of the skin, a yellow color to the skin and eyes, unusual tiredness or weakness, constant headache, unusual joint or low back pain, pain while urinating (passing your water), blood in the urine, difficulty swallowing, swelling of the throat or neck, itching or unusually pale skin.

Allergic Reactions

Call your doctor immediately if you think you may be allergic to the medicine or if you develop a skin rash, hives, itching, swelling of the face or difficulty in breathing. If you cannot reach your doctor, phone a hospital emergency department.

Storage

If for some reason you cannot take all of the medicine, throw away the unused portion by flushing it down the toilet. Do not take or save old medicine.

Miscellaneous

Carry an identification card in your wallet or wear a medical alert bracelet indicating that you are taking this medicine as well as the names and phone numbers of your doctors. If you do not already carry such a card, complete the Medicine Card in this book. Always tell your dentist, pharmacist and other doctors who are treating you that you are taking this medicine.

Did You Know That?

Medical World News reports that lingering throat and mouth infections may be aggravated by the transfer of the bacteria to toothbrushes and subsequent multiplication of the bacteria.

A professor of oral pathology compared the toothbrushes of 10 healthy people and 10 people with mouth and throat infections. He discovered that it takes only 17 to 35 days for a toothbrush to become heavily infected. This is not surprising since bacteria in toothbrushes find moisture, warmth (from a warm bathroom) and food (from the mouth) to grow.

When the oral pathologist suggested that those people with mouth and throat infections start using new toothbrushes every few weeks, they quickly recovered. It may be advisable for people with mouth infections to change their toothbrushes frequently. Depending on the toothbrush, it may be possible to thoroughly clean toothbrushes frequently by putting them through a dishwasher cycle and allowing them to dry completely.

SULFONAMIDE PREPARATIONS (ORAL)

SULFADIAZINE

SULFADIAZINE

SULFADIAZINE-TRIMETHOPRIM
Coptin

SULFAMETHOXAZOLE
Apo-Sulfamethoxazole, Gantanol

SULFAMETHOXAZOLE-TRIMETHOPRIM
Apo-Sulfatrim, Apo-Sulfatrim DS, Apo-Sulfatrim Pediatric, Bactrim, Bactrim DS, Novotrimel, Novotrimel DS, Protrin, Protrin DF, Roubac, Roubac DS, Septra, Septra DS

SULFAPYRIDINE
Dagenan

SULFISOXAZOLE
Apo-Sulfisoxazole, Novosoxazole

SULFONAMIDE-PHENAZOPYRIDINE PREPARATIONS
Azo-Gantrisin, Uro Gantanol

Purpose
This medicine is an anti-infective used to treat certain types of infections.

Allergies/Warnings
If you have ever had an allergic reaction to sulfa drugs, thiazide diuretics (water pills), diabetes medicine that you take by mouth or glaucoma medicine that you take by mouth, tell your doctor and pharmacist before you take any of this medicine.

This medicine should *not* be given to infants under 2 months of age.

How to Use This Medicine

Time of Administration

It is best (but not necessary) to take this medicine on an empty stomach 1 hour before (or 2 hours after) eating food, unless otherwise directed. Take the medicine at the proper time even if you skip a meal. If stomach upset occurs, call your doctor.

Space your doses of the medicine around the clock (throughout the entire day of 24 hours). For example, if you are to take 4 doses each day, space the doses 6 hours apart. This will keep a constant level of the medicine in your body.

How to Administer

Take this medicine with a full glass (8 ounces) of water and try to drink at least 6 to 8 additional glasses of water or other liquids every day unless otherwise directed by your doctor. This will help prevent unwanted side effects on the kidneys and if the medicine was prescribed to treat an infection of the bladder, the extra intake of water will help to wash the bacteria causing the infection out in the urine.

For tablets and capsules:

- Take the medicine with a full glass of water unless otherwise directed.

For liquid medicines:

- If you were prescribed a *suspension,* shake the bottle well each time before pouring so that you can measure an accurate dose.
- If a spoon is used to measure the dose, it is recommended that you use a medicine spoon or an oral liquid syringe, which you can obtain from your pharmacist. *See* How to Administer Medications (page 15).

Special Instructions

Length of Therapy

It is important to take all of this medicine plus any refills that your doctor told you to take. Do not stop taking this medicine earlier than your doctor has recommended even if you begin to feel better. If you stop taking the medicine too soon, the infection may return.

Pregnancy/Breastfeeding

Women who are pregnant or planning to become pregnant should tell their doctor before taking this medicine. This medicine should generally not be taken during the last month of pregnancy.

Women who are breastfeeding should tell their doctor before taking this medicine.

Special Precautions

This medicine may make some people more sensitive to sunlight and various tanning lamps. When you begin taking this medicine, try to avoid too much sun until you see how you are going to react. If your skin does become more sensitive to sunlight, tell your doctor and try not to stay in direct sunlight for extended periods of time. While in the sun, wear protective clothing and sunglasses. You may wish to ask your pharmacist about suitable sunscreen products. Call your doctor if you become sunburned.

If you become dizzy, you should be careful going up and down stairs. Sit or lie down at the first sign of dizziness. Do not drive a car, pilot an airplane, operate dangerous machinery or do jobs that require you to be alert until you know how you are going to react to the drug. Tell your doctor if the dizziness continues.

If you were prescribed AZO-GANTRISIN *or* URO GANTANOL:
- Your urine may turn orange-red in color. This is a temporary effect and will go away after you have finished the medicine. Protect your undergarments while you are taking this medicine as your urine could cause staining of clothing.

Potentially Expensive Drug Interactions

A 32-year-old woman who wore a gas-permeable (hard) contact lens in one eye and a soft contact lens in the other eye developed an acute attack of colitis. She was treated with SULFASALAZINE. During the first 2 days of drug therapy, she did not wear the contact lenses. On the third day, she started wearing the lenses again and within 12 hours, the soft contact lens became stained yellow and the blue of the iris in the eye appeared green when the lens was in place. The hard lens was not stained and the iris was its normal blue

SULFASALAZINE predictably stains the urine orange and has also been reported to color tears yellow to orange. The staining of the soft contact lens in this patient was attributed to the ability of the drug to stain tears which in turn stained the lens.

This was an expensive drug interaction since extended-wear contact lenses cost approximately $250.

Other drugs which have been reported to discolor soft contact lenses are RIFAMPIN (orange staining), EPINEPHRINE HYDROCHLORIDE 2% and EPINEPHRYL BORATE 1% (dense brown staining). During treatment with any of these medicines, soft contact lenses should not be worn. Most eyedrops are labeled to indicate whether they can be used with soft contact lenses, but it is always a good idea to check with the pharmacist before using any eyedrops if soft contact lenses are worn.

When to Call Your Doctor

Call your doctor if your symptoms do not improve within a few days or if they become worse.

Most people experience few or no side effects from this drug. However, any medicine can sometimes cause unwanted effects. Call your doctor if you develop a sore throat, fever, mouth sores, nausea or vomiting, unusually pale skin, unusual bruising or bleeding, swelling of the front part of the neck, difficulty in swallowing, unusual tiredness or weakness, unusual joint or lower back pain, blood in the urine, pain while urinating (passing your water), redness, blistering, peeling or loosening of the skin or a yellow color to the skin or eyes.

Allergic Reactions

Call your doctor immediately if you think you may be allergic to the medicine or if you develop a skin rash, hives, itching, swelling of the face or difficulty in breathing. If you cannot reach your doctor, phone a hospital emergency department.

Storage

Store the medicine in a cool, dark place and keep the bottle tightly closed. Do not freeze the liquid preparation.

If for some reason you cannot take all of the medicine, discard the unused portion by flushing it down the toilet. Do not take or save old medicine.

Refills

Do not go without medicine between prescription refills. Call your pharmacist for a refill 2 or 3 days before you will run out of the medicine.

TETRACYCLINE HCl (ORAL)

ACHROMYCIN V, APO-TETRA, NOVOTETRA, TETRACYN

Purpose

This medicine is an antibiotic used to treat certain types of infections and help control acne.

Your doctor has prescribed this antibiotic for your present infection only. Do not use it for other infections or give it to other people.

Allergies/Warnings

If you have ever had an allergic reaction to TETRACYCLINE or any other medicine or if you have any allergies (for example, asthma, hay fever, or hives), tell your doctor or pharmacist before you take any of this medicine.

This medicine should not be given to children under 12 years of age unless directed by your doctor. TETRACYCLINE may permanently discolor the child's teeth and slow down the growth of the teeth and bones.

How to Use This Medicine

Time of Administration

It is best to take this medicine on an empty stomach 1 hour before (or 2 hours after) meals or food unless otherwise directed. Take the medicine at the proper time even if you skip a meal.

If you develop stomach upset after taking the drug, take it with some crackers (not with dairy products). Call your doctor if you continue to have stomach upset.

Space your doses of the medicine around the clock (throughout the entire day of 24 hours). For example, if you are to take 4 doses each day, space the doses 6 hours apart. This will keep a constant level of the medicine in your body.

How to Administer

For tablets and capsules:

- Take the tablets and capsules with a full glass (8 ounces) of water. This will help prevent irritation of the stomach and esophagus.

For liquid medicines:

- If you were prescribed a *suspension*, shake the bottle well each time before pouring so that you can measure an accurate dose.
- If a spoon is used to measure the dose, it is recommended that you use a medicine spoon or an oral liquid syringe that you can obtain from your pharmacist. *See* How to Administer Medications (page 15).

Do not drink milk or eat cheese, cottage cheese, ice cream or other dairy products 1 hour before or 2 hours after you have taken a dose of this medicine. If taken too close to this medicine, these foods can interfere with the absorption of the medicine and make it less effective.

Special Instructions

Length of Therapy

It is important to take all of this medicine plus any refills that your doctor told you to take. Do not stop taking this medicine earlier than your doctor has recommended even if you begin to feel better. If you stop taking the medicine too soon, the infection may return.

Pregnancy/Breastfeeding

Women who are pregnant or planning to become pregnant should not take this medicine. This medicine could cause permanent discoloration of the infant's teeth and may slow down the normal growth and development of the infant's teeth and bones.

Women who are breastfeeding should tell their doctor before taking this medicine. This medicine may pass into the breast milk and cause discoloration of the infant's teeth and may slow down the normal growth and development of the infant's teeth and bones.

Drug Interactions

Some antacids and laxatives can make this medicine less effective if they are taken at the same time. This includes products that contain aluminum, bismuth, calcium, magnesium, Epsom salt, sodium bicarbonate and baking soda. Check with your pharmacist before you purchase any antacids or laxatives. If you must take certain antacids or laxatives, they should be taken at least 2 hours before or after this medicine.

Iron or zinc pills or vitamins containing minerals can also make this medicine less effective. If you must take iron, zinc or vitamins containing minerals, take them 3 hours before (or 2 hours after) the tetracycline.

There have been some reports that oral contraceptives (birth control pills) may not work as well while taking this medicine. Unplanned pregnancies may occur. Ask your doctor about using another form of birth control while you are taking this antibiotic. Also call your doctor if you develop spotting or breakthrough bleeding since these can be signs of decreased birth control effect.

Special Precautions

This medicine may make some people more sensitive to sunlight and various tanning lamps. When you begin taking this medicine, try to avoid too much sun until you see how you are going to react. If your skin does become more sensitive to sunlight, tell your doctor and try not to stay in direct sunlight for extended periods of time. While in the sun, wear protective clothing and sunglasses. You may wish to ask your pharmacist about suitable sunscreen products. Call your doctor if you become sunburned.

When to Call Your Doctor

Call your doctor if your symptoms do not improve within a few days (or a few weeks or months if you are taking the medicine for acne) or if they become worse.

Most people experience few or no side effects from this drug. However, any medicine can sometimes cause unwanted effects. Call your doctor immediately if you develop severe cramps or burning of the stomach, vomiting, severe watery diarrhea, skin rash, dark-colored tongue, sore mouth or tongue, itching of the rectal or genital areas or, in women, a vaginal discharge that was not present before starting the medicine.

Did You Know That?

TETRACYCLINES should not be taken by pregnant women, infants or children up to 12 years of age.

TETRACYCLINES can stain the teeth of the child if they are given during the time that the baby teeth or permanent teeth are forming. The drugs combine with calcium in the teeth and stain the dentin (the part of the tooth that lies directly beneath the white enamel). The stained dentin shows through the white enamel of the tooth and gives a yellow-gray appearance to the tooth.

If a TETRACYCLINE drug is given to a woman during the last three months of pregnancy or to a baby during the first three months of life, staining of the teeth can occur.

If a TETRACYCLINE drug is given to a child between the ages of 3 months and 8 years, staining of the permanent teeth can occur. The severity of the stain appears to depend on the dose of the antibiotic and the stage of tooth development.

At the present time, there is no treatment which will remove the stain permanently. Some dentists have reported limited success with bleaching techniques and others have placed artificial crowns or plastic materials over the teeth.

The best treatment is prevention.

Allergic Reactions

Call your doctor immediately if you think you may be allergic to the medicine or if you develop a skin rash, hives, itching, swelling of the face

or difficulty in breathing. If you cannot reach your doctor, phone a hospital emergency department.

Storage

Store the tablets and capsules in a cool, dark place and keep the bottle tightly closed. Do not freeze the liquid preparation.

If for some reason you cannot take all of the medicine, discard the unused portion by flushing it down the toilet. Do not take or save old medicine. Outdated tetracycline can cause serious problems.

Refills

Do not go without medicine between prescription refills. Call your pharmacist for a refill 2 or 3 days before you will run out of the medicine.

Outdated Tetracycline

Some TETRACYCLINES decompose with age and/or exposure to light and when improperly stored under high humidity or heat. The resulting product may be toxic to the kidney.

THEOPHYLLINE (ORAL)

ELIXOPHYLLIN, PMS THEOPHYLLINE ELIXIR, PULMOPHYLLINE, QUIBRON -T/SR, QUIBRON-T LIQUID, SLO-BID, SOMOPHYLLIN-T, SOMOPHYLLIN-12, THEOCHRON, THEO-DUR, THEOLAIR, THEOLAIR SR, THEO-SR, UNIPHYL

AMINOPHYLLINE (ORAL)

PALARON, PHYLLOCONTIN, PHYLLOCONTIN-350

AMINOPHYLLINE (RECTAL)

COROPHYLLIN

OXTRIPHYLLINE (ORAL)

CHOLEDYL, CHOLEDYL SA

Purpose

This medicine is used to help open the bronchioles (air passages in the lungs) to make breathing easier and to relieve wheezing and shortness of breath. It is used in the treatment of bronchial asthma, bronchitis, emphysema and other lung conditions.

Allergies/Warnings

If you have ever had an allergic reaction to caffeine or any medicine for lung conditions, tell your doctor and pharmacist before you take any of this medicine.

How to Use This Medicine

Time of Administration

This medicine should be taken with a glass of water.

Many of these medicines can be taken with food but you should check with your pharmacist or doctor for instructions on your particular medicine. Whether you take it with or without food, it is important that you *always take it the same way all the time* so that the same amount of medicine reaches the bloodstream.

Take the medicine in a sitting or upright position. Do not lie down immediately after taking the drug in order to ensure that the medicine reaches the stomach.

For UNIPHYL:

- Most patients only have to take this medicine once a day. Take it with food or within 1 to 2 hours of eating food. It is best to take the medicine later in the day, with or shortly after the evening meal.

Space your doses of the medicine as equally as possible around the clock (throughout the entire day of 24 hours). For example, if you are to take 3 doses each day, try to space the doses as close as possible to 8 hours apart. This will keep a constant level of the medicine in your body. It is very important to always take this medicine at the same time(s) every day. Do not take extra doses without your doctor's approval and try not to miss any doses. If you miss doses, the amount of theophylline in your blood will fall and you will not get the full benefit of this medicine.

Try not to take doses more than 1/2 hour before their scheduled time.

How to Administer

If you were prescribed CHOLEDYL SA, PHYLLOCONTIN, PHYLLOCONTIN-350, QUIBRON-T/SR, SLO-BID, THEOCHRON, THEO-DUR, THEOLAIR SR, THEO-SR, UNIPHYL:

- This medicine is long-acting and must be swallowed whole. Do not crush or chew.

If you were prescribed SOMOPHYLLIN-12:

- These capsules may be swallowed whole or may be opened and the contents sprinkled on a small amount of soft food just before taking. The contents of the capsule should not be chewed or crushed.

- Hold the capsule horizontally just above a spoonful of cool, soft food that is easy to swallow such as applesauce, fruit puree, pudding or ice cream.
- Turn both ends of the capsule in opposite directions and gently pull apart.
- Sprinkle the contents of the capsule onto the food.
- Do not chew the drug/food mixture but swallow it immediately. Then drink some water.
- Do not save or reuse any of the medicine that has been sprinkled on any food.
- If you spill any of the beads while sprinkling, start over to make sure that you get the right dose.

For liquid medicines:

- If a spoon is used to measure the dose, it is recommended that you use a medicine spoon or an oral liquid syringe that you can obtain from your pharmacist. *See* How to Administer Medications (page 15).

For COROPHYLLIN SUPPOSITORIES: *See* How to Administer Medications (page 15).

Special Instructions

Length of Therapy

Do not take this medicine more often or longer than recommended by your doctor. To do so may increase your chance of developing side effects. Do not stop taking this medicine without your doctor's permission. If you suddenly stop taking this medicine, you may have an asthmatic attack. You should discuss the length of therapy with your doctor.

Pregnancy/Breastfeeding

Women who are pregnant, breastfeeding or planning to become pregnant should tell their doctor before taking this medicine.

Drug Interactions

Some nonprescription drugs can aggravate your condition. Do not take any of the following without the approval of your doctor or pharmacist: cough, cold or sinus products; ASA-containing medicines; asthma or allergy products. Read the label of the product to see if there is a warning. If there is, check with your doctor or pharmacist before using the product.

Do not take this medicine at the same time as a nonprescription drug containing aminophylline or theophylline without the approval of your doctor.

Avoid drinking large amounts of coffee, tea, cocoa (chocolate) or cola drinks while you are on this medicine because you could be more sensitive to the caffeine in these beverages.

Do not smoke while you are on this medicine because smoking can make the drug less effective. If you insist on smoking, be sure to tell your doctor so that he or she can take this into consideration when adjusting your doses.

The effect of this medicine can be decreased by a diet low in carbohydrates, high in protein or with a high frequency of charcoal-broiled foods. On the other hand, a diet high in carbohydrates and low in protein can cause unwanted higher levels of the medicine. Check with your doctor if you have any questions about your diet.

Blood tests for theophylline can be made inaccurate by previous ingestions of coffee, tea, cola beverages, chocolate and medicines containing acetaminophen.

Alcohol

Do not drink alcoholic beverages or nonprescription drugs containing alcohol while taking this drug without the approval of your doctor.

Special Precautions

If your mouth becomes dry, drink water, suck ice chips or a hard, sour candy (sugarless) or chew gum (sugarless). Sugarless products are recommended in order to avoid dental problems. You may wish to ask your pharmacist about special solutions, called artificial saliva, that can also be used to help restore moisture in the mouth. It is especially important to brush and floss your teeth regularly if you develop a dry mouth to help prevent gum problems.

In some people, this drug may cause dizziness. This side effect is more common in people over 60 years of age and people with lung conditions. Do not drive a car, pilot an airplane, operate dangerous machinery or do jobs that require you to be alert if you are dizzy or drowsy. You should also be careful going up and down stairs. Sit or lie down at the first sign of dizziness. Tell your doctor if the dizziness continues.

Be sure to keep your appointments with your doctor after you first start taking this medicine. People respond to this drug at different rates and your doctor must examine you in order to determine the best dose for you.

If your doctor wants to check the level of this medicine in your blood (a simple blood test), be sure to tell him or her if you have missed a dose of the medicine in the last 2 days. The test will have to be done another time because it will not be accurate if you have missed taking the drug. Also, be sure to have the blood tests done at the times recommended by your doctor. If the blood test is not done at the correct time, the test results may not be accurate.

Do not change the dose of any other asthma or bronchitis medicines except on the advice of your doctor.

When to Call Your Doctor

Call your doctor if you develop flu symptoms, a fever or diarrhea.

Most people experience few or no side effects from this drug. However, any medicine can sometimes cause unwanted effects. Call your doctor if you develop a skin rash, hives, sore throat, fever, mouth sores, vomiting of blood or coffee-ground material, stomach pain or red or black stools, fast or irregular heartbeats, confusion, unusual tiredness, convulsions or agitation, tremor, difficulty sleeping, restlessness or thirst, headaches, muscle twitching or increased urination (passing your water).

If you are using rectal suppositories, contact your doctor also if you develop burning or irritation of the skin in the rectal area.

Refills

Do not stop taking this medicine without your doctor's approval and do not go without medicine between prescription refills. Call your pharmacist for a refill 2 or 3 days before you will run out of the medicine.

Discuss with your pharmacist the implications of dispensing all your refills for this medicine with the same manufacturer's product. (*See* Generic Drugs, page 12.)

TIMOLOL (OPHTHALMIC)

Timoptic

BETAXOL HCl

Betoptic

LEVOBUNOLOL HCl

Betagan

Purpose

This medicine is used in the treatment of certain types of glaucoma to lower the pressure in the eye. Increased pressure may lead to a gradual loss of vision.

Allergies/Warnings

If you have ever had an allergic reaction to any medicine or if you have bronchial asthma, bronchitis, thyroid problems, diabetes, emphysema or heart problems, tell your doctor and pharmacist before you take any of this medicine.

BETAGAN contains sulfites. Do not use it if you are allergic to sulfites.

How To Use This Medicine

How to Administer

For eye drops: see How to Administer Medications (page 15).

- If more than 1 drop is prescribed, wait 3 to 5 minutes before administering another drop.
- Wait at least 5 minutes before using any other eye drops.

Special Instructions

Length of Therapy

Do not use the eye drops more frequently or in larger quantities than prescribed by your doctor.

Do not stop using the eye drops on your own without talking with your doctor or pharmacist.

Pregnancy/Breastfeeding

Women who are pregnant, breastfeeding or planning to become pregnant should tell their doctor before taking this medicine.

Drug Interactions

Do not use this medicine at the same time as any other eye medicine without the approval of your doctor. Some medicines cannot be mixed.

Special Precautions

If you are wearing contact lenses, you must remove them before using the eye drops. Ask your doctor how long you must wait before reinserting the lenses.

Keep your doctor's appointments regularly so that your doctor can make sure that the medicine is working correctly and that your glaucoma is under control.

If you are using BETOPTIC and your eyes become more sensitive to light, wearing sunglasses may help.

Did You Know That?

Large doses of vitamin C can interfere with the stool blood tests for cancer of the colon.

Consumers are now able to test for cancer of the colon, rectum and anus in the privacy of their own homes. A positive test result for cancer occurs when hemoglobin of the blood is in the stool being tested and a blue color results.

However, these tests may not be accurate if a person has eaten certain foods or is taking medicines that can interfere with the test and give false readings. Large doses (more than 250 mg per day) of vitamin C should be avoided because the drug can cause false negative readings. In other words, vitamin C may prevent the test from turning blue in color even if the person has blood in the stool—and perhaps has colonic cancer.

In contrast, red meats, broccoli, horseradish and cauliflower may interfere with the test and cause false positive readings. Toilet bowl cleaners that have been used prior to the test may interfere with the results of commercial stool blood tests. The person may be unnecessarily alarmed that cancer is present when in reality, the cause of the positive test result was due to one of these other factors.

A positive test does not always mean cancer is present. Any medical condition (such as hemorrhoids, stomach ulcers, gastritis, colitis, diverticulitis and esophageal varices) or medications that can cause stomach bleeding (such as ASA, steroids, and nonsteroidal anti-inflammatory drugs) can be the reason for blood in the stool.

The best advice is to make an appointment with your doctor if you have a positive test reading. It may not be as serious as you think—but then again you may have caught a cancer in the early stages.

The Canadian Cancer Society publishes public education materials on colonic cancer and methods of early detection. Contact your local office to obtain copies of these publications.

When to Call Your Doctor

Contact your doctor if your vision gets worse or if the eye becomes painful or irritated by the medicine for more than a few minutes. Many eye medicines sting and cause tears for a short time immediately after use.

If you were prescribed TIMOPTIC:

- Also call your doctor if you develop unusual tiredness or weakness, slow or irregular heartbeats, wheezing or difficulty breathing, fainting, persistent headaches, confusion, depression, swelling of legs or ankles or sudden weight gain of 5 pounds (2.5 kg) or more.

If you were prescribed BETAGAN:

- Also call your doctor if you develop slow or irregular heartbeats, wheezing, redness of eyes, difficulty breathing or shortness of breath, fainting, swelling of feet, ankles or legs, or sudden weight gain of 5 pounds (2.5 kg) or more. Also call your doctor if you develop unusual tiredness or weakness, confusion, depression or persistent headaches.

If you were prescribed BETOPTIC:

- Also call your doctor if you develop increased sensitivity to light, difficulty sleeping, depression, wheezing or difficulty breathing, fainting, slow or irregular heartbeats, swelling of the legs or ankles, or sudden weight gain of 5 pounds (2.5 kg) or more.

Allergic Reactions

Call your doctor immediately if you think you may be allergic to the medicine or if you develop a skin rash or itching. If you cannot reach your doctor, phone a hospital emergency department.

Miscellaneous

This medicine is for external use only. Do not swallow it.

Carry an identification card in your wallet or wear a medical alert bracelet indicating that you are taking this medicine as well as the names and phone numbers of your doctors. If you do not already carry such a card, complete the Medicine Card in this book. Always tell your dentist, pharmacist and other doctors who are treating you that you are taking this medicine.

TOCAINIDE (ORAL)

TONOCARD

MEXILETINE

MEXITIL

Purpose

This medicine is used to help regulate the heartbeat so that it is strong and steady.

Allergies/Warnings

If you have ever had an allergic reaction to any local anesthetic or any other medicine or have a history of epilepsy (seizures), tell your doctor and pharmacist before you take any of this medicine.

How To Use This Medicine

Time of Administration

It is very important that you take this medicine exactly as your doctor has prescribed. Do not miss any doses and take the medicine even if you feel well. Do not take extra doses without your doctor's approval.

Take the medicine at the same times every day so that you have a constant level of the medicine in your body.

How to Administer

Take the medicine with food (*See* Special Precautions below).

Special Instructions

Pregnancy/Breastfeeding

Women who are pregnant or planning to become pregnant should tell their doctor before taking this medicine.

This medicine should not be used in women who are breastfeeding.

Drug Interactions

It is important that you obtain the advice of your doctor or pharmacist before taking any other prescription or nonprescription medicines that can excite the heart (including certain pain relievers, sleeping pills, tranquilizers, or medicines for depression, cough/cold or sinus products, asthma or allergy products, or diet medicines).

There are other drug interactions which can occur. If you are taking any other medicines, be sure to check first with your pharmacist or doctor.

For MEXILETINE:

- Avoid large amounts of foods or drugs that can increase the acidity (e.g. cranberry juice, meats, fish, eggs, gelatin products, prunes, plums, ASA, vitamin C, etc.) or alkalinity (e.g. citrus fruits and juices, milk and milk products, most vegetables, high doses of antacids, baking soda, etc.) of the urine.

For TOCAINIDE:

- Avoid large amounts of food and drugs (e.g. citrus fruits and juices, milk and milk products, most vegetables, high doses of antacids, baking soda, etc.) that increase the alkalinity of the urine.

Special Precautions

This medicine sometimes causes lightheadedness, dizziness, nausea, numbness and tremor. It may help to take the medicine with some food if these side effects occur. If food does not help, call your doctor. It may be necessary to change your dosing schedule.

Your doctor will want to do blood tests, especially during the first six months of treatment.

If your mouth becomes dry, drink water, suck ice chips or a hard, sour candy (sugarless) or chew gum (sugarless). Sugarless products are recommended in order to avoid dental problems. You may wish to ask your pharmacist about special solutions, called artificial saliva, that can also be used to help restore moisture in the mouth.

It is especially important to brush and floss your teeth regularly if you develop a dry mouth to help prevent gum problems.

In some people, this drug may cause dizziness, drowsiness or blurred vision. Do not drive a car, pilot an airplane, operate dangerous machinery or do jobs that require you to be alert if you are dizzy or drowsy. You should also be careful going up and down stairs. Sit or lie down at the first sign of dizziness. Tell your doctor if these problems continue.

When to Call Your Doctor

Call your doctor if you develop a sore throat, fever or chills, mouth sores, coughing, wheezing, difficulty breathing, tremors, fast heartbeats, unusual bruising or bleeding, a yellow color to the skin or eyes, confusion, depression, nightmares, hallucinations, changes in vision or hearing, fainting, unusual sweating, clamminess, muscle or joint pain, heartburn, stomach pain, neck pain, constipation, diarrhea, difficulty urinating, severe nausea, vomiting, or sudden weight gain of 5 pounds (2.5 kg) or more.

The appearance of tremors, i.e. mild shaking of the hands, etc. may mean that the highest dose you can tolerate has almost been reached. Tell your doctor.

Allergic Reactions

Call your doctor immediately if you think you may be allergic to the medicine or if you develop a skin rash, hives, itching, swelling of the face or difficulty in breathing. If you cannot reach your doctor, phone a hospital emergency department.

Refills

Do not stop taking this medicine without your doctor's approval and do not go without medicine between prescription refills. Call your pharmacist for a refill 2 or 3 days before you will run out of the medicine.

Miscellaneous

Carry an identification card in your wallet or wear a medical alert bracelet indicating that you are taking this medicine as well as the names and phone numbers of your doctors. If you do not already carry such a card, complete the Medicine Card in this book.

Always tell your dentist, pharmacist and other doctors who are treating you that you are taking this medicine.

TRETINOIN (TOPICAL)

STIEVAA, VITAMIN A ACID

Purpose

This medicine is used to treat mild to moderate acne. Its use is presently being investigated in the treatment of sun-damaged skin.

Allergies/Warnings

Tell your doctor and pharmacist if you are allergic to TRETINOIN or any vitamin A medicine.

How to Use This Medicine

Time of Administration

The medicine is usually applied once a day before going to bed.

How to Administer

For cream and gel:

- Each time you apply the medicine, wash your hands and gently cleanse the skin area well with a mild soap and water unless otherwise directed by your doctor. Pat the skin gently with a clean towel until dry. Wait about 20 to 30 minutes to be sure the skin is completely dry.

- Apply a small amount of the drug to the area under treatment and gently massage into the skin. Only the medicine that is actually touching the skin will work. A thick layer is not more effective than a thin layer. Do not bandage unless directed by your doctor. After applying this medication, you may notice a slight stinging sensation or feeling of warmth. This is normal.
- Do not use the drug more frequently or in larger quantities than prescribed by your doctor. Overuse of this medicine may cause increased skin irritation and bleeding.
- Wash your hands thoroughly after applying the cream or gel.

For solution:

- Cleanse the skin area well with water unless otherwise directed. Pat the skin with a clean towel until the skin is completely dry. (This may take 20 to 30 minutes.)
- Apply the solution using the applicator that comes with the bottle. After applying this medication to the area under treatment, you may notice a slight stinging sensation or feeling of warmth. This is normal.
- Do not use the drug more frequently or in larger quantities than prescribed by your doctor. Overuse of this medicine may cause increased skin irritation and bleeding.
- Wash your hands thoroughly if you applied the solution with your fingertips.

Special Instructions

Length of Therapy

It may take up to 6 to 10 weeks before you receive the full benefit of this medicine.

Pregnancy/Breastfeeding

Women who are pregnant, breastfeeding or planning to become pregnant should tell their doctor before using this medicine.

Drug Interactions

Do not use this medicine at the same time as any other acne product or product that is abrasive, causes peeling of the skin or contains alcohol unless directed by your doctor. Examples of such products include abrasive soaps and cleansers, soaps and cosmetics that are drying, astringents or products with spices or lime in them.

Usually it is all right to continue using cosmetics (as long as they are not too drying), but it is a good idea to check with your doctor first. Some cosmetics can be extremely drying and this could cause problems. Always remove cosmetics before a new dose of the medicine is applied.

Helpful Tips to Reduce Nausea and Vomiting from Chemotherapy

Patients who are receiving chemotherapy may find the following dietary suggestions helpful in reducing nausea and vomiting:

- Eat small meals frequently throughout the day to keep your stomach from feeling too full at any one time.
- Chew your food well so that it will be easier for your body to digest it.
- Eat slowly so that only small amounts of food enter your stomach at any one time.
- Avoid drinking liquids at mealtime to prevent filling up your stomach. Instead, drink liquids one hour before or after eating.
- Try to drink clear, cool, unsweetened beverages, such as apple juice.
- Before you go for your chemotherapy treatment, eat a light meal, such as soup and crackers.
- Try not to lie down flat for at least two hours after eating. However, it may be helpful to rest after eating since this will help your body digest the food.
- If the smell of food causes nausea, try to stay out of the kitchen.

Special Precautions

While using this medicine, your skin may become more sensitive to sunlight. Do not use sunlamps and wear protective clothing. Check with your doctor if you must work outside in the sunlight. It may be wise to use sunscreens with an SPF of 15 or higher. Also call your doctor if you get sunburned.

When you apply this medicine, you may have a mild stinging sensation or redness. This is not unusual. At first, your acne may even seem to get worse. This is due to the effect of the medicine on deep acne lesions that could not be seen previously. After a few days, you can expect some peeling to occur.

Your skin may become more sensitive to wind or cold temperatures.

Dress warmly.

Do not apply this medicine to chapped, windburned or sunburned skin or to open cuts or wounds.

Keep this preparation away from the eyes, eyelids, mouth or inside the nose. If you should accidentally get some in your eyes, wash it away with water immediately.

When to Call Your Doctor

Call your doctor if the condition for which you are using this medicine becomes worse or if the medicine causes itching or severe burning or redness for more than a few minutes after application. When you first start using the medicine, be prepared for some redness, dryness and scaling of the skin at the place the medicine was applied.

Also call your doctor if you develop blistering or crusting, swelling of the skin or darkening or lightening of treated areas.

Miscellaneous

This medicine is for external use only. Do not swallow it.

TRIAMTERENE (ORAL)

DYRENIUM

TRIAMTERENE-HYDROCHLOROTHIAZIDE

APO-TRIAZIDE, DYAZIDE, NOVOTRIAMZIDE

Purpose

This medicine is used to help the body get rid of excess fluids and to decrease swelling. The medicine does this by increasing the amount of urine and is commonly called a *water pill* or *fluid pill*. It is commonly used to treat high blood pressure and other medical conditions.

Allergies/Warnings

Be sure to tell your doctor or pharmacist if you are allergic to any medicine.

How To Use This Medicine

Time of Administration

Try to take this medicine at the same time(s) every day so that you have a constant level of the medicine in your body.

When you first start taking this medicine, you will probably urinate (pass your water) more often and in larger amounts than usual. Therefore, if you are to take 1 dose each day, take it in the morning after breakfast. Do not initially take a dose at bedtime or you may have to get up during the night to go to the bathroom.

If you are to take more than 1 dose each day, take the last dose approximately 6 hours before bedtime so that you will not have to get up during the night to go to the bathroom. This effect will usually decrease after you have taken the drug for a while.

How to Administer

Take this medicine with food, meals or milk if it upsets your stomach. If stomach upset continues, call your doctor.

Special Instructions

Length of Therapy

For patients with high blood pressure:

- High blood pressure (hypertension) is a long-term condition and it will probably be necessary for you to take the drug for a long time even if you feel better. If high blood pressure is not treated, it can lead to serious problems such as heart failure, strokes, blood vessel problems or kidney problems.

It is very important that you take this medicine as your doctor has directed and that you do not miss any doses. Otherwise, you cannot expect the drug to keep your blood pressure down or remove excess fluid.

Pregnancy/Breastfeeding

Women who are pregnant or planning to become pregnant should tell their doctor before taking this medicine.

This medicine can pass into the breast milk and women should not breastfeed while they are on this drug.

Drug Interactions

Some nonprescription drugs can aggravate high blood pressure. Do not take any of the following without the approval of your doctor or pharmacist: cough, cold, or sinus products; asthma or allergy products since they may increase your blood pressure. Read the label of the nonprescription drug product to see if there is a warning. If there is, check with your doctor or pharmacist before using the product.

Alcohol

Be careful drinking alcoholic beverages while taking this medicine because it could make the possible side effect of dizziness worse.

Special Precautions

If this medicine causes dizziness or lightheadedness, you should be careful going up and down stairs and you should not change positions too rapidly. Lightheadedness is more likely to occur if you stand up suddenly—this is due to blood collecting in the legs and lasts for a few seconds. Therefore, get up from a sitting or lying position more slowly and tighten and relax your leg muscles or wiggle your toes to help promote circulation. In the morning, get out of bed slowly and dangle your feet over the edge of the bed for a few minutes before standing up. Sit or lie down at the first sign of dizziness. Do not drive a car, pilot an airplane, operate dangerous machinery or do jobs that require you to be alert if you are dizzy. Tell your doctor if you have been dizzy.

In order to help prevent dizziness or fainting, your doctor may also recommend that you avoid strenuous exercise, standing for long periods of time (especially in hot weather), hot showers, hot baths, Jucuzzis or saunas. People more than 65 years of age may be more sensitive to the side effect of dizziness.

This medicine does not cause your body to lose potassium as some other types of water pills do. Therefore, it is not usually necessary for you to eat foods rich in potassium. In fact, too much potassium while you are taking this medicine could be harmful. Call your doctor if you develop any of the warning signs of too much potassium: irregular heartbeats, numbness or tingling in the hands, feet or lips, confusion, difficulty breathing, unusual tiredness or weakness, unexplained nervousness, weakness or a feeling of heaviness in the legs. Since not all patients develop these symptoms, your doctor may want to check your blood occasionally to see if the potassium level is normal.

Do not use salt substitutes, low-salt milk or low-salt soups without the approval of your doctor. They may contain large amounts of potassium, which could affect the way you respond to this medicine.

This medicine may make some people more sensitive to sunlight and various tanning lamps. When you begin taking this medicine, try to avoid too much sun until you see how you are going to react. If your skin does become more sensitive to sunlight, tell your doctor and try not to stay in direct sunlight for extended periods of time. While in the sun, wear protective clothing and sunglasses. You may wish to ask your pharmacist about suitable sunscreen products. Call your doctor if you become sunburned.

This medicine may cause your urine to turn pale-blue.

If you are a diabetic and were prescribed APO-TRIAZIDE, DYAZIDE *or* NOVOTRIAMZIDE:

- This medicine may cause your blood sugar to rise. Carefully test your blood or urine for sugar while you are taking this medicine. Call your doctor if you think your blood sugar is higher than normal or harder to control.

News about ASA

ASA has been approved "to reduce the risk of death and/or nonfatal myocardial infarction (heart attack) in patients with a previous infarction or unstable angina pectoris." This new approved use for ASA was based on the results of clinical studies reported in the *Journal of the American Medical Association.* The studies involved more than 12,000 patients with heart attacks or angina (chest pain). ASA treatment was associated with a reduction in the risk of death within 12 weeks in 20% of the heart attack patients and 50% of the patients with angina. The majority of the patients were males and the use of ASA therapy in women is still being investigated.

The best dose of ASA in these conditions has not yet been established. Any person who has had a heart attack or has angina should not self-treat with ASA but should follow his doctor's advice. ASA can interact with many other medications and serious problems could occur if a person self-medicated with ASA while on one of these other medications.

When to Call Your Doctor

Most people experience few or no side effects from this drug. However, any medicine can sometimes cause unwanted effects. Call your doctor if you develop sore throat, fever, skin rash, mouth sores, nausea or vomiting, dry mouth (or if you become very thirsty), bright red tongue, cracked corners of the mouth, weakness, irregular pulse, shortness of breath, stomach pain, headaches, swelling of the legs or ankles or a sudden weight gain of 5 pounds (2.5 kg).

Also call your doctor if you become sick or develop persistent vomiting or diarrhea.

If you were prescribed APO-TRIAZIDE, DYAZIDE *or* NOVOTRIAMZIDE:

- Also call your doctor if you develop sharp joint pain, muscle weakness, unusual bruising or bleeding, a yellow color to the skin or eyes or dark-yellow colored urine.

Allergic Reactions

Call your doctor immediately if you think you may be allergic to the medicine or if you develop a skin rash, hives, itching, swelling of the face or difficulty in breathing. If you cannot reach your doctor, phone a hospital emergency department.

Refills

Do not stop taking this medicine without your doctor's approval and do not go without medicine between prescription refills. Call your pharmacist for a refill 2 or 3 days before you will run out of the medicine.

VALPROIC ACID
DEPAKENE

DIVALPROEX SODIUM
EPIVAL

Purpose

This medicine is used to help control seizures. It is commonly used in the treatment of epilepsy.

Allergies/Warnings

If you have ever had an allergic reaction to an anticonvulsant or seizure medicine, tell your doctor and pharmacist before you take any of this medicine.

Also tell your doctor if you have any liver problems.

How to Use This Medicine

Time of Administration

It is very important that you take this medicine exactly as your doctor has prescribed. Do not miss any doses and take the medicine even if you feel well. Try to take this medicine at the same time(s) every day so that you will have a constant level of medicine in your body. This is the only way that you can receive the full benefit of the medicine. If you forget to take this medicine, the amount of medicine in your blood will decrease and you may have seizures.

How to Administer

Take this medicine after food if it upsets your stomach. Call your doctor if you continue to have stomach upset or if you develop nausea, vomiting, diarrhea or constipation.

For DEPAKENE 500 mg capsules *and* EPIVAL tablets:

- This medicine has a special coating and should be swallowed whole. Do not chew or break the capsules open.

For DEPAKENE syrup:

- If a dropper, oral liquid syringe or special measuring spoon is used to measure the dose and you do not fully understand how to use it, *see* How to Administer Medications (page 15).

Special Instructions

Length of Therapy

Do not stop taking this medicine suddenly without the approval of your doctor. It usually will be necessary for your doctor to slowly reduce your dose since your body will need time to adjust. You could develop seizures if you suddenly stopped taking the medicine.

Pregnancy/Breastfeeding

Women who are pregnant or planning to become pregnant should tell their doctor before taking this medicine.

Women should not breastfeed without their doctor's approval. This medicine can pass into the breast milk and cause side effects in the infant.

Drug Interactions

It is important that you obtain the advice of your doctor or pharmacist before taking any other prescription and nonprescription medicines including pain relievers, sleeping pills, tranquilizers, medicine for seizures, muscle relaxants, anesthetics, anticoagulants (blood thinners), medicines for depression or medicines for allergies. Combining this medicine with some of these drugs could cause drowsiness or dizziness.

There are other drug interactions that can occur. If you are taking any other medicines, be sure to check first with your pharmacist or doctor.

Alcohol

Do not drink alcoholic beverages while taking this drug without the approval of your doctor because the combination could cause drowsiness. One drink may have the same effect that 2 or 3 drinks normally would have.

Special Precautions

Be sure to keep your doctor's appointments so that your doctor can check your progress. This is especially important during the first few months of therapy when the doctor will decide the best dose of this medicine for your condition.

This medicine may cause dizziness, drowsiness or blurred vision in some people. If you become dizzy, you should be careful going up and down stairs. Sit or lie down at the first sign of dizziness. Do not drive a car, use a sewing machine, operate dangerous machinery or do jobs that require you to be alert until you know how you are going to react to the drug. Tell your doctor if you are dizzy, drowsy or have blurred vision.

If this medicine is for a child, do not let him or her ride a bike, climb trees, etc. until you can determine how he or she is going to react to this medicine. Children could hurt themselves if they participated in these activities when they were dizzy.

Avoid swimming alone or taking part in high-risk sports in which a sudden seizure could cause injury.

This medicine can cause weight gain and, less frequently, hair loss.

For patients with diabetes:

- This medicine can cause the test for urinary ketones to be falsely high. Check with your doctor.

When to Call Your Doctor

Most people experience few or no side effects from this drug. However, any medicine can sometimes cause unwanted effects. Call your doctor if you develop a sore throat, fever, or mouth sores, skin rash and itching, swollen glands, unusual bruising or bleeding, changes in vision, fast eye movements, muscle or joint pain, menstrual irregularity (in women), swelling of the hands or feet, loss of appetite, vomiting, tremors or shaking, light-colored stools, yellow color to the skin or eyes, or if you become "hyper," confused or depressed.

Call your doctor if you have an increase in the frequency of seizures.

Allergic Reactions

Allergic reactions to this medicine are very uncommon. Call your doctor immediately if you think you may be allergic to the medicine or if you develop a skin rash, hives, itching, swelling of the face or difficulty in breathing. If you cannot reach your doctor, phone a hospital emergency department.

Refills

Do not stop taking this medicine without your doctor's approval and

do not go without medicine between prescription refills. Call your pharmacist for a refill 2 or 3 days before you will run out of the medicine.

Miscellaneous

Carry an identification card in your wallet or wear a medical alert bracelet indicating that you are taking this medicine as well as the names and phone numbers of your doctors. If you do not already carry such a card, complete the Medicine Card in this book. Always tell your dentist, pharmacist and other doctors who are treating you that you are taking this medicine.

WARFARIN POTASSIUM (ORAL)

ATHROMBIN-K

WARFARIN SODIUM

COUMADIN, WARFILONE

Purpose

This medicine is used to treat or help prevent harmful blood clots from forming in the blood vessels. It is commonly called a blood thinner.

Allergies/Warnings

If you have ever had an allergic reaction to any blood thinner, tell your doctor and pharmacist before you take any of this medicine.

How to Use This Medicine

Time of Administration

Take this medicine exactly as your doctor has prescribed. Try to take the medicine at the same time every day and do not miss any doses. If you miss a dose, do not take extra tablets without your doctor's approval because overtreatment may cause serious bleeding problems.

How to Administer

It is best to take this medicine with a glass of water. Do not take it with food or other drugs unless otherwise directed because there are many possible interactions that could occur.

Special Instructions

Length of Therapy

Do not take any more of this medicine than your doctor has prescribed and do not stop taking this medicine suddenly without the approval of your doctor.

After you stop taking the medicine, it will take your body some time to eliminate the drug and return to normal. Your doctor or pharmacist will tell you how long you must follow these instructions after you have stopped taking this medicine.

Pregnancy/Breastfeeding

Women who are pregnant or planning to become pregnant should tell their doctor before taking this medicine. This medicine should not be taken during certain stages of pregnancy.

Women who are breastfeeding should tell their doctor before taking this medicine. This medicine can pass into the breast milk.

Drug Interactions

Do not start or stop taking any drugs you are currently taking without first consulting with your doctor. Many medicines can increase or decrease the effect of this drug. This includes both prescription and nonprescription medicines, especially pain relievers, sleeping pills, tranquilizers, medicine for seizures, muscle relaxants, anesthetics, medicines for depression or medicines for allergies. Always check with your pharmacist before you take or buy *any* nonprescription products.

Do not treat yourself with any product containing ASA or salicylate. This includes many pain killers, drugs for fever, cold medicines and antacids. ASA may interact with this medicine and cause serious bleeding problems.

Do not take any vitamin or health food supplements, especially those containing vitamin K, without the approval of your doctor or pharmacist.

Alcohol

It is best to avoid alcoholic beverages while you are taking this medicine. However, your doctor may feel it is safe for you to have an occasional drink. Small amounts of wine or beer may be safe. Brandy, cognac, whiskey or gin could be dangerous.

Special Precautions

Regular blood tests, called prothrombin times or PT's, are necessary in order for your doctor to prescribe the correct dose for you. Your dose may change from time to time depending on these tests.

Do not change your normal diet and do not eat unusually large amounts of foods high in vitamin K such as fish, fish oils and leafy, green vegetables (broccoli, turnip greens, cauliflower, alfalfa sprouts, carrot tops, cabbage, lettuce, watercress, asparagus), or change your diet without telling your doctor. Certain foods can affect the way you will respond to this medicine and your dose may have to be adjusted.

If you have a tendency to cut yourself while shaving, you may wish to use an electric razor to avoid possible bleeding.

You may wish to use a soft-bristled toothbrush to help prevent bleeding of the gums while brushing the teeth.

Do not donate blood because the presence of this medicine in the blood could cause problems in the recipient.

Try to avoid contact sports or activities in which you could become injured because this could result in internal bleeding or severe bruises.

Did You Know That?

If you go to more than one doctor or pharmacy, you should tell each one what medicines you are taking.

This should include both prescription and nonprescription drugs as both types of drugs could interfere with a new medicine that the doctor may prescribe for you.

The Medicine Card in this book is an excellent way to keep a record of all your medicines. Simply show it to every doctor and pharmacist you visit.

When to Call Your Doctor

If your body gets more medicine than it needs, bleeding may occur. Call your doctor if you notice any unusual signs of bleeding that you cannot explain, for example, nosebleeds, unusual bruising without any obvious cause, heavy menstrual bleeding (in women), bleeding from the gums after brushing the teeth, eye hemorrhage, heavy bleeding from cuts, red or black stools, red or dark-brown urine or blood in the urine, stomach cramps, back pain, vomiting or coughing up of blood or material that looks like coffee grounds.

Call your doctor if you develop stomach or back pain, joint pain, chest pain, unusual headaches, changes in vision, constipation or diarrhea, loss of appetite, unusual weight gain, swelling of the feet or ankles, loss of hair, dizziness, a skin rash, unexplained sore throat, fever or mouth sores, chills, a yellow color to the skin or eyes, difficulty urinating (passing your water) or unusual tiredness. Also call your doctor if you fall or hit your head.

Did You Know That?

Large amounts of broccoli have been reported to interfere with the action of warfarin, a blood thinner used to help prevent blood clots.

Warfarin is an anticoagulant, commonly called a "blood thinner." It is used to help prevent clots from forming in the blood vessels. The dose of warfarin must be carefully adjusted so that the person has just the right amount in the bloodstream. If the dose is too low, clots could form. If the dose is too high, the person could start bleeding and hemorrhage.

Vitamin K is used as an antidote if the patient has too high a blood level of warfarin. There are also some foods that contain high amounts of vitamin K, e.g. turnip greens, broccoli, lettuce, cabbage. For this reason, patients are warned not to eat unusually large amounts of leafy, green vegetables or change their diets without checking with their doctor. Small amounts are not likely to cause problems.

One patient was not responding to warfarin and it was learned that she had been having both broccoli soup and raw broccoli salad for lunch almost every day. Now she is undergoing treatment on a broccoli-free diet. Another patient had been eating at least 1 pound of broccoli daily for several years. Once broccoli was eliminated from her diet, she responded to the drug treatment.

Allergic Reactions

Call your doctor immediately if you think you may be allergic to the medicine or if you develop a skin rash, hives, itching, swelling of the face or difficulty in breathing. If you cannot reach your doctor, phone a hospital emergency department or Emergency Medical Service.

Refills

Do not stop taking this medicine without your doctor's approval and do not go without medicine between prescription refills. Call your pharmacist for a refill 2 or 3 days before you will run out of the medicine.

Do not change brands of this medicine without your doctor's approval. The dose you need could be different with different brands.

Miscellaneous

Carry an identification card in your wallet or wear a medical alert bracelet indicating that you are taking this medicine as well as the names and phone numbers of your doctors. If you do not already carry such a card, complete the Medicine Card in this book. Always tell your dentist, pharmacist and other doctors who are treating you that you are taking this medicine.

APPENDIX A

Foods Rich in Potassium

If you have been instructed by your doctor to eat foods rich in potassium, this chart may be helpful. In most cases, you will want to select a food that is also low in calories and low in sodium.

Foods	Average Portion	Potassium (in mg)	Calories	Sodium (in mg)
FRUITS				
Orange	1 medium	360 mg	95	0.8
Grapefruit	1 cup	380 mg	75	1.0
Banana	1 medium	630 mg	130	0.8
Strawberries	1 cup	270 mg	55	1.2
Avocado	1/2	380 mg	275	3.4
Apricots	3 medium	500 mg	55	0.7
Dates	1 cup	1390 mg	500	1.8
Watermelon	1/2 slice	380 mg	95	1.0
Cantaloupe	1/2 melon	880 mg	75	46.0
Raisins	1 cup	1150 mg	425	34.0
Prunes	4 large	240 mg	90	2.4
JUICES				
Orange	8-oz glass	440 mg	105	9.0
Grapefruit	8-oz glass	370 mg	130	1.0
Prune	8-oz glass	620 mg	170	5.0
Pineapple	8-oz glass	340 mg	120	1.2
MEAT				
Hamburger	3 oz	290 mg	310	92.0
Beef (chuck)	3 oz	310 mg	260	44.0
Beef (round)	3 oz	340 mg	200	58.0
Rib roast	3 oz	290 mg	270	92.0
Turkey	4 oz	350 mg	300	46.0
VEGETABLES				
Tomato	1 medium	340 mg	30	4.5
Artichoke	1 medium	210 mg	30	22.0
Brussel sprouts	1 cup	300 mg	35	11.0

Reference: Merck Sharp & Dohme Canada Limited, Dorothy L. Smith, Medication Guide for Patient Counseling, second edition, page 815, 1982.

APPENDIX B

General Instructions for Patients with Diabetes

- Keep a regular schedule of daily activities. Eat, exercise and take your medicine at approximately the same time every day.
- The diet that your doctor has prescribed has been carefully planned especially for you. It is to your advantage to follow it very closely. These medicines will not work effectively if you do not follow your diet. This is especially important if you are overweight.
- Take special care of your feet. Some people with diabetes are prone to foot infections that can lead to serious problems.
  - Wash your feet daily and dry them well.
  - Check your feet daily for minor injuries and athlete's foot. Tell your doctor immediately.
  - Wear clean shoes and stockings and choose shoes that fit well.
  - If you develop corns or calluses, soak your feet in lukewarm water for about 10 minutes. Then rub them off gently with a pumice stone. Never use a knife to cut corns or calluses on your feet. Do not use commercial corn removers or commercial arch supports.
  - Soften dry skin by rubbing with oil or lotion.
  - Trim your toenails straight across with a file or a nail cutter. Do not cut your own toenails if your eyesight is poor.
  - Do not wear garters or socks with tight elastic tops. Do not sit with your knees crossed.
  - Do not warm your feet with a hot water bottle or a heating pad. Use loose bed socks instead. If your feet are cold, numb or tingling under normal conditions, tell your doctor. Your circulation may bc poor and your doctor can offer advice.
  - Test bath water temperature with your hands and not your feet since your feet may not be sensitive to heat.
  - Call your doctor if you injure your toes or feet. Cuts and scratches in the diabetic person can become infected easily and take longer to heal. Do not apply iodine or strong antiseptics to the feet at any time.
- Know the signs of *hypoglycemia* (low blood sugar). When this happens, your urine or blood sugar will bc negative. Hypoglycemia may occur if you delay or skip a meal, exercise too much, become sick or emotionally upset, take too much insulin, drink alcohol or take certain drugs.

If you develop sweating, shaking, drowsiness, headache, excessive hunger, nausea, nervousness, chills, cold sweats, cool pale skin, confusion or unusual tiredness or weakness, eat or drink any of the following *immediately:*

- A commercial sugar product (e.g. Monoject Insulin Reaction Gel) for insulin reactions.
- 2 sugar cubes or 2 teaspoons of sugar dissolved in water.
- 4 ounces orange juice.
- 4 ounces regular ginger ale, cola beverage or any other sweetened carbonated beverage. Do not use low-calorie or diet beverages.
- 2 to 3 teaspoons honey or corn syrup.
- 4 Lifesaver candies.

Artificial sweeteners are of no use.

- Call your doctor if this does not relieve your symptoms in about 15 minutes. If you cannot locate your doctor, call a neighbor, a friend or an emergency medical service and tell them your concern.
  Always carry sugar cubes or hard candy in case you have a hypoglycemic (low blood sugar) reaction.
- Call your doctor immediately if you develop any of the following symptoms of *hyperglycemia* (high blood sugar): high urine sugar, acetone in the urine, drowsiness, loss of appetite, unusual thirst, fast breathing, nausea, vomiting, confusion, a flushed dry skin, increase in urination (passing your water more often than usual) or a fruity odor to the breath. These symptoms may occur if you miss a dose of medicine, overeat or if you have a fever or an infection.
- Carry a supply of glucagon with you if your doctor has prescribed it for you.

If you would like more information about diabetes, contact your local chapter of the Canadian Diabetes Association.

APPENDIX C

Tips to Detect Tampering

As a result of the tampering scares, several pharmaceutical manufacturers are using different types of sealing techniques so that the consumer can detect any tampering of the capsules. Lilly has developed a double-banded gelatin seal so that it is next to impossible to separate the two parts of the capsule. Warner-Lambert is using a thermal sealing technique and a flattened capsule shape which reduces the surface area that can be gripped and makes it nearly impossible to pull the two sections apart. R.P. Scherer and Sterling are using a special machine that seals capsules by sonic waves.

Not every company is using special sealing techniques on its capsules. As a safety measure, it is always a good idea to inspect all nonprescription drug products before using them. Some things to look for include:

- Check the outer covering of the container for any breaks or indications of being unwrapped or opened.
- Is the cap on the container tight?
- Do the lot numbers on the outer and inner packages match?
- Is the protective seal on the bottle in place?
- Is the container full?
- Do all the tablets/capsules have the same appearance? Are they all the same color?
- Are any of the capsules dented?
- Are the two halves of the capsules lined up correctly so that any imprint matches perfectly? Many capsules have half an imprint on each half of the capsule so that when the two sections are put together the imprint matches perfectly.
- Is there any unusual or disturbing odor coming from the medicines?

If there is *anything* unusual about the package or medication inside it, take the product to the pharmacist and have it checked.

About the Author

Dorothy L. Smith is an internationally recognized pharmacist, author and consultant. A graduate of the University of Saskatchewan, she has held teaching appointments with the colleges of pharmacy at the University of British Columbia and the University of Toronto, and presently holds a cross appointment at Georgetown University School of Medicine.

In 1983, Dr. Smith founded the Consumer Health Information Corporation, a privately owned company dedicated to the development of patient education programs and publications. Dr. Smith has 17 years of experience in patient counseling and has won awards for her work in patient education. She has written several books, including a textbook for health professionals, *Medication Guide for Patient Counseling,* and the "Patient Advisory Leaflets" distributed by pharmacists to patients across Canada.